Handbook of
Nonpathologic Variations in Human Blood Constituents

Handbook of
Nonpathologic Variations in Human Blood Constituents

Richard W. Richardson, B.Sc., M.C.B.
Formerly Head of Biochemistry Department
Coventry Hospitals
Coventry
United Kingdom

CRC Press
Boca Raton   Ann Arbor   London   Tokyo

Library of Congress Cataloging-in-Publication Data

Richardson, Richard W., M.C.B.
   Handbook of nonpathologic variations in human blood constituents / Richard W. Richardson
     p.   cm.
   Includes bibliographical references and index.
   ISBN 0-8493-8664-0
   1. Blood—Analysis.   2. Reference values (Medicine).   I. Title.
   [DNLM: 1. Blood Chemical Analysis—methods.   2. Analysis of Variance.   QY 450 R524h 1994]
   616.07'561—dc20
   DNLM/DLC
   for Library of Congress   93-37925
                                                                             CIP

© 1994 by CRC Press, Inc.

No claim to original U.S. Government works
International Standard Book Number 0-8493-8664-0
Library of Congress Card Number 93-37925
Printed in the United States of America   1 2 3 4 5 6 7 8 9 0
Printed on acid-free paper

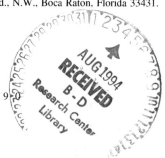

Preface

Information about nonpathologic variation in the concentration of blood constituents can be found throughout the medical and scientific literature. General textbooks give mainly qualitative accounts, whereas more detailed works that give quantitative information often only deal with a section of the subject, such as children or the elderly, and do not cover the whole subject.

In this book I collect reports of nonpathologic changes of some of the substances most frequently analyzed in clinical laboratories. I hope that the information will be useful to readers who are not clinical chemists and as a reference for clinical chemists as well.

Changes may be due to a number of factors, such as the use of different units, differences in accuracy and precision, statistical difference within a group of subjects, physiological or dietary change, analytical interference, or the effect of drugs. A general, mainly qualitative account is given in the early chapters, including references to internationally agreed upon recommendations for the standardization of units and for the conditions for sample collection.

Later chapters give a detailed account of quantitative changes in the blood level of specific substances. Many references from the whole period of development of clinical chemistry are given, which should give a historical perspective that may be of interest. It is sometimes surprising to find the changes that were known to the earliest workers, and to find that in some instances, the information seems to have been rediscovered later. The literature reports are sometimes conflicting or inconclusive; I hope that some readers will be stimulated to attempt to resolve the differences or clarify the facts.

Most of us use some terms loosely; for instance, "normal range" is often used as a convenient phrase. When used in this book, it is intended to correspond to a health-associated 95% reference interval. The term "plasma" will be used to mean the fluid obtained form anticoagulated samples, and "serum" to mean the fluid obtained after coagulation.

My thanks are due to a number of people who have contributed to the writing and production of this work.

Sincere thanks are due to Miss Margaret Adams, Administrator of the Warwickshire Postgraduate Medical Centre, and to the Librarians of the Centre for their help over several years, and to Colin Lynch and Brian Gee of the Coventry Public Health laboratory for the figures. I wish to record my thanks to the American Association for Clinical Chemistry Press for permission to quote extensively from Paediatric Clinical Chemistry, Reference (Normal Values), 3rd Edition, edited by Samuel Meites.

Thanks are due to the CRC Press staff, in particular to David Grist, who has constantly helped and encouraged me. Without him the book would not have been produced.

Finally, I would be grateful for information on any errors and omissions in this work, which are solely my responsibility.

Richard W. Richardson
Coventry, March 1994

Abstract

Information scattered throughout the medical and scientific literature about nonpathologic changes in the concentration of blood constituents is collected in this book. The variations may be statistical, methodological, physiological, or due to age, alcohol, smoking, or drugs, and must be taken into account by clinicians when interpreting laboratory results.

About 1500 references covering the whole period of development of clinical chemistry are given, to enable those interested to obtain further information and to give a historical perspective.

Some previously unpublished results from the author's laboratory are included, of levels in healthy subjects of different sex and age, and the distribution of serum bilirubin obtained from over 3000 hospital staff.

This book will help medical and laboratory staff in their work, and should be included in the libraries of medical schools, postgraduate medical centers, medical, surgical, pediatric, obstetric, and laboratory departments, and will be useful for those studying for qualifications in clinical chemistry, clinical pathology, medicine, and other medical specialties.

The Author

Richard W. Richardson was Head of the Biochemistry Department from 1956, and Co-ordinator of the Pathology Group of Departments of the Coventry Hospitals from 1980, until his retirement in 1989.

He graduated from the University of London in 1947 with a B.Sc. degree in Chemistry, and obtained the degree of Master of Clinical Biochemistry in 1962.

After some experience in analytical chemistry in industry, he received his early training in Clinical Chemistry from 1951–1956 at Dudley Road Hospital, Birmingham, before moving to Coventry. A Founder Member of the Association of Clinical Biochemists, he is a past Chairman of the West Midlands Branch and was a Fellow of the Royal Institute of Chemistry until his retirement as a practicing Clinical Chemist. He has also been elected an Honorary Member of the Coventry and Warwickshire Postgraduate Medical Centre.

During his career, he has published a number of papers on clinical chemistry subjects and supervised students working for research degrees. He has lectured to students of Biological Sciences and Laboratory Technology at the Coventry Polytechnic and has been a member of the Research Committee of that institution.

Contents

Chapter 16—Glucose

Handbook of Nonpathologic Variations in Human Blood Constituents

Chapter 1

UNITS, RANGES, AND ANALYSIS

INTRODUCTION

There are reports of blood analysis in the literature during the 19th century; Berzelius reported protein levels as early as 1831.[1] However, body fluid analysis as an aid to the investigation and treatment of disease has mainly developed during the 20th century. Techniques have been developed so that the volume of the sample now required is usually small, and with the use of automatic analyzers, many analyses can be made quickly.

As noted by Zilva et al.,[2] "the clinician has a great many tests at his disposal. If used critically these often provide helpful information: if used without thought the results are at best useless, and at wors[t] misleading and dangerous."

When considering the results of chemical analysis of body fluids, it is useful to start from a knowledge of the levels in persons free from disease, so that a comparison can then be made with the levels in sick individuals, to assist in diagnosis and prognosis and to assess the effect of treatment. As the amount of any constituent varies among healthy individuals, it is necessary to consider the likely range of values.

Early work used ranges based on maximum and minimum values found in a group of subjects; although those studied were considered "normal," the criteria for normalcy were frequently inadequately defined. Some early figures for the composition of human blood are quoted in the textbook by Hawk and Bergeim in 1927;[3] they recognized that ranges could vary according to the method of analysis, as different ranges were given for the estimation of blood glucose by different methods.

By the 1930s a normal-range concept based on statistical theory using standard deviations, and later percentiles, rather than maximum–minimum values, began to be used. Attempts have been made to clarify the definition of ranges found in healthy subjects, and a useful historical review is given in the book by Martin et al.[4]

Many factors have been found to affect the level of substances in blood, including changes related to factors such as

1. Food: diet, fasting, meals
2. Posture: standing, sitting, lying, resting in bed
3. Time: diurnal and circadian rhythms, seasons
4. Individual characteristics: height, mass, race, blood type, blood pressure
5. Age: newborn, puberty, menopause
6. Sex: male, female
7. Physiology: ovulation, menstruation, pregnancy, lactation
8. Environment: latitude, exposure to hot and cold
9. Activity: exercise, stress, weightlessness
10. Collection of specimen: site of collection, use of tourniquet, effect of anticoagulants
11. Analytic method
12. Drug ingestion: therapeutic, alcohol, tobacco

This list is not exhaustive and is given here to illustrate that many factors can potentially alter blood composition and need to be considered when establishing criteria for interpretation. Standardization of the collection procedure will minimize variance. This may be particularly important when studying sequential measurements in an individual.

1

Clinicians and laboratory workers are often aware that there is some effect associated with a given factor, but they may be unsure of the quantitative change and whether any change is significant. Most will, for instance, recognize that excessive stasis, when performing venipuncture, can affect blood composition, but the extent of the quantitative effect is less well known.

Consideration of nonpathological changes in blood composition should enable clinicians to derive more useful information from test results. A figure outside the range for healthy people may mean that the patient is ill, but it is also possible, as pointed out by Statland,[5] that there is another explanation:

1. The result may be a statistical outlier.
2. The patient may be demographically different from the reference population.
3. The preparation of the sample, or method of analysis, may be different from that of the reference population.
4. The patient may have been engaged in activities, prior to specimen collection, that caused the value to be outside the limits.

In this book I attempt to help answer the question: what should we conclude when it is reported that the level of a patient's blood constituent is outside the accepted level in healthy persons?

NORMAL RANGES AND REFERENCE INTERVALS

The expression "normal range" is frequently used by both clinicians and laboratory staff when discussing laboratory results, and ranges are often issued for use as a guide to the interpretation of results. These ranges are often not adequately defined and may have been taken from textbooks that do not give a clear indication of the population from which the ranges originated. Significant variation can be found between figures in different textbooks, and in one textbook different ranges are quoted on consecutive pages.[6] Some of the variation between publications can be explained statistically, but other factors may contribute to the differences:

1. The subjects sampled may have originated from unrepresentative sections of the total population.
2. Differences in subgroups may not have been considered; for example, there may be a variation in the proportion of males to females or in the age distribution.
3. The methods used may give different results.
4. Consideration may not have been given to the effect of meals, posture, or diurnal change.

WHAT IS "NORMAL"?

King, in 1946,[7] defined the "normal value" as the amount of a constituent present in the body fluid or excreta of a healthy human being. Although this is a useful starting point, it does not take into account the variation between different groups of people, nor does it define the word "healthy". Clinical and laboratory staff often use "normal" with a meaning similar to "nonpathological", and there has been confusion caused by an assumption that the distribution is also "normal" or gaussian, as used by statisticians. Attempts have been made to overcome the confusion, by using terms such as "the usual range" or "cut-off points", or by avoiding such terms altogether.

Current terminology is based on the suggestions of Grasbeck and Saris,[8] who considered that a well-defined nomenclature and recommended procedures should be established and that the term "reference interval" should replace "normal range". Use of the term "reference interval" implies that the interval was derived in a clearly defined way, details of which are available. This concept enables values to be established for specific groups and used for different purposes. The ideas of Grasbeck and Saris have been developed by both national and international bodies, and a number of definitions and procedures have been agreed upon.[9-16]

METHODS OF EXPRESSING REFERENCE INTERVALS

For any particular substance, most subjects have values near the middle of the frequency distribution; thus, limits obtained using the total range from the highest to the lowest will depend upon the number of subjects used. This procedure will underestimate the range in small samples and may give limits that are uselessly wide if large samples are used. It is now usual to determine limits by statistical analysis of the results obtained, with ranges containing 95% of the appropriate population frequently, but not always, used. Many clinicians interpret laboratory results by considering a figure unremarkable if it is within the range and significant if it is considerably outside the range. Borderline results are interpreted according to the clinical picture, and the test may be repeated if any doubt remains.

Wooton and King attempted to develop this approach by calculating 80 and 98% limits representing mean $\pm 1^1/_2$ SD and mean $\pm 2^1/_2$ SD of a gaussian population.[17] They suggested that values outside 98% limits were significant and values between 80 and 98% limits were borderline, but this attempt to quantify the approach has been little used in practice.

It has often been assumed that when the frequency distribution of an analyte concentration is unimodal and not skewed, it is gaussian and that the 95% limits can be defined as mean ± 2 SD. In practice few distributions are precisely gaussian, although some are sufficiently close for the statistics to be used. The distributions of some analytes, such as sodium, are leptokurtic, and of others, platykurtic. The distribution of some analyte values, particularly enzymes, is skewed; in these cases a gaussian distribution often appears if the logarithm is used.

To avoid making any assumptions about the shape of the frequency curve, many workers prefer to use the percentile method and take limits from the 2.5th to the 97.5th percentile. The main disadvantages of this are that larger numbers of samples are required and that the range is sensitive to outliers. Herrara gives details of the procedure for estimating percentiles and determining their precision.[18]

UNITS OF MEASUREMENT

The numerical value obtained for a chemical analysis will vary according to the units used. The use of different units can produce problems if a patient is investigated in different hospitals, and confusion can occur when attempting to compare published work. To standardize the units of measurement, recommendations of the Section of Clinical Chemistry of IUPAC, made in 1966[19] based on the SI units adopted in 1960, have been introduced throughout the world.

The main change in clinical laboratories is the use of molar, rather than mass, units. The use of molar concentrations for drug levels in blood is not obligatory, although they are used in some laboratories. This is surprising, as it may be thought that the molar concentration would relate better to drug activity. An Expert Panel of the International Federation of Clinical Chemistry (IFCC), however, reiterating the recommendations to use SI units in 1990,[20] said that the inter- and intrapatient relationships between a drug administered and measured in body fluids is so variable that the need to express them in the same units has little or no relevance.

In this book, figures given in other units in the original work have been converted to the recommended SI units. There may be small differences introduced due to the rounding of significant figures, but there is no alternative in order to obtain meaningful comparisons.

Enzyme Units

Estimations of enzyme activity in body fluids have been made since the earliest work in clinical chemistry, often using arbitrary units defined by the originator of the method used. Comparison of results is difficult due to the different conditions used. In an attempt to standardize, the adoption of an "international unit" based on the rate of reaction was proposed in 1961.[21] The Commission on Clinical Chemistry of IUPAC and IFCC, in 1966, recommended this unit for adoption in clinical chemistry, leaving the temperature of the assay and the concentration of the reagents to be defined. In general, the use of reagent concentrations that give the greatest activity results in the maximum differentiation between normal and abnormal specimens. Exceptions are the assay conditions chosen for the estimation of hydroxy butyric dehydrogenase in serum, to give the maximum difference between the activity of heart enzyme and the activity of isoenzymes from other tissues.

The Katal

The SI unit of the catalytic activity of an enzyme is the rate of reaction of one mole per second. The special (non-SI) name "katal" is recommended, in the specific context of enzymes and clinical chemistry, by the IFCC Expert Panel on Enzymes.[22]

$$1 \text{ IU} = 1 \text{ } \mu\text{mol/min} = 16.7 \text{ nmol/s} = 16.7 \text{ katal.}$$

Large series of enzyme levels in blood have not been expressed in katals, and since few clinical laboratories yet use these units, the conversion will not be made in this book. If required, the calculation to convert from IU is easy.

TEMPERATURE FOR ENZYME ASSAY

Several temperatures for the assay of enzyme activity in body fluids have been used. Temperatures of 25 and 37°C are probably the most common, although 30, 32, and 35°C have all been proposed. The rate of reaction increases with temperature, usually doubling between 25 and 37°C. Other factors, such as optimal reagent concentration, buffer pH, and absorption curves, may also be temperature dependent.

IFCC Recommendations

The Expert Panel on Enzymes of the Committee on Standards of the IFCC made a number of recommendations to be applied to the consideration of official IFCC methods.[22] With as few exceptions as possible, 30.00°C should be used. Proposals have been made for the selection of agreed reference methods, terminology, and nomenclature and for the consideration of optimal conditions.

COMPARISON OF DIFFERENT ENZYME METHODS

Literature references to changes in serum enzyme activity involve the use of different methods, and this makes comparisons difficult. Some workers relate the figures to the upper-range limit (URL) for the method concerned. In this approach there are imperfections that must be recognized, as not all ranges will be determined by the same statistical procedure. So care must be taken when interpreting small changes. Until sufficient work has been done using standard methods, the procedure is useful and will be used in this book if comparisons are necessary.

ANALYTIC CONSIDERATIONS

When comparing results by different methods, imprecision and inaccuracy must both be considered, as they both affect the measured reference intervals.

DEFINITIONS

Accuracy is the relation between the best estimate of a quantity and its true value. The numerical difference between the mean of a set of replicates and the true value is termed the "inaccuracy" of a method and is commonly called "bias."

Precision is the agreement between replicate measurements and has no numerical value. This is usually expressed mathematically as the standard deviation (SD) or coefficient of variation (CV) and should be termed the "imprecision" of a method.

"Sensitivity" is the ability of an analytical method to detect small quantities and is expressed as the "detection limit," defined as the smallest single result that can be distinguished from a suitable blank with a stated probability.

Bias in a method will result in bias in the measured reference interval. An extreme example is the range for blood glucose found by the now-little-used Folin and Wu method, which is about 1 mmol/L higher than the range found using a more specific method. There are other examples, and they can often be demonstrated by studying results from quality-assurance schemes.

Greater imprecision in a method will give rise to a wider range for the reference interval. Analyses of a blood constituent of a group of subjects show a variance that can be expressed as a standard variation s_{obs} that includes an analytic variation s_a and a biologic variation s_b:

$$s_{obs} = \sqrt{s_a^2 + s_b^2}$$

Gowenlock gives various calculations[23] to show the effect of these factors:

Analytic error as % of biologic variation	Change in observed variance (%)
20	2.0
25	3.2
30	4.4
40	7.7

Using the maximum acceptable between-laboratory variation (proposed by Tonks) of 25% of the reference interval, the reference limits would be about 12% greater than if there was no analytic variation. Both possible bias and variation in analytic precision must be borne in mind when comparing results with ranges found in different laboratories or in the same laboratory at different times.

INTERFERENCE WITH ANALYSIS

Hemolysis, bilirubin, and lipemia

Methods may be affected in different ways by factors that interfere with analysis and give variations in the results. Either an affected method must be developed to minimize any error, or the effect must be taken into account and a correction made if possible. Removal of protein, either by precipitation or by the introduction of a dialysis stage, frequently eliminates the problem. However, the direct reacting methods used in discrete analyzers are often subject to error, and in some commercially available instruments, a correction is incorporated. Another cause of error relating to hemolysis is due to a constituent having a higher concentration in cells than in serum. Attempts have been made to use correction factors based on the hemoglobin content of serum, but in general, in these cases it is preferable to avoid hemolysis.

Drugs

Potential interference in the analysis, from drugs and their metabolites present in serum, must also be considered. This will be discussed in detail later.

STORAGE AND TRANSPORT OF SPECIMENS

It is not always possible for samples to be analyzed immediately on collection; so it is necessary to be aware of the stability of substances analyzed in body fluids. Any changes can often be delayed by the use of suitable preservatives and temperatures. Cooling the sample with ice as soon as it is collected is necessary for a number of substances such as ACTH, PTH, and glucagon. Acid phosphatase activity is only stable for 15 min at room temperature, and samples should be placed on ice on collection. After separation, serum acid phosphatase activity is stable for up to 1 week if the pH is adjusted to about 5.

Not all substances are more stable if frozen. LDH activity in serum, particularly from the isoenzymes LD_4 and LD_5, is unstable at low temperatures, and potassium and phosphate increase more quickly in the serum of unseparated blood when it is cold rather than at room temperature. Temperature affects the stability of some protein fractions.[24] Ceruloplasmin is less stable after 8 and 12 weeks at $-70°C$ than at 4 and $-20°C$. Lipemic sera give higher blanks in immunonephelometric estimations when they have been stored frozen than when they have been stored at $4°$, making low concentrations difficult to estimate. Estimation by radial diffusion methods is not affected.

Breakdown of glucose and ethanol in blood can be delayed by adding sodium fluoride as an enzyme inhibitor (see Chapter 16). Analysis for amino acids should use plasma from an oxalate/fluoride specimen, since amino acids are unstable in serum at room temperature. Bilirubin is affected if serum is exposed to light. It may be advantageous not to separate the cells from the serum — the bilirubin will then be protected by the cells from UV light.

For most substances, glass or plastic containers can be used, but others, such as calcitonin and ACTH, are adsorbed onto glass; in these cases collection must be into plastic tubes.

An indication of the stability of a number of frequently assayed serum and urine constituents is given by Wilding et al.,[25] and this paper can be consulted for further information.

Chapter 2

SELECTION, PREPARATION, AND STANDARDIZATION

SELECTION

THE HEALTHY SUBJECT

A useful reference population for the interpretation of laboratory analyses would be healthy individuals defined in a specific way. However, no definition of "health" is completely satisfactory. The constitution of the World Health Organization (WHO) defines health as a "state of complete physical, mental, or social well-being and not merely the absence of disease or infirmity." However, practically, health is relative and may be conceptually different in different countries and in the same country at different times and at different ages. The problem is summed up by Pryce,[26] who wrote,

> I presume that by healthy they mean free from dental caries, alopecia, sinusitis, presbyopa myopia, reduced auditory acuity, diminished expiratory volume, neurosis, allergy, etc., which rules out anyone over the age of 20 years. If they include immaturity, that excludes anyone under the age of 20 years; and if they also include possible heterozygotes for known diseases, that excludes the whole of mankind several times over.

Frequently, a person is considered healthy by ignoring some of the factors mentioned by Pryce and by attempting to exclude some possible pathologic conditions. As a disease develops, it may be incipient, full blown, receding, etc., and it is not surprising that laboratory findings from diseased individuals overlap with those obtained from subjects considered healthy.[27]

There are some conditions, such as hemoglobinopathies and red cell enzyme deficiencies, that exist in a high proportion of the population of certain communities. Homozygote subjects are considered to have the disease, but in a number of conditions, heterozygotes show no pathologic manifestation. Should heterozygotes be included in a population used to determine the reference interval for a substance with no apparent link with the abnormality?

A group under the chairmanship of Gräsbeck[10] considered the problem of selection of "healthy" individuals and proposed the selection of subjects at random from the population, with inclusion or rejection on the basis of a health examination and a health questionnaire. Berg tested these proposals[28] and found that only 41 of 237 subjects would be acceptable according to the recommended criteria. Later, Gräsbeck agreed that the criteria were too rigid due to an acceptance, at the time, of the idea of absolute health.[29] This work illustrates the difficulties of determining healthy individuals and leads to the consideration of a need to define groups of individuals according to the use proposed for the intervals determined.

In clinical diagnosis, we may consider that part of the distribution curve for healthy subjects that provides the least overlap with values in the relevant diseased population. It is therefore important to obtain a satisfactory definition of disease and also to recognize that there may be subjects without symptoms, who are beginning to show pathologic changes in organs and tissues. The inclusion of a small proportion of subjects who are not healthy may not have a serious effect if results are evaluated statistically, but in some groups, such as the elderly, the proportion may be greater, and this needs consideration.

SAMPLE GROUPS

Ideally, a reference population of healthy subjects should be obtained by sampling the total population, with inclusion or exclusion based on stated criteria. In practice a potential bias may be introduced, since true random sampling may be difficult for logistic reasons. Some groups may not be a true random sample of the general population, but may be conveniently available. Possible bias must always be considered when using reference intervals derived from such groups.

It is pointed out in the IFCC recommendations[12] that the criteria to be applied for the exclusion of a reference individual will be determined by the use to which the reference values are put. It is suggested that well-identified groups, such as pregnant women, women taking oral contraceptives, drinkers, smokers, and obese individuals, should be considered for exclusion from a reference sample group of apparently healthy persons. Individuals suffering from systemic disease and pathophysiologic disorders should be excluded, although the precise definition may be difficult. Nothing restricts the definition of a state of good health, but it is important to define the state of health required for inclusion.

Many studies, particularly in early works, have used groups of hospital workers or medical students. Ranges obtained in this way can be misleading, since such highly selected groups may not be representative of the general population. Even in such selected groups, ranges obtained can be more acceptable if simple factors such as age and sex are taken into account. Samples taken from healthy hospital staff working normally and not admitting to ill health have been used by the author for many years to establish ranges; some examples of the results obtained are given in this book. Subjects were not fasted, and pregnant subjects or those suffering from conditions requiring constant therapy were excluded. Results were usually separated into male and female categories and into 5-year age groups, with ranges given from the 2.5th to the 97.5th percentile.

Some workers have obtained samples from blood donors, as such subjects may be considered to represent the general population. It could be argued that blood donors are a self-selected group and need not therefore be typical of the population as a whole. A greater criticism is that the possible effect of blood donation on blood constituents has not always been taken into account. Donors are usually rejected if blood hemoglobin is low, and it is possible that this exclusion may distort the ranges obtained.

A definite variation, depending on whether samples were taken before or after a donation, was found by Flynn et al.[30] Differences were infrequently found in serum urea, sodium, and chloride, but significant changes were noted in potassium. The effect of the donation was related to the predonation level. Subjects with original levels of serum potassium above the mean tended to show a fall, whereas those with original levels below the mean tended to show a rise.

SIZE OF THE REFERENCE SAMPLE

The number required for the satisfactory determination of a reference interval has been discussed for many years. Scott, in a study in 1927 of blood sugar in rabbits,[31] showed that in a series of 1000 tests, about 50 were required to give an acceptable mean. Copeland believed that only 10 to 20 samples were required for a "reasonable approximation" of the normal value,[32] whereas Reed et al. considered the number of samples required to be 120,[33] but recognized that sometimes this number would be inadequate. Martin et al. stated that at the Rhode Island Hospital they considered 300 samples to be an optimal number,[4] but preferred 500. Lott et al. studied a number of blood constituents[34] and concluded that approximately 200 samples were required to obtain 95% reference limits at a 99% confidence level, by a nonparametric method. If data followed a gaussian distribution, about 120 would suffice.

The number of samples required will depend upon a number of factors, such as

1. The size of acceptable error
2. The frequency of other errors
3. The differences that are clinically acceptable

4. The variability in measurement
5. The statistical method used — whether nonparametric or gaussian

In practice, the number required probably needs to be considered in each specific case.

PREPARATION

A number of nonpathologic factors affect blood composition, and the need to standardize conditions must be considered when collecting specimens for analysis. It has been pointed out[35] that there is no simple system that will meet the requirements for all analytes and that a method of collection and storage that may be appropriate for one may be invalid for another. In practice this results in the common problem of inappropriately collected specimens.

POSTURE

Blood composition changes within 30 min when a person moves from a standing to a lying position, due to an increase in circulating blood volume as a result of reduced diuresis.[36] Hemodilution may be greater in ill subjects such as those with edema or abnormal serum protein levels.[37] Concentrations of all proteins change, and there is also an effect on substances that are bound to protein. Changes are on the order of 10%,[38] although the level of some substances may change by greater amounts. Plasma renin activity doubles within 40 min of rising, and a failure to collect samples after a subject has been supine overnight can give misleading results. Noradrenalin doubles within 3 min of a 60° tilting of healthy individuals and then remains constant.[39] Angiotensin II is similarly affected. Prolonged bed rest may have a different effect. For example, serum calcium, which falls when a subject lies down, may rise after the person has spent more than 7 days lying, due to mobilization of calcium from bone.

STRESS

The intermediary metabolism of lipids and carbohydrates is affected by stress, resulting in increases in serum triglyceride, cholesterol, cortisol, glucose, catecholamines, growth hormone, and nonesterified fatty acids. There may also be an increase in serum prolactin, especially in women, and a fall in serum testosterone. Levels may be affected by the stress of venipuncture, particularly in children. In addition, possible hyperventilation can alter blood levels of gases and other substances affected by alkalosis.

A rarely considered, but potential, factor affecting levels of blood constituents is the effect of recent coitus. Changes up to 60 min after coitus were studied by Stearns et al.[40] No change was observed in serum testosterone, follicle-stimulating hormone (FSH), luteinizing hormone (LH), estradiol, or progesterone, but an eightfold increase in serum prolactin was found in two of six women surveyed. There was no change in serum growth hormone, suggesting a separate control mechanism. Possible causes for the increase in serum prolactin were considered to be the stress of coitus or the effect of breast stimulation.

MEALS AND DIET

Changes in blood levels soon after a meal may be due to an increase caused by transporting nutrients, such as with glucose or lipids, or due to metabolic changes, as with phosphate.

The nature of the meal may have an effect. A high-fat meal may result in an increase in serum alkaline phosphatase activity, due to an influx of intestinal phosphatase, whereas high-meat intake may increase serum creatinine. Caffeine increases both catecholamines and nonesterified fatty acid.

An extended fast affects some blood constituents. After a 48-h fast, there may be a 24% increase in serum bilirubin, a 50% increase in glucagon, a 25% increase in triglyceride, and a 15% increase in insulin. There can be a decrease in blood glucose, which is most pronounced in healthy women, in whom it may be as low as 2.5 mmol/L.[41] It is clear that the optimum time of collection from a fasting specimen is not the same for all analytes.

There may also be an effect due to the previous diet. Diets may be taken for therapeutic reasons or due to life style, e.g., vegetarian, low fat, weight reducing, etc. The effect of a low-fiber, high-protein, high-fat diet, common in Western countries, has been shown to be associated with higher levels of sex hormones and lower levels of sex-hormone-binding globulin in serum.[42]

Consideration must also be given to possible differences in blood composition due to giving human or cow milk to neonates.

EXERCISE

When blood is taken for analysis, the amount of recent exercise taken by the patient will usually, at most, be a short walk to the clinic. So the effect on serum constituents will be small, although in a list of 24 analytes, McLaughlan and Gowenlock[43] suggested that significant changes can occur in albumin, GOT, creatinine, glucose, phosphate, potassium, total protein, urate, and urea.

The effect of severe exercise is greater and may be important when attempting to interpret changes in a patient taken ill during events such a marathon run or similar energetic activity. Peak levels may occur sometime after the exercise. Ahlberg and Brouhult found that for creatine kinase and lactic dehydrogenase, the highest levels were not found until the next day,[44] and for ornithine carbamyl transferase, the highest level occurred on the seventh day after exertion. They also noted that peak enzyme levels were much lower in trained subjects after physical conditioning.

Galteau and Siest, using standardized exercise on a cycloergonometer,[45] found increases in serum phosphate, cholesterol, creatinine, total protein, and albumin, and a decrease in serum urea, although not all of the changes were statistically significant. Some changes were found to vary in amount with the age of the subject.

Changes after strenuous exercise were reviewed by Statland and Winkel,[46] who found (apart from changes in enzymes, proteins, and substances bound to protein) increases in a number of hormones and related blood constituents, including thyroxine, triiodothyronine, thyroid-stimulating hormone (TSH), insulin, glucagon, human growth hormone (HGH), estrogen, androgen, renin, angiotensin, aldosterone, and catecholamines.

Muscle work from the common practice of exercising the hand when collecting specimens may result in an increase in protein and protein-bound substances, due to an increase in local hydrostatic pressure.

SMOKING

The concentration of a number of blood constituents is affected by smoking tobacco. An increase in carboxyhemoglobin is related to the inhalation of gases, and increases in catecholamines, cortisol, and nonesterified fatty acids may be related to the effect of nicotine. Hemoglobin concentration and the number of erythrocytes and leukocytes are greater in the blood of smokers; serum gastrin and alpha$_1$ antitrypsin are about 20% higher, and levels of cadmium and the tumor markers placental alkaline phosphatase and carcinoembryonic antigen are doubled. Small changes in other serum constituents can be demonstrated by studying large groups of subjects. Dales investigated 57,352 white, and 9812 black, men and women[47] and found significantly different mean levels of albumin, glucose after 75-g glucose, urate, cholesterol, and creatinine in smokers, compared with nonsmokers.

ALCOHOL

Consumption of ethyl alcohol has been shown to affect the serum concentration of a number of substances. Freer and Statland showed increases in serum gamma-glutamyltransferase

(GGT) and glutamic-pyrovic transaminase (GPT) and decreases in aspartate aminotransferase (GOT),[48] but no constant effect on LDH, 60 h after alcohol ingestion. The same workers later studied longer-term effects[49] and found a number of individual responses, with serum GGT increasing by up to 25% in seven of eight subjects. Rollason et al. found that 25 of 50 subjects who stated that they took six or more alcoholic drinks per day had serum GGT above the "normal" range for the laboratory,[50] compared with 6 of 38 of those who claimed to be teetotalers. Increases in serum enzymes may be related to the induction of liver enzymes.

There is a decrease of blood glucose and bicarbonate and an increase in urate and lactate within 24 h of taking alcohol.[41] Serum cholesterol and triglycerides are increased some days later. Even moderate ethanol consumption in healthy subjects significantly alters the level of blood constituents and must be considered when interpreting results and standardizing collection conditions.

BIOLOGIC RHYTHMS

Consideration of changes in blood composition due to circadian or nychthermal rhythms is complicated by concurrent changes due to food and stress. Changes may be exogenous when the change is a direct response to the environment and disappears if the environmental factor becomes constant. Changes may be endogenous when the change is an inherent property of the organism. Periodicity of about 24 h is linked to alternate light and dark and to the sleeping–waking cycle; changes may be inverted if there is a reversal of the sleeping–waking pattern. Hypothalamic-pituitary hormonal systems have a pattern of secretion related to the 24-h sleeping–waking pattern in humans.[51]

Growth hormone is secreted in substantial amounts during the last few hours of sleep at night, whereas prolactin shows progressively higher values during the night, with a peak at the end of the sleep period. Cortisol secretion patterns have been shown to be episodic, with a greater clustering of episodes during the latter part of the sleep period, giving the highest serum cortisol levels soon after waking. Episodes decline in frequency as the day progresses, giving the lowest serum levels at about midnight. Variation in this pattern can be of diagnostic importance if changes are absent.

Other changes include variation in serum thyroxine and phosphate, which in an individual may cover the whole of the reference interval for the relevant population, and variation in serum iron and testosterone, with the highest levels in the morning. There is also a small circadian rhythm in TSH, although changes may not be significant.

MENSTRUAL CYCLE

The variation in hormone secretion during the menstrual cycle affects the blood concentration of a number of substances. Serum progesterone levels are low during the follicular phase and rise sharply after ovulation, reaching a peak 5 to 9 days later and then declining during the late luteal phase if pregnancy does not occur. The gonadotrophins LH and FSH show a large increase in serum concentration associated with ovulation, and serum estradiol varies considerably during the menstrual cycle, with an ovulatory peak and high levels during the midluteal phase. Varley et al. quote the ranges found by a number of workers.[52] The concentrations of a number of other substances vary during the cycle. Mean serum prolactin is reported to be about 50% higher in the luteal phase than in the follicular phase.[53] Albumin falls during the middle of the cycle and then rises, and aldosterone, amino acids, vitamin C, cholesterol, magnesium, and creatine phosphokinase (CPK) are all reported to change in concentration during the cycle.

DRUGS

The level of blood constituents can be affected in a number of ways by drug therapy. The presence of a drug or its metabolite in blood may interfere with the analytic method, giving a false result. The drug may have a toxic effect on the kidney, liver, or other organ affecting blood constituents, or levels may be affected due to interference of the drug with metabolism, either as a desired, intended effect or as a possibly undesired side effect. The IFCC Expert Panel on Drug Effects in Clinical Chemistry has considered these effects, and seven of their recommendations are collected in a single publication.[54]

In the well-known work by Young et al.,[55] first published in 1975 and last revised in 1990,[56] with a supplement in 1991, interference with analysis is found in about 20% of the quoted references of the effect of drugs on laboratory tests. The effect may vary according to the method used. For instance, paracetamol interferes with the estimation of glucose by glucose oxidase methods, but not by hexokinase methods. Many commonly used drugs have kidney and liver effects that mimic many of the naturally occurring diseases of these organs. About 2% of patients hospitalized with jaundice are said to have a drug-induced disease.[57]

The effect of a drug may vary with the age of the patient. Children with paracetamol overdose are much less liable to have liver damage than adults, and elderly people are, in general, more affected by drug toxicity than younger subjects are.

Physiologic and metabolic effects may result in a change in blood composition, in a number of ways:

1. The drug may be given to alter a blood constituent, e.g., to reduce cholesterol, glucose, or urate.
2. The metabolism of a drug may have an effect, e.g., as when one metabolic path of isoniazid leads to an increase in blood ammonia.
3. There may be a physiologic effect, e.g., pethidine, codeine, and morphine causing constriction of the Oddi's sphincter, leading to increased amylase and lipase in the blood.
4. Enzyme induction may occur in the liver. Over 200 drugs have been identified as liver enzyme inducers. It frequently may not be clear whether the increase is due to enzyme induction or toxicity.
5. Other factors may affect blood constituents, such as inhibition or stimulation of synthesis, interference with secretory mechanisms, or competitive protein binding.

The effect of a drug frequently causes a shift in the median of the distribution of a blood constituent, compared with that for a similar untreated population. The change may sometimes be statistically significant, but not clinically important.

In some cases only a proportion of subjects are affected, due to idiosyncrasy, genetic sensitivity, or another cause, and in others, only patients with the particular disease being treated are affected, and not healthy persons or others without the disease.

ORAL CONTRACEPTIVES

More than 100 *in vivo* effects due to oral contraceptives have been reported in clinical laboratory tests. Changes are usually caused by physiologic alteration rather than by interference with analysis, and most are due to the estrogen component and often resemble changes occurring in pregnancy. Generally, products containing less estrogen give a smaller alteration in analytic results.[58] Many reports in the literature refer to the effect of early, higher-dose preparations; so care must be taken when interpreting changes in subjects taking lower doses.

SOURCES OF INFORMATION ON DRUG EFFECTS

A number of publications list literature references regarding the effect of drugs on laboratory constituents.[55,56,59,60] All of these works give both positive and negative information concerning these effects. In this book the author has used many of these references. The reader is also referred to the references for information concerning nephrotoxic, hepatotoxic, and other pathologic effects. This book is concerned with nonpathologic changes, although the differentiation may be difficult. Frequently, a published work gives inadequate information, e.g., the method of analysis is not given, or a statement is made, such as "measured by routine laboratory methods." There are often discrepancies between reports that may be due to factors such as different methods of analysis and differences in the route of administration, dose given, or duration of treatment.

STANDARDIZATION

Consideration must be given to the various factors affecting blood levels, as the importance will vary according to the constituent. For samples for the production of reference intervals, this should be taken into account. Samples should also be collected under conditions similar to those expected when collecting specimens for observation. Frequently, fasting for a particular time is suggested, and an optimum time, which may vary among analytes, is chosen. Body posture may be important, and exercise, stress, alcohol, caffeine, drugs, and other factors must be taken into consideration.

Frequently, a number of substances are estimated on the same sample; so recommendations have been made to standardize specimen collection. IFCC recommendations list factors that need to be taken into account[13] and refer to several national recommendations. The procedure suggested by the Scandinavian Society[10] requires, on the day before collection, ordinary food intake, and alcohol restricted to not more than the equivalent of one bottle of beer. Proposals have been made for standardization of the collection, treatment, and storage of specimens, and recommendations have been made for ambulatory subjects, for bedridden subjects, for outpatients giving fasting specimens in the morning, and for outpatients giving specimens in the afternoon after a light breakfast. Recommendations for the collection of skin-puncture blood from infants and children were made later.[61] The term "skin puncture" was suggested by Meites and Levitt[62] to avoid the less-suitable term "capillary blood". They point out that although capillary blood predominates in skin punctures, traces of interstitial fluid are likely to be present and cannot be ignored.

Further recommendations were made by Meites,[63] who said that collection should be done by adequately trained personnel and that collection should be monitored to ensure that the number of hemolyzed specimens is not excessive. He quoted work showing that serum hemoglobin does not exceed 200 mg/L in infants over 13 days old; so no visible hemolysis should be present. In the first 13 days of life, erythrocytes are more fragile, and hemolysis is more likely, with not more than 5% of samples showing visible hemolysis if the collection is satisfactory. Skin puncture is somewhat dangerous, and can lead to osteomyelitis. This danger is reduced by using recommended techniques.

Small, but significant, differences have been reported in skin puncture samples, compared with venous specimens, with serum potassium, protein, and calcium a little lower, and glucose, LDH, and aldolase reported to be a little higher.[64] Possible variation must be taken into account when interpreting results.

The results from a reference group must be examined to establish subgroups that show significant differences. There are a number of possibilities that should be considered.

SEX

There are often significant differences in the level of blood constituents between males and females. Differences are often linked to muscle mass or hormone pattern and may not occur in children and the elderly.

AGE

There are changes during the neonatal period as the baby adapts to an independent existence. When collecting samples, the number of hours since birth should be recorded, and suitable reference groups should be used. It may be necessary to take note of differences between those born full term and those born prematurely, taking into account variation in the length of gestation. Dietary differences may also be important, as some babies are breast-fed and others receive various formula milk products. In the very-low-birth-weight infant, a combination of immature organs and diminished reserves will lead to disturbances of biochemical functions and to changes in the levels of blood constituents.[65] Prior to puberty, levels are similar in boys and girls for most constituents, but in older children, consideration should be given to the degree of maturation. Instead of relating to chronologic age, ranges may need to relate to a sexual maturity rating, growth rate, or skeletal age.

As people age, endocrine and other changes occur, and there is a gradual change due partly to life style and partly to organ deterioration. An increase in interindividual variation can also be expected, as there is a decreased ability to maintain homeostasis. If values are found to change with age, the question must be asked whether this is due to inadvertant inclusion of values caused by disease. For instance, is the increase, with age, of the upper limit for urea and urate in apparently healthy individuals due to deterioration of function and is this the same as the beginning of a disease? It is also important to avoid attributing to age fluctuations due to other factors, such as change in body weight.

MENOPAUSE

Hormonal changes at menopause give rise to a number of changes in blood constituents. Thus, it may be necessary to consider separate reference intervals for pre- and postmenopausal subjects of the same age. This is often not easy, as changes develop over time. For instance, serum FSH may increase 13-fold, and LH threefold, within a year of the cessation of menses, with maximum levels occurring 3 to 5 years later.

PREGNANCY

Many changes in blood composition develop during pregnancy, and reference intervals must be obtained for healthy women with uncomplicated pregnancies, at various stages of gestation. Changes in pregnancy are reviewed by Young[66] and Lind.[67]

RACIAL AND GENETIC DIFFERENCES

Inherited differences in blood levels are known for a number of substances, and it may often be difficult to separate the influence of environment from that of heredity. Socioeconomic conditions and location of residence may affect levels; it is not always possible to translate reference intervals from one country to another.

BODY MASS

A number of blood constituents have been found to correlate positively with an individual's body mass. It has been recommended that over- and underweight subjects should be excluded from the reference intervals.[10] The problem is in defining the degree of obesity warranting exclusion. The Scandinavian Society recommends exclusion if a subject is 20% or more over the mean weight for the group, and overweight for exclusion is suggested as more than 89 kg in Norway, more than 97 kg in Finland, more than 104 kg in Denmark, and more than 111 kg in Sweden. The effect of using different figures in different communities on the reference intervals is not stated.

OTHER SUBGROUPS

Some constituents of blood are said to vary according to the social class of the individual, but findings have been confusing. It is possible that differences are related to life style.

There is also said to be a correlation between some blood levels and blood pressure.

Blind people often demonstrate features of hypoadrenalism,[66] with low levels of urinary keto- and oxysteroids, reduced serum glucose and calcium, and high levels of serum urea and creatinine. Little attention appears to have been given to these as a subgroup or to the possible difficulties in interpretation of results from blind or partially sighted people.

A number of changes in blood composition are found after acclimatization to altitude, and in the cases of substances such as hemoglobin, bicarbonate, CO_2, and erythrocyte count, reference intervals will be different in patients living at high altitudes.

To summarize, when determining reference intervals consideration should be given to the following conclusion of the IFCC Expert Panel:[12]

> Production of reference values from any population or individuals requires appropriate selection and often subclassification. This can only be made by careful description of the characteristics of the reference individuals and by the application of clearly stated criteria.

Chapter 3

CALCIUM

Calcium in blood is mainly present in plasma, with little found in the red cells. Ultrafiltration followed by estimation of free ions in the filtrate suggests that about 45% of plasma calcium is protein bound.[68] Most of the remainder is present as ionized calcium, with a small amount in the form of nonionic complexes mainly combined with organic acids.

ANALYTIC CONSIDERATIONS

METHOD DIFFERENCES
Early work on serum calcium levels in healthy and diseased subjects must be viewed with caution, since the methods used were often based on the procedure of Clark and Collip.[69] Although inaccuracies in this method were pointed out by MacIntyre in 1957,[70] it was still considered an acceptable reference method until about 1970.

Bold[71] and Gosling[72] reviewed methods of estimating serum calcium. Both noted that the narrow reference interval in healthy subjects puts a greater demand on the analytic system than on most estimations in clinical chemistry.

Some methods frequently used in literature references are

1.	Precipitation as oxalate and titration with $KMnO_4$ (Clark & Collip method)	Inaccurate due to coprecipitation of Mg and loss of Ca during washing
2.	Emission and atomic absorption flame photometry	Atomic absorption suggested for use as a reference method[73]
3.	Titration with a chelating agent, such as EDTA, using a photometric or photometric end point	Useful for pediatric work, as small volumes are used
4.	Fluorimetric measurement of calcein complex	Also useful for small volumes
5.	Measurement of color with cresolphthalein complexone (CPC)	Used in many laboratories using either continous-flow or discrete methods of analysis

Gosling gives figures from the UK External Quality Assessment Scheme for 1982 to 1984, giving bias and imprecision for the most frequently used methods (Table 1). Compared with atomic absorption methods, CPC methods show a positive bias, and EDTA titration methods show a negative bias. The acceptable analytic error is calculated by Gosling to be 0.02 to 0.04 mmol/L, and external quality assurance schemes suggest that only a minority of laboratories consistently achieve this standard.

SI UNITS
Serum calcium is expressed in the literature both in mass units and in milliequivalents. To convert to SI units,

$$\text{serum mmol / L} = \frac{\text{mg / 100 mL}}{4}$$
$$= \frac{\text{mEq / L}}{2}$$

TABLE 1.
Bias and Imprecision for the Most Frequently Used Methods
for Serum Calcium Estimation[a]

Method group	Mean cv (%)	Bias at overall mean value (mmol/L)		
		2.00	2.60	3.20
Atomic absorption spectroscopy	3.4	0.000	0.000	0.000
O-cresolphthalein				
manual/discrete	3.4	+0.010	+0.035	+0.055
continuous flow	2.4	−0.040	+0.015	+0.075
Automatic titration	2.5	−0.075	−0.075	−0.040

[a] From Gosling, P., *Ann. Clin. Biochem.*, 23, 146, 1986. With permission.

INTERFERENCE WITH ANALYSIS

HEMOLYSIS
Titration Methods

Henry stated[74] that hemolysis interferes with the end point of some titration methods. Alexander,[75] using titration with EGTA and calcein as an indicator, found no interference with 0.3 g/L serum hemoglobin, and a reduction of 1% with 0.6 g/L, of 5% with 2 g/L, and 9% with 3 g/L.

Fluorimetric Methods

Meites found that up to 3 g/L of serum hemoglobin did not affect a proposed standard method utilizing fluorimetry of the calcium/calcein complex.[76]

CPC Methods

Hemolysis does not affect estimations using a continuous-flow analyzer.[77] Directly reacting methods are affected, and Corns noted several factors relevant to methods of correction used in different instruments.[78]

1. Hemolysate plus premixed alkaline reagent

   Oxyhaemoglobin persists. Considerable spectral interference found at 575 nm in AMP, glycine, and diethylamine buffers.

2. Hemolysate plus acid reagent with buffer added later

   A hemoglobin derivative is formed with 575-nm absorption greater than that of acid hematin.

3. Hemolysate plus alkaline buffer followed by adding CPC reagent

   Results are buffer dependent. Oxyhemoglobin persists with AMP and glycine buffers. A derivative similar to that formed with acid reagent is formed with diethylamine buffer.

Using the Technicon RA 1000 (Technicon Instruments Corp., Tarrytown, NY), a reading is taken at 550 nm in acid reagent, and a further reading is taken after adding AMP buffer. Correction will be inadequate due to the different absorbance of two hemoglobin derivatives. The correction in the Beckman Astra 8 (Beckman Instruments Inc., Fullerton, CA) would be adequate, as a reading is taken after adding sample to diethylamine buffer and again after adding CPC reagent. In the Dupont ACA (Du Pont Diagnostics, Wilmington, DE), sample is added to CPC in glycine buffer, and readings taken at 570 and 600 nm. Under these conditions, oxyhemoglobin will be present, and the correction will be inadequate.

BILIRUBIN

Serum bilirubin of more than 40 μmol/L has been reported to reduce apparent serum calcium estimated by fluorimetric methods using calcein.[75,79] Mann and Green found the effect to be much less than previously reported[80] and attributed this to the availability of better-quality calcein. They compared analysis by a fluorimetric method using a Corning titrator (Corning Glass Works, Science Products Division, Corning, NY) with atomic absorption spectroscopy and found a difference of less than 4% at serum bilirubin of 400 μmol/L. It was concluded that interference is not serious if satisfactory-quality calcein is used.

OTHER INTERFERING SUBSTANCES

Fluorescence is depressed by salicylates and sulfonamides, and methods using fluorescence of the calcium/calcein complex cannot be used for the analysis of constituents from patients taking these drugs.[76] It has been reported that there is no effect on *o*-cresolphthalein methods.[77]

Olthuis et al. showed[81] that palmitic and stearic acids interfere with the EDTA titration method using murexide as an indicator and considered that the method could not be used if serum free fatty acid was more than 1.5 mmol/L.

Amino phenol is not used therapeutically, but is a possible metabolite of *N*-acetyl *p*-amino phenol. Singh et al. found that 0.1 mmol/L added to serum increased apparent serum calcium[82] by 0.1 mmol/L when estimated using a Technicon SMA 12/60 analyzer. Addition of 1.0 mmol/L increased the level by 3.4 mmol/L.

PREANALYTIC ERROR

COLLECTION OF THE SPECIMEN

Although factors such as the time since eating, and posture, are known to have some effect on constituent levels, in normal medical practice the specimen for serum calcium is frequently collected without any special preparation of the patient. Changes in disease are often small, and ideally, fasting specimens taken under standard conditions should be used.

Most laboratories use serum from a clotted specimen of blood. Plasma from tubes containing oxalate, edetate, or citrate, which prevent clotting by binding calcium, cannot be used.

Lacher and Elsea found that the commercially available product Liposol (Biosol Ltd., Ann Arbor, MI), used to decrease lipemia, affected serum calcium.[83] The mean serum calcium of 26 randomly selected sera shaken with Liposol fell from 2.250 to 2.102 mmol/L.

VENOUS STASIS

Laboratory workers have been aware for many years that excessive pressure from a tourniquet, when collecting samples, is likely to result in falsely high serum calcium results. Early work using the Clark and Collip method[84-86] has been confirmed by Berry et al.,[119] who found that serum calcium rose by from 0.025 to 0.200 mmol/L after a sphygmomanometer cuff had been in place for 15 min at a pressure of 90 mm of mercury. Serum-ionized calcium did not change, suggesting that the effect was due to an increase in serum protein.

It is frequently suggested that specimens for serum calcium should be taken without the use of a tourniquet, but the quantitative effect of restricting blood supply is not usually given. Assuming that the change shown by Berry et al. can be applied universally and that the change is linear with time, then an increase of up to approximately 0.05 mmol/L in serum calcium is possible with normal collection procedures.

CONTAMINATION

There have been a number of reports of analytic error due to contamination with calcium.

Glassware

Calcium in tap water is a potential contaminant. Pybus recommends that all glassware to be used should be washed overnight in alkaline detergent, soaked in molar hydrochloric acid, and finally washed several times in deionized water.[86a]

Bark Corks

Serious errors can be introduced by the leaching of calcium from bark corks used to stopper collection tubes.[87]

Vacuum Collection Tubes

A spurious increase in serum calcium, up to 2%, was found in vacuum collection tubes, by Foster et al.[88] Contamination was found to vary between and within lots, by Pragay et al.[89] A reinvestigation some years later found that 3 to 7 mg of calcium per tube could be obtained with one wash with deionized water.[90] Helman et al. considered that for some tubes the stopper was the source of contamination.[91]

Heparin

Batches of lithium heparin collection tubes were found by Hallsworth et al. to be contaminated.[92]

Anticoagulant

Fitzpatrick et al. warned of possible contamination with potassium edate transferred on a syringe tip that had been rested on the side of a blood-count tube.[93]

Wooden Applicator Sticks

Joseph found an increase in serum calcium after 3-min contact with sticks used to remove fibrin.[94] The increase was 0.2 mmol/L after 30 min.

Filter Paper

Some filter papers contain significant amounts of calcium and should be checked if used to filter solutions used in calcium estimations.

SAMPLE STABILITY

There are conflicting reports of the effect on serum calcium of the storage of samples before analysis (Table 2). It seems likely that some specimens deteriorate on storage, others are stable, and that reconstituted lyophilized serum behaves differently.

A thorough mixing of frozen samples is essential, as there is a concentration gradient, with the highest calcium concentration at the bottom of the tube.[98]

The storage of serum in polystyrene analyzer cups can result in adsorption of calcium if the loss of carbon dioxide results in an increase in serum pH.[99] Adsorption is much less in polypropylene containers. Samples should be stored at 4°C in tightly capped containers.

Overnight storage in tubes containing polyester gel separators had little effect on mean serum calcium,[100] but there was poor correlation with specimens treated normally, with comparisons in the range of 0.34 mmol/L higher to 0.20 mmol/L lower.

Heating to 56°C

Only a small change in calcium is found on heating serum or plasma to 56°C for 30 min to minimize the risk from HIV-positive samples (Table 3). Houssein et al. considered the

TABLE 2.
Effect of Storage on Serum Calcium

Reference	Reported effect
95	Reconstituted lyophilized serum was stable for 19 days at 10°C.
	Deep frozen samples were satisfactory at the end of a 22-day study.
96	There was a significant increase in the apparent calcium level after the 2nd day in separated serum kept at 37°C to simulate transport by post.
	At 4°C there was a significant increase after 12 days.
	All except one sample were stable when frozen for 33 days.
97	Samples of serum were kept frozen for from 3 months to $2^1/_2$ years.
	Some showed no change, whereas others showed large falls in apparent serum calcium level.

TABLE 3.
Effect on Calcium of Heating Serum or Plasma to 56°C for 30 min

Reference	Reported effect
101	Analysis using Technicon SMAC
	Mean increase in serum calcium of 0.08%
102	Analyzed using Technicon SMA
	Heparinized plasma mean decrease 3.4%
	Serum increase 0.9%
	Analyzed using Beckman Astra 8
	Heparinized plasma mean decrease 1.3%
	Serum decrease 2.8%
103	No significant change using heparinized plasma
104	No significant change using heparinized plasma

change to be significant statistically,[102] but not of importance clinically. In view of the suggestion that acceptable analytic error should be less than 1 to 2%, the error introduced may not always be acceptable.

PHYSIOLOGIC CHANGES

POSTURE
There is a fall in serum calcium when a person moves from the upright to the prone position, which is related to the fall in serum protein. The findings of several workers are shown in Table 4. Many published ranges for serum calcium in healthy people are based on studies of ambulatory subjects often sitting for a short, but variable, time before sample collection. The conditions of collection need to be standardized to obtain satisfactory ranges, and the differences need to be considered when interpreting results from patients who were lying prone when the samples were collected.

MEALS
Although early reports suggested that serum calcium is not altered after a meal,[108,109] later investigators found a small change. Wills found a change during the day of 0.200 to 0.475 mmol/L in 12 subjects taking meals normally,[110] but in three subjects fasted during the day, the maximum change was about 0.125 mmol/L from the average for the person concerned. These findings were considered to suggest that any changes were due to meals.

Seamonds et al., who found an increase in serum calcium after meals of 0.02 to 0.05 mmol/L in four subjects,[111] showed that the increase was related to increased alkalinity of the blood.

TABLE 4.
Change in Serum Calcium on Moving From Lying to an Upright Position
(in mmol/L)

Reference	Reported effect		Mean	Corrected for protein Mean
105	Fall of 5% or about 0.10 after subject prone for 30 min			
106	Mean fall of 0.07 in men and 0.09 in women, after subject prone for 1 h			
107	Lying in bed overnight		2.44	2.44
	followed by standing for 45 min, walking for 10 min,		2.52	2.47
	and sitting for 20 min followed by lying for 1 h		2.46	2.46

TABLE 5.
Serum Calcium in Subjects Immobilized for Long Periods
(in mmol/L)

Reference	Subjects	Reported effects
116	Four healthy men in plaster casts for 4 weeks	Before, 2.65–2.80 After, 2.68–3.18 Each subject had at least one value more than 3.00
117	Five healthy volunteers rest in bed 24 or 30 weeks	Mean increase 0.05 Unaffected by phosphate administration
118	Four healthy men rest in bed 12 days	Mean before, 2.218 Mean after, 2.321 No rise seen until 7th day

DIET

It has been known for many years that a high-fiber diet results in a negative calcium balance, leading to lower serum calcium.[112] The change has usually been ascribed to the phytate content of whole wheat, but binding of metal ions to fiber has been observed.[113] Heaton and Pomare found a mean fall of 0.075 mmol/L in serum calcium of 14 subjects given 18 to 100 g of bran (median 38 g) daily for 4 to 9 weeks.[114] Reinhold et al. gave three volunteers in Iran a diet containing 2.5 g of phytic acid for 60 days[115] and obtained a fall of about 0.2 mmol/L.

IMMOBILIZATION AND BED REST

Several groups have demonstrated mean increases in serum calcium of 0.05 to 0.10 mmol/L in immobilized subjects (Table 5). Occasionally, the level exceeded that found in healthy individuals.

EXERCISE

Paradoxically, vigorous exercise also produces an increase in serum calcium (Table 6). Changes observed in the hematocrit suggest that the changes are explained by a fall in plasma volume. The more modest exercise involved in walking to a clinic is unlikely to affect serum calcium levels significantly, but it would be wise for specimens to be taken under standard conditions, including a period of rest before collection.

HYPERVENTILATION

Due to the change in blood pH, hyperventilation would be expected to lead to a change in serum calcium. Mostellar and Tuttle found the mean serum calcium increased from 2.26 to 2.33 mmol/L after hyperventilating for 60 min,[122] followed by a fall to 2.16 after a 60-min

TABLE 6.
Change in Serum Calcium after Exercise

Reference	Subjects	Sex	Age	N	Change in % mean	
119	Healthy young men exercise to the limit of their capacity	M			+10.00	Individual increase up to 17% (A fault in this work was that specimens before exercise were taken with subjects lying down)
120	Fasting subjects exercised for 12 min	M	20–30	18	+7.30	
			30–40	47	+8.80	
			40–50	88	+6.80	
		F	20–30	34	+10.16	
			30–40	48	+12.40	
			40–50	28	+14.40	
121	Volunteers exercised for 20 min	M			+7.00	

TABLE 7.
Reports of Variation of Serum Calcium During the Year

Reference	Location	Reported effect
124	Uppsala, Sweden	31 subjects. Mean 0.20 mmol/L; higher in spring Analysis by Clark and Collip method
125	United States	13 males and 13 females. Variation between months, but no consistent pattern
126	Kyoto City, Japan	4 males, Dec–Feb mean 2.68 ± 0.13 mmol/L 4 males, Jun–Aug. mean 2.51 ± 0.09 mmol/L Analysis by Clark and Collip method
97	England	10 male and 10 female. No significant change over 2 years Analysis by an atomic absorption method
127	England	No change in serum calcium during the year, but change in serum 25 hydroxy cholecalciferol
128	Sweden	0.02–0.04 mmol/L; higher in summer
129	England	No seasonal or long-term trends found in laboratory means over 6 years. Any variation explained by changes in laboratory practice

recovery period. Seamonds et al. gave the results of an experiment on a healthy subject in whom serum calcium of 2.38 and blood pH of 7.38 before hyperventilating changed to serum calcium of 2.55 mmol/L and blood pH of 7.61 after 25 min of hyperventilating.[111]

Hyperventilation will not normally be a problem, but occasionally it may need to be taken into account if the subject is emotional or, as with a child, is frightened of venipuncture.

SEASONAL CHANGES

As long ago as 1927, Bakwin and Bakwin reported that serum calcium in infants was higher in summer than in winter,[123] with an increased incidence of tetany and rickets in winter. A number of groups have since studied changes in serum calcium during the year, due to the potential link between exposure to sunlight and vitamin D metabolism. Reports are conflicting (Table 7), with some finding no seasonal changes, and others claiming that there is a mean rise of about 0.02 mmol/L in spring and summer.

Iwanani et al. investigated the possibility that seasonal variation was related to changes in the ambient temperature.[126] Two subjects lived in a room at 30°C for 16 h each day. There was little change in serum calcium for 4 days, and then the level fell about 0.02 mmol/L. In a study by Hodkinson et al., a group of 25 elderly patients with no exposure to sunlight had mean serum calcium of 2.22 mmol/L,[130] whereas in 78 elderly patients with varying amounts of exposure to sunlight, the mean was 2.30 mmol/L. A sunlight exposure score showed a positive correlation. A different finding was reported by Lester and Wills,[97] who found no relationship between serum calcium and exposure to bright sunlight in the previous 3 months in ten males and ten females, ages 24 to 51.

Although the published work is not conclusive, it seems possible that serum calcium is higher in summer than in winter and that this may be related to changes in ambient temperature or to exposure to sunlight.

RANGE IN HEALTHY SUBJECTS

CORRECTION FOR SERUM PROTEIN

When interpreting serum calcium, it is necessary to take into account the protein level, as variations in the protein level have effects on serum calcium. Correction factors have been used, and care must be taken, when comparing reference intervals from different workers, to note if adjustment to a standard protein or albumin level has been made.

Some methods make corrections using plasma specific gravity as an indication of protein concentration.[86,131] This does not take into consideration other substances affecting specific gravity, such as urea, glucose, and lipid, and also relies on an estimation less precise than an assay for protein or albumin. Other methods[132,133] correct using total protein or albumin.[134,135] The use of albumin is based on the report[136] that 81% of serum protein-bound calcium is held by albumin. Correction to albumin does not take into account alterations in globulin, possible abnormal binding of calcium, or method differences. Published correction factors differ widely, and this may, in some cases, reflect the different populations studied.[137] Whether a single correction factor can be used for all patients has been questioned.[138] A single factor may not even be satisfactory for an individual patient, as it may change with blood pH. Walker and Payne responded[139] to a suggestion that changes caused by use of a tourniquet when collecting samples could be corrected by stating that forearm exercise before collection would give a variable production of lactate and that the lowering of blood pH would alter the calcium/albumin relationship. The difficulties in correcting for protein levels have driven most clinical chemists to use unadjusted serum calcium results and take into account changes in protein levels, as appropriate.

In the literature, there is reasonable agreement about the range of serum calcium levels in healthy adults when possible differences in method are taken into account. The findings of several large series are shown in Tables 8 and 9, and ranges found by other workers using extraction from hospital records are shown in Tables 10 and 11. Correction for serum protein was not made in any of the studies shown. The lower levels found in hospital patients can probably be explained by the proportion confined to bed. In males there is a fall with age to about 50 to 55 years, and an increase after 50 years in women. When noted, most reports state that the distribution is approximately gaussian.

It is interesting to compare the published ranges from studies of large numbers of subjects with ranges given in textbooks over the past 60 years (Table 12). At first, ranges were probably based on the Clark and Collip method, and the earliest textbooks give a figure for the lower end of the range of about 2.25 mmol/L. Most recent textbooks give a figure of 2.10 to 2.20 mmol/L, which compares well with figures derived using CPC methods. The top end of the range is given as about 2.75 mmol/L in the early books, and in recent textbooks the top end varies from 2.50 to 2.70 mmol/L, with a few quoting different ranges for males and females.

WITHIN-INDIVIDUAL VARIATION

Table 13 shows results from a number of studies of the variation of serum calcium during a number of weeks in individuals, using standardized methods of collection. The range that

TABLE 8.
Serum Calcium in Healthy Men (in mmol/L)

Age (years)

Reference		<20	21–25	26–30	31–35	36–40	41–45	46–50	51–55	56–60	61–65	66–70	>70
140[a]	Mean		2.41		2.40		2.38		2.36		2.35		2.32
	Range		2.27–2.55		2.26–2.54		2.24–2.52		2.23–2.50		2.21–2.50		2.18–2.47
141[b]	N		96		721		1268		1112		415		105
	Mean		2.51		2.50		2.49		2.48		2.47		2.48
	Range		2.32–2.70		2.29–2.71		2.28–2.69		2.28–2.67		2.27–2.68		2.23–2.72
142[c]	Mean	2.48		2.45		2.43		2.41		2.41			
143[d]	N	527		1381		692		320		163			
	Mean	2.48		2.44		2.43		2.41		2.41			
	Range	2.31–2.68		2.27–2.64		2.23–2.64		2.23–2.65		2.22–2.61			
Coventry[e]	N	137	245	247	218	218	208	163	143	137	57		
	Mean	2.44	2.43	2.41	2.41	2.40	2.37	2.37	2.38	2.37	2.37		
	Range	2.27–2.61	2.27–2.60	2.25–2.57	2.23–2.57	2.21–2.59	2.17–2.57	2.21–2.53	2.19–2.54	2.19–2.54	2.20–2.54		

[a] Direct titration with EDTA. 298 Caucasian men over 20 years old in good health.
[b] Emission flame photometry. 3600 men from a well-persons' clinic.
[c] Cresolphthalein complexone method using a continuous-flow analyzer. Approximately 500 male blood donors.
[d] Cresolphthalein complexone method using Technicon AA2 analyzer. Healthy persons, supine, exclusions based on clinical examination, health questionnaire, overweight, and medication.
[e] Cresolphthalein complexone method on American Monitor discrete analyzer. Healthy hospital staff, as described in Chapter 2.

TABLE 9.
Serum Calcium in Healthy Women[a] (in mmol/L)

Reference		<20	21–25	26–30	31–35	36–40	41–45	46–50	51–55	56–60	61–65	66–70	>70
140[b]	Mean		2.35		2.36		2.36		2.36		2.36		2.36
	Range		2.21–2.50		2.20–2.51		2.21–2.51		2.21–2.51		2.21–2.51		2.21–2.47
141[c]	N		72		193		283		278		229		39
	Mean		2.49		2.46		2.46		2.50		2.51		2.39
	Range		2.28–2.70		2.28–2.65		2.25–2.68		2.30–2.70		2.30–2.72		2.27–2.69
142[d]	Mean	2.46		2.42		2.40		2.44		2.45			
143[e]	N	537		1093		543		276		80			
	Mean	2.43		2.39		2.40		2.40		2.45			
	Range	2.27–2.62		2.22–2.60		2.19–2.60		2.19–2.61		2.28–2.69			
Coventry[f]	N	698	602	332	327	254	245	162	123	79	12		
	Mean	2.40	2.38	2.37	2.36	2.36	2.35	2.36	2.39	2.38	2.39		
	Range	2.21–2.57	2.21–2.55	2.20–2.53	2.19–2.54	2.19–2.54	2.16–2.54	2.19–2.53	2.18–2.53	2.18–2.58	2.22–2.56		

Column spanning note (from the original brace structure): for references 140[b] and 141[c], each pair of age groups (21–25/26–30, 31–35/36–40, 41–45/46–50, 51–55/56–60, 61–65/66–70) shares one value; for references 142[d] and 143[e], the shared values span (26–30/31–35, 36–40/41–45, 46–50/51–55, 56–60/61–65).

a   Methods are as given in Table 8.
b   278 Caucasian women in good health.
c   1100 women from a well-women's clinic.
d   Approximately 500 female blood donors.
e   Healthy persons, supine, exclusions based on clinical examination, health questionnaire, overweight, and medication.
f   Healthy hospital staff, as described in Chapter 2.

TABLE 10.
Reference Intervals Derived from Hospital Records for Serum Calcium in Males (in mmol/L)

Reference		<20	21–25	26–30	31–35	36–40	41–45	46–50	51–55	56–60	61–65	66–70	>70
144[a]	Mean	2.43	2.38	2.38	2.38	2.38	2.33	2.33	2.33	2.33			
145[b]	Mean		2.60	2.60	2.55	2.55	2.50	2.50	2.50	2.50	2.50	2.50	
	Range		2.30–2.80	2.30–2.80	2.35–2.80	2.35–2.80	2.35–2.75	2.35–2.75	2.25–2.85	2.25–2.85	2.30–2.80	2.30–2.80	
146[c]	Mean	2.42	2.40	2.40	2.40	2.40	2.38	2.38	2.36	2.36	2.36	2.36	2.33
	Range	2.21–2.63	2.20–2.61	2.20–2.61	2.16–2.65	2.16–2.65	2.14–2.62	2.14–2.62	2.11–2.61	2.11–2.61	2.16–2.56	2.16–2.56	2.14–2.52
147[c]	Mean		2.38	2.38	2.36	2.36	2.35	2.35	2.34	2.34	2.33	2.33	2.30
	Range		2.15–2.61	2.15–2.61	2.15–2.57	2.15–2.57	2.13–2.56	2.13–2.56	2.12–2.56	2.12–2.56	2.10–2.56	2.10–2.56	2.06–2.53

[a] Estimated using CPC method on Technicon SMA 12/60 analyzer.
[b] Estimated using CPC method on Technicon SMA 12/60 analyzer.
[c] Method not given.

TABLE 11.
Reference Intervals Derived from Hospital Records for Serum Calcium in Females (in mmol/L)

Reference		<20	21–25	26–30	31–35	36–40	41–45	46–50	51–55	56–60	61–65	66–70	>70
144	Mean	2.38	2.30	2.30	2.30	2.30	2.30	2.30	2.30	2.30	2.30	2.30	
145	Mean		2.50	2.50	2.50	2.50	2.50	2.50	2.50	2.50	2.55	2.55	
	Range		2.20–2.75	2.20–2.75	2.35–2.75	2.35–2.75	2.25–2.75	2.25–2.75	2.25–2.85	2.25–2.85	2.30–2.85	2.30–2.85	
146	Mean	2.38	2.38	2.38	2.38	2.38	2.38	2.38	2.39	2.39	2.38	2.38	2.38
	Range	2.19–2.58	2.16–2.60	2.16–2.60	2.16–2.59	2.16–2.59	2.20–2.56	2.20–2.56	2.18–2.60	2.18–2.60	2.17–2.59	2.17–2.59	2.15–2.60
147	Mean		2.35	2.35	2.34	2.34	2.34	2.34	2.37	2.37	2.35	2.35	2.37
	Range		2.14–2.56	2.14–2.56	2.12–2.55	2.12–2.55	2.12–2.55	2.12–2.55	2.14–2.60	2.14–2.60	2.12–2.59	2.12–2.59	2.09–2.53

TABLE 12.
Range Given in Textbooks for Serum Calcium in Healthy Subjects

Reference	Range mg/100 mL	Range mmol/L	Comment
148	9.0–11.5	2.25–2.88	
149	9.0–11.0	2.25–2.75	
150	9.0–11.5	2.25–2.88	
7	9.0–11.0	2.25–2.88	
151	8.5–11.5	2.13–2.63	"During infancy and early childhood, average values approach upper limits of range"
152	9.0–11.5	2.25–2.88	
153	9.0–11.0	2.25–2.75	Range in random sample of women 8.5–10.5 mg/100 mL (2.13–2.63 mmol/L)
154	9.0–11.0	2.25–2.75	States 8.5–10.5 mg/100 mL (2.13–2.63) using EDTA titration
155		2.12–2.62	Gives range in molar units
156	9.4–11.0	2.35–2.75	
157	8.5–10.5	2.13–2.63	
158		2.30–2.60	
159		2.20–2.70	Increase of 0.5–1.0 mg/100 mL (0.13–0.25 mmol/L) after meals
160		2.10–2.55	Children 2.20–2.70 mmol/L Newborn 2.25–2.65 mmol/L
161		2.10–2.50	Children 2.20–2.70 mmol/L
43		2.25–2.65	Range in inpatients 2.15–2.60 mmol/L
162		2.10–2.65	Atomic absorption method

TABLE 13.
Variation of Serum Calcium Within Individuals

Reference	Subjects	N	Analytic variation SD (mmol/L)	Analytic variation cv (%)	Mean personal variation SD (mmol/L)	Mean personal variation cv (%)
163	Fasting samples taken weekly for 10–12 weeks with minimal stasis from healthy subjects	68	0.071	2.71	0.043	1.64
164	Fasting samples taken weekly for 10 weeks from healthy male physicians. All samples analyzed on same day.	10	0.76	2.96	0.40	1.53
165	Five samples taken within 3 weeks from healthy male students 21–27 years old					1.7

might be expected in an individual is approximately ±0.08 mmol/L from the mean for that person when analytic variation has been excluded.

THE ELDERLY

Ranges found by several workers in the elderly are shown in Table 14. Levels appear similar to those found in 50- to 60-year-old subjects.

TABLE 14.
Serum Calcium in the Elderly (in mmol/L)

References	Subjects	Males age (years) 65–74		75+		Females age (years) 65–74		75+	
		Mean	SD	Mean	SD	Mean	SD	Mean	SD
166	500 nonfasting subjects sampled randomly from the population and excluding the acutely ill. Analysis by a continuous-flow method	2.410	0.113	2.360	0.085	2.450	0.125	2.408	0.140
		2.390	0.100[a]	2.355	0.100[a]	2.435	0.128[a]	2.390	0.145[a]
167	90 subjects, age 63–94, excluding 17 with disease initially or within 6 months and 11 taking thiazides	Mean 2.40	SD 0.125			Range 2.20–2.675			
168	1403 elderly men and 639 elderly women fasted[b] for 2 h	Mean 2.375 5–97.5th percentile 2.175–2.500				Mean 2.375 5–95th percentile 2.200–2.550			

[a] Corrected as indicated by Dent.[165]
[b] No significant difference found in those on medication.

TABLE 15.
Effect of Menopause on Serum Calcium[a] (in mmol/L)

Reference	Subjects	Concentration	
		Mean	SD
169	9 patients before oophorectomy	2.360	
	3 and 6 months after	2.565	
	11 patients after hysterectomy	No change	
142	Blood donors		
	age 36–45, premenopause	2.400	
	Postnatural menopause	2.420	
	Posthysterectomy	2.420	
	age 46–55, premenopause	2.400	
	Postnatural menopause	2.430	
	Posthysterectomy	2.460	
170	62 women over 35 years of age attending for minor complaints		
	Premenopause	2.360	0.08
	Postnatural menopause	2.430	0.06
	Postbilateral oophorectomy	2.440	0.09

[a]   CPC method of analysis used by each group.

EFFECT OF MENOPAUSE

A number of studies have been made of serum calcium at menopause, as estrogens are known to affect bone metabolism. The findings shown in Table 15, combined with the change with age found in women in Table 9, suggest that there is a small rise in serum calcium of about 0.03 to 0.05 mmol/L after natural menopause, a hysterectomy, or a bilateral oophorectomy.

CHILDREN

Table 16 shows ranges found by various groups for serum calcium in childhood. Most agree that there is a fall at puberty in girls and that mean levels in childhood are probably a little higher than in adults.

NEONATES

The frequent presence of factors affecting serum calcium makes a study during the neonatal period difficult. Low serum protein and frequent acidosis in premature infants, in infants of diabetic mothers, and in infants subject to a period of asphyxia may cause changes in the first 4 days of life, and variation in the type of feed begins to affect serum calcium by the fifth day of life.

Meites quotes ranges from 19 reports on the level in full-term newborn infants,[174] with "nor-mal" defined as the absence of any specific disease associated with calcium. He states that this definition requires clinical, as well as statistical, support for the upper and lower limits. The analytic method used can be a source of differences in ranges reported. Despite this, any direction of change can be detected. Serum calcium falls during the first days of life, and breast-fed babies have higher serum calcium than bottle-fed babies (Table 17). Despite dilution of cow milk because of the high protein content, the phosphorous is twice that in human milk, raising the serum phosphorous of infants on artificial feeds and predisposing them to hypocalcemia.[179]

The range in premature infants is 0.25 to 0.50 mmol/L lower than in full-term infants. Whereas the level in full-term neonates reaches adult levels within 2 weeks, this level may not be attained in premature infants for a month or more.[174]

TABLE 16.
Serum Calcium in Children

Reference		Age (years)																		Adult
		1	2	3	4	5	6	7	8	9	10	11	12	13	14	15	16	17	18	
171[a]	Male mean	2.475		2.450				2.450			2.425			2.350		2.400				
	Female	2.475		2.475				2.450			2.450			2.400		2.400				
	Range male and female	2.200–2.280		2.150–2.750				2.150–2.750			2.150–2.750			2.150–2.750		2.175–2.750				2.250–2.750
172[b]	Mean male											2.520	2.520	2.570	2.580	2.450	2.470	2.440		
	Mean female											2.520	2.500	2.530	2.560	2.380	2.450	2.400		
143[c]	N Male							1716					1087				595			
	Male Mean							2.46					2.49				2.51			
	Male Range							2.29–2.66					2.32–2.69				2.32–2.71			
	N Female							1591					998				516			
	Female Mean							2.49					2.49				2.48			
	Female Range male and female							2.32–2.67					2.32–2.69				2.29–2.67			
173[d]	Male 50 percentile					2.42	2.45	2.42	2.45	2.45	2.42	2.45	2.45	2.48	2.47	2.47	2.45	2.45		
	Male 2.5–97.5 percentile					2.27–2.57	2.27–2.59	2.32–2.57	2.27–2.54	2.30–2.57	2.30–2.59	2.27–2.59	2.32–2.59	2.32–2.59	2.27–2.62	2.32–2.62	2.32–2.57	2.32–2.62		
	Female 50 percentile					2.45	2.47	2.45	2.45	2.47	2.45	2.45	2.47	2.47	2.45	2.45	2.42	2.40		
	Female 2.5–97.5 percentile					2.32–2.64	2.35–2.67	2.32–2.67	2.30–2.62	2.35–2.67	2.32–2.57	2.32–2.62	2.32–2.59	2.30–2.67	2.30–2.67	2.30–2.59	2.25–2.57	2.27–2.54		

a 837 healthy children 6 months to 16 years old. Fingerstick specimens with hemolyzed samples excluded.

b 111 healthy children from 2 schools near Vienna. Samples taken each year from age 11 to 18 years. Analysis on Greiner GSA analyzer.

c Heparinized plasma from fasting French children 4–18 years of age. Exclusions based on clinical examination, health questionnaire, overweight, and medication. Analysis using cresolphthalein complexone method on Technicon SMA II analyzer.

d About 3600 mainly Caucasian children from a screening program in Marshfield, U.S. Fasting serum analyzed using Technicon SMAC analyzer. Transcription error for 50 percentile of males age 13 and 17 years in original publication corrected by Dr. Haas in a personal communication.

TABLE 17.
Serum Calcium in Neonates (in mmol/L)

Reported values for method of feeding

Reference	Methodology	Day	Breast-fed Mean	Breast-fed Range	Adapted cow milk[a] SMA Mean	SMA Range	S26 Mean	S26 Range	Unadapted cow milk[b] Half cream Mean	Half cream Range	Full cream Mean	Full cream Range
175	Method not given	cord	2.75	SD 0.23								
		0–2	2.57									
		3–5	2.44	0.17								
		6–10	2.59	0.20								
176	Analysis by flame photometry	6	2.650	2.200–3.025	2.575	1.925–3.125	2.575	2.325–3.050	2.400	1.750–2.775	2.400	1.850–2.725
177	Full-term babies with normal birth weight. Up to 11 in each group. Analysis by atomic absorption spectroscopy	1	2.27	1.45–2.15[c]				1.800	1.45–2.15[d]			
		2	1.875	1.30–2.45				2.150	1.85–2.45			
		3	2.325	1.80–2.80				2.000	1.45–2.85			
		4	2.150	1.80–2.55				1.850	1.50–2.10			
		5	2.075	0.60–3.15				1.900	1.60–2.25			
		6	2.150	1.60–2.55				2.150	1.50–2.85			
		7	2.225	1.70–2.85								
178	Sample taken 2.5–3 h after a feed. Analysis by atomic absorption spectroscopy	5–7	2.550	2.025–3.175					Babies with no convulsions		2.325	1.800–3.000[e]
									Babies with convulsions		1.575	0.925–1.975

a   Cow milk modified to phosphorus content nearer to human milk.
b   Evaporated or dried milk.
c   No differentiation between bottle- and breast-fed at first day of life.
d   Type of artificial feed not stated.
e   Evaporated cow milk.

TABLE 18.
Serum Calcium in Neonates of Different Racial Groups (in mmol/L)

Reference	Methodology		N	Day	Mean	SD
					Reported values	
180	Analysis using	Caucasian	11	6	2.310	0.32
	cresolphthalein	Black	11	6	2.440	0.19
	complexone method	Asian	11	6	2.120	0.34
181	Full-term babies	Caucasian				
	Analysis by EDTA	Male		1	2.090	
	titration method			2	1.960	
				3	1.940	
				4	2.040	
		Female		1	2.163	
				2	2.060	
				3	2.040	
				4	2.090	
		Black	166			
		Male		1	2.240	
				2	2.140	
				3	2.110	
				4	2.190	
		Female		1	2.240	
				2	2.140	
				3	2.170	
				4	2.140	

Racial differences in serum calcium in neonates have been reported (Table 18). No explanation has been given for these findings.

CONCLUSION

Serum calcium in healthy subjects varies with age. The range 2.25 to 2.60 mmol/L probably represents 95% limits for young, healthy ambulatory males. Healthy ambulatory females of the same age probably have a range of 2.20 to 2.55 mmol/L.

There is a fall in serum calcium with age in adult males, which does not continue beyond the age of about 55 years. After an increase at menopause, the level does not change with increasing age in women.

The figure given for the top of the range in healthy subjects, in a number of textbooks, is too high. Levels fall during the first days of life, increasing after the fourth or fifth day. A fall in serum calcium at puberty in girls leads to different levels in men and women.

RANGE DURING PREGNANCY

It has been known for many years that serum calcium falls during pregnancy. Widdows, in 1923,[182] noted a fall during the last months of pregnancy and a rise directly after giving birth. Most work shows a decline in serum calcium in each trimester,[183,184] although one group found little change until the third trimester.[185] Pitkin and Gebhardt noted a steady fall in serum calcium from 8 weeks of pregnancy until the lowest levels at 32 to 36 weeks.[184] There was then a small rise, which continued until term. Various explanations have been suggested for the changes. The view in the 1920s appears to attribute the fall in serum calcium to the demands of the fetus and suggests that as a consequence, extra milk was required by the mother.[182] Others thought that the fall was due to the increased estrogen and adrenal steroid production,[185] known to have a hypocalcemic effect. Pitkin et al. have shown that the fall in serum calcium

TABLE 19.
Serum Calcium and Albumin During Pregnancy[a]

Stage of pregnancy		Serum calcium (mmol/L)	Albumin (g/L)
Trimester	First	2.33 ± 0.08	42.6 ± 3.5
	Second	2.23 ± 0.08	37.0 ± 3.8
	Third	2.18 ± 0.10	34.2 ± 3.1
6 weeks post partum		2.35 ± 0.12	46.0 ± 3.6

[a]   From Pitkin, R.M., et al., *Am. J. Obstet. Gynecol.*, 133, 781, 1979. Estimation on heparinized plasma, using a continuous-flow analyzer.

TABLE 20.
Serum Calcium in Mother and Fetus[a] (in mmol/L)

	Fetus		Mother	
Weeks of pregnancy	Mean	Range	Mean	Range
15–18	2.15	2.03–2.30	2.42	2.30–2.55
19–22	2.22	2.07–2.37	2.34	2.27–2.40
23–26	2.15	2.01–2.29	2.32	2.23–2.40
27–30	2.32	2.24–2.39	2.30	2.21–2.40
32–34	2.31	2.20–2.43	2.25	2.20–2.30
35–38	2.39	2.23–2.55	2.24	2.19–2.29

[a]   From Moniz, C.F., et al., *J. Clin. Pathol.*, 38, 468, 1985.

TABLE 21.
Median Serum Calcium[a] during Pregnancy in Asians from the Indian Subcontinent and White-Skinned Caucasians in the United Kingdom (in mmol/L)

	Asian		Caucasian	
Weeks of pregnancy	N	Serum calcium	N	Serum calcium
10–20	11	2.29	18	2.36
21–30	11	2.30	10	2.39
31–40	10	2.30	15	2.36
During labor	11	2.27	12	2.72

[a]   From Okonofua, F., et al., *Ann. Clin. Biochem.*, 24, 22, 1987. Estimation using Technicon SMACanalyzer.

is almost exactly parallel to the fall in serum albumin (Table 19).[186] They also claim that serum ionic calcium does not change during pregnancy, although Tan et al. earlier had reported a fall,[185] using measurement with calcium electrodes. An interesting study by Moniz et al. of maternal and fetal samples obtained for prenatal diagnosis from 344 pregnancies subsequently found to be normal showed that serum calcium was higher in the mother during the first two trimesters,[187] but higher in the fetus in the later weeks of pregnancy (Table 20). This is supported by earlier reports[188,189] that cord serum calcium is 0.10 to 0.40 mmol/L higher than maternal serum calcium at term.

Racial differences in serum calcium during pregnancy have been reported. Table 21 shows lower levels found during pregnancy in mothers from the Indian subcontinent, compared with white-skinned mothers in the United Kingdom.

OTHER CHANGES

BODY WEIGHT

There are conflicting reports on the relationship between serum calcium and body weight. Goldberg et al. found no relationship,[191] whereas Munan et al. reported that in female subjects, serum calcium varied inversely with body weight.[192]

DRUGS THAT AFFECT SERUM CALCIUM

DRUGS USED TO TREAT HYPERCALCEMIA
Phosphate

Oral phosphate has been used to treat patients with hyperparathyroidism,[193,194] and although Dent commented on the fear of formation of renal stones and extraskeletal calcification,[195] Goldsmith and Ingbar later reported similar treatment of patients without ill effect.[196]

Sulfate

Although there are reports of treatment with sulfate,[197,198] it is not clear whether the better state of hydration resulting contributed to the improvement found.

EDTA

A fall in serum calcium can be achieved with EDTA, but there is a severe toxic effect (renal tubular damage), which makes the treatment inadvisable.[199,200]

Calcitonin

There is little change in serum calcium in healthy subjects given calcitonin,[201] but falls of 0.1 to 0.4 mmol/L occur within 3 h in some patients treated.[201,202] The effect may only last for 24 to 48 h, and it may be prolonged by simultaneous administration of glucocorticoid.[203] It has been suggested that since not all cases respond, an alternate treatment should be used if there is no response within 6 h.[204]

Glucocorticoids

The reduction of serum calcium was used as the basis for a test for hyperparathyroidism by Dent.[205] A reduction was found in hypercalcemia of various causes, but not in those with hyperparathyroidism. Despite the unpredictability and short-term reduction, steroids have frequently been used in the management of severe hypercalcemia.[204]

Diphosphonates

Bone resorption is inhibited by diphosphonates, and they have been given intravenously to treat hypercalcemia, and orally to treat Paget's disease.

Intravenous Treatment

Serum calcium returned to normal within 5 to 10 days in 10 hypercalcemic patients treated with etidronate (ethane hydroxyphosphonate) and 21 treated with clodronate. (dichloromethylene diphosphonate).[206] The fall is quicker and greater with pamidronate (amino hydroxypropylidene phosphonate).[207]

Oral Treatment

No change in serum calcium is found using etidronate.[208-210] Eight hundred to 3200 mg of clodronate daily was found to give a mean fall of 0.33 mmol/L in corrected fasting serum calcium after 5 months of treatment.[211]

TABLE 22.
Serum Calcium in Patients Taking Various Anticonvulsants (in mmol/L)

Reference	Subjects	Therapy	Range mean	Comment
213	75 male, 85 female age 16–70 years mean age 36 years	Taking one or more of: phenytoin phenobarbitone primidone pheneturide	1.875–2.650 Less than 2.25 in 30 of 160	Est. Auto analyzer Corrected for protein by Dents method.
	Controls 40 male, 42 female mean age 34 years		2.250–2.625	Effect related to high dosage and individual drugs in order: pheneturide primidone phenytoin phenobarbitone
214	48 adult patients compared with 38 controls matched for age and sex	Taking either: phenytoin or phenytoin phenobarbitone and phenytoin	**Mean** Phenytoin 2.395 + phenobarbitone 2.332 controls 2.445	
215	31 patients compared with matched controls	Taking carbamazepine for 20.5 ± 10 months dose 758 ± SD 468 mg/d Serum carbamazepine 26.4 ± 11.5 µmol/L	On carbamazepine 2.34 (3 of 31 less than 2.10) controls 2.44	Est. Technicon SMAC Serum albumin not significantly different in two groups
Coventry (Unpublished results from author's laboratory)	Samples from in- and outpatients submitted for drug levels	Patients taking drugs for varying periods	Phenytoin 4 of 22 lower than range in healthy subjects Phenobarbitone + phenytoin, 4 of 17 lower than range healthy subjects	Analysis by CPC method on AmericanMonitor "Parallel" analyzer

Gallium Nitrate

Warrell et al.[212] gave gallium nitrate to 24 patients with cancer-related hypercalcemia and serum calcium of more than 3.0 mmol/L (200 mg/m^2 body surface area per day intravenously for 5 days). Eighteen patients became normocalcemic.

OTHER HYPOCALCEMIC DRUGS
Anticonvulsants

Groups of patients taking anticonvulsants, either as single drugs or as multiple therapy, show reduced mean serum calcium levels (Table 22). Most levels are below the mean for age and sex, but only about 20% are below the range in healthy subjects. Anticonvulsants appear to influence vitamin D metabolism by inducing hepatic microsomal enzymes. It is suggested that serum calcium should be monitored regularly in patients treated for long periods, due to the possibility of osteomalacia.[216]

Asparaginase

Hypocalcemia was found in 21 of 27 children and 59 of 99 adults treated with asparaginase, by Oettgen et al.,[217] who concluded that the changes were associated with reduced serum albumin levels.

Barbiturates

Barbiturates used as hypnotics affect serum calcium in a way similar to phenobarbitone used to treat epilepsy.[218]

Cimetidine

Although Sherwood et al. claimed that cimetidine reduced PTH in the blood of patients with hyperparathyroidism,[219] and consequently serum calcium is reduced, other groups found no significant change.[220,221] Fisken and Wilkinson found no change when 1.6 g of cimetidine was given orally for 8 weeks,[222] but noted a mean fall of 0.14 mmol/L 48 h after intravenous administration.

Cisplatin

A renal tubular defect mainly affecting magnesium develops in patients treated with cisplatin, and occasionally symptoms of tetany occur. Schilsky and Anderson reported that 2 of 51 cases developed tetany, with serum calcium less than 2 mmol/L.[223]

Digoxin

A study by Tishler et al. found low serum and platelet calcium in patients taking digoxin.[224]

Sex	N	Group	Age (years)	Mean serum calcium (mmol/L)
M	11	Digoxin intoxication	47–96	2.040
F	13			
M	11	Digoxin treatment	55–81	2.095
F	5			
M	5	Control subject	20–71	2.215
F	16			

The different ages and sex ratios in the groups may have contributed to the differences.

Enfluane

A small decrease in serum calcium after anesthesia with enfluane was reported by Eqilmez et al.[225] No quantitation or other details were given, and it is possible that the change is related to mild alkalosis.

Ethylene Glycol

Poisoning by ethylene glycol was reviewed by Vale et al.[226] About 1% of ingested ethylene glycol is metabolized to oxalate, which combines with calcium and may lead to hypocalcemia.

Fluoride

Low serum calcium has been reported after poisoning with sodium fluoride.[227] Larsen et al. gave five healthy fasting subjects 60 mg of sodium fluoride and noted a fall of about 0.05 mmol/L during the next 3 h.[228] Pretreatment levels were regained after 24 h.

Gastrin

A mean fall in serum calcium of 0.175 mmol/L was found in five healthy males given 0.15 μg/kg/h of human gastrin, by McQuire et al.[229]

Gentamicin and Capreomycin

Drug-induced secondary hyperaldosteronism with hypokalemia and hypomagnesemia in four patients on a number of antituberculosis drugs was considered to be due to gentomicin, by Holmes et al.[230] Two of the patients were also hypokalemic, with serum calcium of 2.00 and 2.15 mmol/L. The same group later reported similar findings in 3 of 67 patients treated with capreomycin.[231]

Glucagon

Birge and Aviol gave intravenous glucagon over 4 h.[232] In seven healthy subjects mean serum calcium fell by 0.11 mmol/L, and in 11 with hyperparathyroidism, mean serum calcium fell by 0.17 mmol/L. Londono et al. found a mean fall of 0.33 mmol/L 1 h after subcutaneous injection of 1 mg of glucagon in "normal" children.[233]

Glucose

Serum calcium was found to fall by up to 0.25 mmol/L during a glucose tolerance test.[234] No details were given of the analytic procedure.

Interleukin-2

Twelve patients were given 100,000 units per kilogram of body weight every 8 h for 5 days to treat metastatic melanoma and renal and colorectal cancer, by Textor et al.[235] Mean serum calcium fell from 2.425 to 2.150 mmol/L, due to a corresponding fall in serum albumin.

Licorice and Carbenozolone

Both carbenoxolone and its parent substance, licorice, have an aldosterone-like effect, and most reports concerned with severe hypokalemia produced note changes in serum calcium. The earliest reports involved long-term treatment with *p*-amino salicylic acid flavored with licorice to mask the unpleasant taste,[236,237] carbenoxolone to treat gastric ulcers.[238,239] Cases have been reported of hypocalcemia in subjects who have eaten large amounts of licorice over long periods. One was said to have eaten 30 to 40 g daily for 9 months,[240] and another, $3^1/_2$ lb weekly for 15 to 20 years.[241]

Methyl Dopa

A single case has been described with serum calcium of 1.76 mmol/L and features of malabsorption related to methyl dopa therapy.[242]

Mithramycin

Serum calcium was found to fall in some patients given mithramycin as an antitumor drug.[243,244] The drug is no longer used in antitumor therapy, but can be used in emergency treatment for hypercalcemia.[204] The fall in serum calcium is said to average 0.70 mmol/L over 48 h and to be maintained for several days. Perlia et al. found that a single dose of 25 µg/kg body weight gave an immediate fall in serum calcium in 24 of 32 cases, with falls in others after further injections.[245]

Estrogens

Bone resorption is inhibited by estrogen, and a number of groups have reported consequent effects on serum calcium. Postmenopausal women given ethinyl estradiol daily or treated with percutaneous estradiol cream[246] showed falls in mean serum calcium of 0.07 to 0.08 mmol/L. Treatment with oral estradiol[247] and mestranol[248] gave a mean fall of 0.03 mmol/L.

McPherson et al. reported similar changes in blood donors taking oral contraceptives,[142] compared with other female blood donors of the same age, but did not state the dose or type of oral contraceptive used.

Some patients with metastases from breast carcinoma obtain temporary suppression of metastases by estrogen therapy. A few have estrogen-dependent metastases, and in these, serum calcium may increase very rapidly. Kennedy et al. noted 9 cases in 361 patients with advanced breast carcinoma[249] and later suggested that the presence of hypercalcemia could be used to detect estrogen dependence.[250] Increases of serum calcium to 4 or 5 mmol/L, after treatment with stilbestrol, have been reported.[244,251,252]

Probucol

A small fall of about 0.1 mmol/L in mean serum calcium has been reported after treatment of diabetic subjects with the cholesterol-lowering drug probucol.[253] No change was found in a nondiabetic group.

Purgatives

Tetany associated with hypocalcemia has occasionally been described in cases of chronic purgative abuse.[254] The mechanism is uncertain, but could be linked with the mild steattorrhea noted in some patients.

Rimiterol and Salbutamol

Small falls in serum calcium have been found during intravenous treatment with the selective B_2-adrenoceptor stimulants rimoterol and salbutamol. Phillips et al.[255] noted a mean fall of 0.12 mmol/L after giving up to 0.7 μg/kg/min of salbutamol over 90 min, and a mean fall of 0.89 mmol/L after up to 0.44 μg/kg/min of rimiterol over 60 min.

Salicylate

A small effect on serum calcium in patients taking large amounts of aspirin was found by Routh and Paul.[256] No change was noted after 2 × 325 mg of aspirin, or 2 × 325 mg each 4 h for 3 days, but after giving 2 × 650 mg of aspirin each 4 h, serum calcium fell by 0.05 to 0.18 mmol/L. Levels returned within a week of stopping aspirin intake.

Streptozotocin

Stanley et al. reported a fall in serum calcium in patients with malignant islet cell tumor treated with streptozotocin,[257] but gave no figures. Laryea et al.,[258] on treatment of a similar case with hypercalcemia, found a fall from 3.00 to 2.25 mmol/L.

Thyrotrophin-Releasing Hormone (TRH)

Serum calcium declines after administration of TRH. Röjdmark et al. gave 0.2 mg intravenously and found a fall of 0.19 ± 0.03 mmol/L in patients with primary hypothyroidism,[259] 0.10 ± 0.02 in euthyroid patients with various diseases, and 0.08 ± 0.02 in healthy subjects after 90 min. The effect was not caused by a direct influence on the kidney or by the major calcium regulatory hormones.

DRUGS THAT INCREASE SERUM CALCIUM

Aluminum Hydroxide

In a study designed to compare the absorption of aluminum in healthy subjects with those with renal failure, Cam et al. gave five normal subjects 100 mL of aluminum hydroxide gel per day for 28 days.[260] Mean serum calcium increased from 2.37 to 2.42 mmol/L.

Cellulose Phosphate

Although Young lists cellulose phosphate as increasing serum calcium without changing calcium balance,[56] in the reference given,[261] it was found that on treating 18 patients with probable absorptive hypercalciuria, with cellulose phosphate there was no change in serum calcium.

Diethyl Stilbestrol

It has already been noted that although serum calcium usually falls following estrogen therapy, some cases of breast cancer treated show very rapid increases.

Lithium

Treatment with lithium salts raises serum calcium by up to 0.3 mmol/L.[262,263] The level returns to normal within 4 weeks when lithium is discontinued. No treatment is required.[264]

Nisolpidine

A mean increase in serum calcium of 0.10 mmol/L has been reported in a group of hypertensive diabetic patients given 10 to 20 mg of nisolpidine for 12 weeks.[265] Although the mean level increased, the level remained within the normal range in all 14 patients at all times.

Propranolol

One group reported a small mean increase in serum calcium of 0.085 mmol/L in 131 hypertensive subjects given propranolol.[266]

Secretin

Intravenous secretin (3 units/kg/h) given to five healthy subjects increased mean serum calcium by 0.32 ± 0.04 mmol/L after 90 min.[267] The mechanism for the effect is not clear.

Tamoxifen

Several groups have noted hypercalcemia in patients with metastases given tamoxifen, as would be expected, since it is an estrogen antagonist. Although Henningsen and Amberger suggested that 20% of treated cases become hypercalcemic,[268] Veldhuis found this in three of the first five cases treated.[269] Kiang and Kennedy reported hypercalcemia in only 2 of 61 patients treated.[270]

Theophylline

An increase in serum calcium has been reported in subjects with theophylline toxicity and in some with subtherapeutic levels. McPherson et al. found that 11 of 60 hospitalized patients with theophylline toxicity had hypercalcemia. In three others there was a significant fall after theophylline was discontinued,[271] although the original level was within the normal range.

Five healthy volunteers were given theophylline for 1 week. Therapeutic levels were only achieved in one subject. After 2×200 mg/day, there was no change, but after 2×400 mg of theophylline per day, mean serum calcium increased by 0.15 mmol/L.

Thiazides and Related Diuretics

There is a fall in urine calcium in patients on a normal diet and taking thiazide diuretics that gives a positive calcium balance leading to a rise in serum calcium. An initial fall in serum calcium due to increased calcium excretion during the first acute phase of action has been noted.[272]

Seitz and Jaworski found that serum calcium increased by 0.075 to 0.200 mmol/L after 3 days,[273] and 0.175 to 0.250 mmol/L after a week, in healthy and hypertensive subjects given hydrochlorthiazide. Lindy and Tarssanen found a mean increase of 0.11 mmol/L in 36 hypertensive patients treated with thiazides for at least 3 months,[274] compared with the mean serum calcium of a control group. A Veterans Administration Study Group found mean serum calcium increased by 0.085 mmol/L in a group of black hypertensives and by 0.065 mmol/L in a similar group of white subjects.[266]

In a study of 783 patients with hypercalcemia (more than 2.60 mmol/L) identified from laboratory records, Harrup et al. considered that 23 were explained by thiazide treatment.[275] Chlorthalidone increased serum calcium by 0.05 to 0.38 mmol/L in 30 of 39 hypertensive patients given 50 mg daily by Palmer.[276] Six showed levels above the upper limit.

Vitamin A

A number of cases of hypercalcemia due to excessive administration of vitamin A have been reported. Katz and Tsagournis reviewed 11 cases in the literature[277] and gave details of another case.

Frame et al. reported three interesting cases.[278] One, a 7-year-old boy, had been given

85,000 units per day, with a vitamin D intake of less than 1500 units. Serum calcium fell from 3.48 to 2.53 mmol/L after discontinuing vitamin A for 3 weeks.

Another was a 16 year old who wanted to be an airline pilot and took 100,000 units daily in an attempt to improve night vision. Serum calcium fell from over 3.00 to 2.43 mmol/L after a month without the vitamin.

The third was a door-to-door salesman of vitamin preparations, who took at least 25,000 units of vitamin A daily without excessive intake of vitamin D. Serum calcium fell from 3.15 mmol/L to normal on discontinuing vitamin A.

Vitamin D

Although treatment with vitamin D would be expected to increase serum calcium, the earliest reports concerning the use of large amounts to treat arthritis suggested that the toxic effects were insignificant. This was later shown to be incorrect, and it was noted that symptoms of hypervitaminosis D will usually occur if 100,000 units daily are taken for some time.[279,280]

The rate of fall of serum calcium on stopping the vitamin varies with the preparation given. Kanis and Russell calculated the half-life of the fall in serum calcium after stopping the drug.[281]

Drug	Mean half-life of decrease (days)
1.25 Dihydrocholecalciferol	1.5
Hydroxycalciferol	3.4
Calciferol	29.5
Dihydrotachysterol	44.0

The rapid reversal found with 1.25 dihydroxycholecalciferol and hydroxycalciferol was thought to make them preferable when treating patients in whom hypercalcemia was thought to be troublesome.

Chapter 4

INORGANIC PHOSPHATE

Phosphate is present in blood as

1. Inorganic phosphate: $H_2PO_4^-$ and HPO_4^{2-} ions in equilibrium. The proportion of each ion depends on pH.
2. Ester phosphate: glycerophosphate, nucleotide phosphate, etc.
3. Lipid phosphate: lecithin, cephalin, and sphingomyelin

There is a similar concentration of inorganic phosphate in cells and plasma, but there are higher levels of both ester phosphate and lipid phosphate in blood cells. Ultrafiltration of plasma followed by estimation of free ions in the filtrate suggests that about 14% of plasma inorganic phosphate is protein bound.[68]

In clinical work the most frequently estimated phosphate compound in blood is serum inorganic phosphate. Although not accurate, this is often referred to as serum phosphate or phosphorus. To avoid confusion, the term inorganic phosphate should be used.

ANALYTIC CONSIDERATIONS

Most methods for the estimation of serum inorganic phosphate are based on the reaction of phosphate with molybdate. The complex formed is either measured directly using the absorption at 340 nm or is reduced to molybdenum blue for quantitation.

Probably the first color method was designed by Taylor and Miller in 1914, who precipitated phosphomolybdate and, after redissolving, obtained a color by phenyl hydrazine reduction. Bell and Doisey later modified the procedure to avoid the precipitation step.[282]

In many manual methods, protein is first precipitated with trichloracetic acid. Care must be taken to ensure that conditions do not encourage splitting of inorganic from organic phosphate, which would yield falsely high results.

There have been a number of reducing agents used.[283] In a frequently used early method, Fiske and Subbarow used 1,2,4, amino sulfonic acid in a sulfite mixture.[284] One problem was that the reagent had to be prepared freshly for use, as it was unstable. Stannous chloride was introduced by Kuttner and Cohen,[285] but a difficulty was that the color did not follow Beer's law. Gomorri used metol (*p*-methyl amino phenol sulfate) in a method that had a number of advantages,[286] such as a stable color that conformed to Beer's law, and stable reagents. Power used this reagent as the basis for a proposed standard method.[287]

When continuous-flow analyzers were introduced, methods used were similar in principle to the manual procedures. Lawrence, for instance, used the molybdate reaction followed by reduction with stannous chloride.[288] Use of discrete analyzers led to consideration of other methods, such as the reaction of phosphomolybdate with malachite green, said by Weissman and Pileggi to be the most sensitive reagent for serum inorganic phosphate estimation.[289]

However, quality control surveys suggest that most laboratories use methods based on the measurement of the phosphomolybdate or phosphomolybdovanadate complex or their reduction products.

ACCURACY AND PRECISION

External quality control schemes show that there is little difference in mean results obtained for serum inorganic phosphate estimated by different methods. Precision varies with the method used. Table 23 shows average figures for between-batch precision, given by Wiener.[290]

TABLE 23.
Mean Between-Batch Precision of
Serum Inorganic Phosphate Estimation by Different Methods[a]

Method	Precision (mmol/L)
Continuous-flow analyzers	
Reduction of phosphomolybdate	0.030
Measurement of phosphomolybdate complex at 340 nm	0.030
Reduction of phosphomolybdovanadate	0.045
Discrete analyzers	0.045
Reduction of phosphomolybdate	
Measurement of phosphomolybdate complex at 340 nm	0.045
Manual methods	
Reduction of phosphomolybdate after protein precipitation	0.050
Measurement of phosphomolybdate complex at 340 nm after protein precipitation	0.065
No protein precipitation	0.075
Reduction of phosphomolybdovanadate	0.070

[a]   From Wiener, K., in *Varleys Practical Clinical Chemistry,* 6th ed., Glowenlock, A. H., Ed., London, Heineman, 1988, 617.

SI UNITS

To convert from mass to molar units,

$$\text{serum mmol} / L = \frac{\text{mg} / 100 \text{ mL}}{3.1}$$
$$= \frac{\text{mEq} / L}{1.8}$$

Since at pH 7.4 the anion exists as two species, its concentration cannot be expressed as a single molar equivalent, and it is probably more correct to use the term "milliatom", rather than "millimol", to recognize that the phosphate anion is measured as phosphorus.

INTERFERENCE WITH ANALYSIS

HEMOLYSIS

Assessment of the effect of hemolysis on serum inorganic phosphate estimation is complicated by the increase due to the rapid breakdown of organic phosphate found in red cells. Inorganic phosphate of hemolysates can double in 24 h at 5 to 7°C, as a result of enzyme action.[291] Bryden and Roberts[292] found an average increase of 0.03 mmol/L per gram per liter of hemoglobin added as hemolysate.

BILIRUBIN

Pesce and Boudourian, using a method measuring the phosphate–molybdate complex at 340 nm,[293] reported that analysis of specimens from infants with serum bilirubin of more than 50 μmol/L gave falsely high results compared with analysis by the Fiske and Subbarow method. The error was due to turbidity not found with serum from infants with lower serum bilirubin. No turbidity was found using lyophilized sera with bilirubin of more than 120 mmol/L or when unconjugated bilirubin was added to serum from an infant.

TABLE 24.
Effect of Mannitol on the Estimation of Serum Inorganic Phosphate
by Various Methods

Reference	Method	Effect
294	Fiske and Subbarow method on urine	Mannitol interferes at more than 5 g/L Normally considered no interference in determination on serum
295	Analysis using Technicon SMA 12/60	No effect at 4.45 g/L, serum mannitol considered diagnostic
296	Dupont ACA using metol	Mannitol above 25 mmol/L interfered with end-point method No effect on a kinetic method using phenylene diamine
297	Dupont ACA	Interference confirmed
	Continuous-flow method with ferrous sulfate reduction	No effect
298	Dade "Paramax"	Low result
	American Monitor "Parallel"	No interference

OTHER INTERFERING SUBSTANCES

Mannitol, given to reduce cerebrospinal and intraocular fluid pressure by producing an osmotic diuresis, interferes with the molybdate reaction, and falsely low inorganic phosphate levels are found with some analytic procedures, in its presence (Table 24)

El-Dorry et al. reported that the antihistamine promethazine,[299] a phenothiazine derivative interfered with the Fiske and Subbarow method, as a complex is formed with phosphomolybdate. Experiments used urine, and it was not stated whether serum levels would interfere.

One and a half g/L of sulfadiazine, when added to serum, is said to increase serum inorganic phosphate when estimated by a phosphomolybdate method using the Technicon SMAC analyzer.[300] No information is given on the quantitative effect.

Estimation of serum inorganic phosphate using the Dacos analyzer (Coulter Electronics Ltd., Luton, U.K.) is affected by the presence of macroglobulins in serum.[301] In this instrument, serum is diluted with distilled water, and macroglobulin precipitates (Sia test), giving a high blank reading. A flag is given for hemolysis, although none is present.

PREANALYTIC ERROR

COLLECTION OF THE SPECIMEN

The sample for estimation of serum inorganic phosphate is frequently collected without any special preparation of the patient, although changes following meals and the diurnal variation, suggest that it would be better if the sample was taken from a fasting subject at a fixed time of day. After collection, serum must be separated as soon as possible in order to avoid changes that occur when serum or plasma remains in contact with cells (Table 25).

ANTICOAGULANTS

Higher levels of inorganic phosphate are found in serum compared with those found in heparinized plasma (Table 25). The higher level in serum may be derived from platelets during the clotting process.

Other problems occur when using anticoagulants. Commercial preparations of heparin have been reported to be contaminated with phosphate introduced during preparation. McKeown et al., in 1955, found that six commercial preparations studied contained sufficient contamination to give apparent inorganic phosphate levels of about twice the actual amount.[303] It is

TABLE 25.
Changes in Serum and Plasma Inorganic Phosphate After Collection[a]

Serum	Level (mmol/L)
Separated 1 h after collection	1.11
Separated 2 h after collection	1.10
Separated 3 h after collection	1.09
Heparinized plasma	
Immediately	1.06
2 h after collection	1.00

[a] From Carothers, J. E., et al., *Clin. Chem.*, 22, 1909, 1976. With permission.

TABLE 26.
Stability of Inorganic Phosphate in Serum

Reference	Stability given
307	Stable for a week
308	Stable for at least 8 h at room temperature
	Stable overnight at 4°C
	Stable for at least 1 year if frozen
309	Level increases after 3 days at 23°C
310	Stable if serum is frozen

unlikely that modern preparations of heparin contain similar contamination, but it is advisable to check for suitability. Oxalated or citrated plasma cannot be used, as oxalate and citrate complex with molybdate to prevent full color development.[304]

VENOUS STASIS

About 14% of inorganic phosphate is protein bound, and the effect of excessive venous stasis would be expected to be about a third of the effect on serum calcium, or an increase of up to about 0.015 mmol/L. There are no reports that such an effect exists, but for interpretation of results, any possible change can be disregarded.

CONTAMINATION

Detergents frequently contain large quantities of phosphate.[305] Thus, it is important that glassware should be cleaned satisfactorily and checked for possible contamination before use.

SAMPLE STABILITY

After collection of a blood sample, there is at first a fall of up to 5% in serum inorganic phosphate, due to passage of phosphate ions into cells to be used for phosphorylation of glucose.[302] The level then increases as organic phosphates existing mainly in the red cells are hydrolyzed by phosphatases and leak through the cell walls. It was recognized by Howland and Kramer in 1921[306] that false results would be obtained if serum was not separated from cells as soon as possible. Once separated, inorganic phosphate in serum is stable for several days (Table 26). Any increase due to a breakdown of organic phosphate in serum is insignificant.

Heating to 56°C

A small but significant decrease in serum and plasma inorganic phosphate is found on heating the sample to 56°C to minimize the risk from HIV-positive samples (Table 27). Ball found no change when B-propriolactone was used to treat the sample.[312]

TABLE 27.
Effect of Heating Serum and Plasma Inorganic Phosphate
to 56°C to Minimize the Risk from HIV

Reference		Effect
101	Serum	Decrease 1.3%
311	Plasma	Decrease 1.0%
312	Plasma	Decrease 5%

TABLE 28.
Changes in Serum Inorganic Phosphate Following a Standard Meal

Reference	Subjects	Method	Change
109	16 male and 16 female subjects 19–67 years of age	Estimation by Fiske and Subbarow method	Mean fall 45 min after standard breakfast 0.08 mmol/L
110	4 subjects	Estimation by continuous-flow analyzer	Mean fall 2 h after breakfast 0.03 mmol/L

PHYSIOLOGIC CHANGES

MEALS

There is a fall in serum inorganic phosphate following meals. Table 28 shows changes found following a standard meal. In view of the effect of alkalosis, the level may be influenced by the postprandial alkalinity of blood.

The change following administration of glucose is much greater. It has been known for many years that blood inorganic phosphate falls after glucose administration. Harrop and Benedict, in 1924,[313] noted a fall to about two thirds of the basal level 60 min after oral intake of 200 g of glucose. Intravenous glucose also produces a fall. In an experiment on a subject with no apparent abnormality of carbohydrate metabolism, Hartman and Bolliger found a reduction of about 20% after an intravenous administration of 35 g of glucose.[314] The decrease is due to insulin release, which shifts the anion from plasma to the tissues.[315]

DIET

The level of serum inorganic phosphate in the nonfasting steady state is highly dependent on the amount of phosphate in the diet. At a normal intake of about 1200 mg/day of phosphate, the mean serum inorganic phosphate level is about 1.16 mmol/L.[316]

EXERCISE

Physical activity increases serum inorganic phosphate (Table 29). A greater effect has been noted in men than in women and in older subjects.[120] It is possible that the change is related to the acidosis produced.

MENSTRUAL CYCLE

Frank and Carr reported that the mean serum inorganic phosphate is 0.1 mmol/L lower at the menses than in the intermenstrual period.[125] The change was not consistent, and the collection procedure was not standardized. Pulkkinen and Willman were not able to confirm this finding.[318] If any change exists, it is too small to affect the interpretation of the results.

TABLE 29.
Effect of Exercise on Serum or Plasma Inorganic Phosphate

Reference	Type or exercise	Method	Changes found		
				Men	Women
			Age	Mean increase	Mean increase
120	Exercise for	Analysis using	20–30	6.25%	6.17%
	12 min on	Technicon SMA	30–40	7.33%	5.86%
	a bicycle	12/60 analyzer	40–50	9.40%	7.31%
	ergonometer				
121	Exercise for	Estimation by	Before exercise mean 1.19 mmol/L		
	12 min on	Fiske and	After exercise mean 1.38 mmol/L		
	a bicycle	Subbarow method	Returned to preexercise level		
	ergonometer		within 20 min		
317	Marathon run	Phosphotungstate			Mean
	by five trained	method on	Before		0.86 mmol/L
	distance	heparinized	10.5 km		1.41
	runners	plasma	26.25 km		1.57
			End		1.43
			(31.5–42 km;		
			not all finished)		
			20–30 h later		0.99

ALKALOSIS AND ACIDOSIS

Large falls in serum inorganic phosphate are found in subjects who induce respiratory alkalosis by hyperventilating. In an experiment, described by Haldane in 1924,[319] in which he hyperventilated for 1 to 1½ h until tetany was produced, the level fell from 0.97 to 0.32 mmol/L. In a number of similar experiments, the level fell to below 0.40 mmol/L in each case. Experiments by Mostellar and Tuttle[320] and Seamonds et al.[111] gave similar results. Haldane also demonstrated a rise when 6% carbon dioxide was breathed to induce respiratory acidosis.

Falls in serum inorganic phosphate have also been obtained after inducing metabolic alkalosis. Mostellar and Tuttle gave 11 healthy adults 3.5 to 4.5 mEq/kg body weight sodium bicarbonate intravenously and found a change from a mean of 1.10 to 0.82 mmol/L.

EFFECT OF SUNLIGHT

The attempt by Hodkinson et al. to investigate possible changes in serum calcium related to levels of exposure of elderly patients to sunlight,[130] described earlier, also included results of the effect on serum inorganic phosphate. The mean level in males with no sunlight exposure was 0.75 mmol/L compared with an average of 0.84 mmol/L for all males. No figures were given for female subjects.

RANGE IN HEALTHY SUBJECTS

WITHIN- AND BETWEEN-PERSON VARIATION

Reasonable agreement is shown in most large studies of serum inorganic phosphate in healthy adults (Tables 30–33). The lower ranges found may be due to the use of heparinized plasma. Only Hitz, who took specimens in the morning from fasting subjects, standardized the conditions. Similar levels are found in males and females, 20 to 50 years old, but after 50 years, there is a fall in men and a rise in women. There is a small rise of about 0.1 mmol/L after natural menopause or hysterectomy (Table 34), and this may explain the increase found in older women.

Studies in the elderly[124,166,167] confirm the small fall in serum inorganic phosphate with increasing age in men, and the higher levels in women than in men, in older age groups.

TABLE 30.
Serum Inorganic Phosphate in Healthy Males[a] (in mmol/L)

Reference		<20	21–25	26–30	31–35	36–40	41–45	46–50	51–55	56–60	61–65	66–70	>70
140[b]	Mean		1.130		1.095		1.060		1.030		1.000		0.960
	Range		0.82–1.44		0.79–1.40		0.76–1.37		0.72–1.34		0.69–1.30		0.65–1.27
141[c]	N		96		721		1268		1112		415		105
	Range		0.74–1.53		0.75–1.55		0.77–1.52		0.78–1.52		0.78–1.52		0.72–1.61
	Mean		1.130		1.150		1.130		1.130		1.150		1.170
142[d]	Mean	1.064		1.015		0.990		0.980		0.950			
321[e]	N			1197			1081				216		
	Mean			0.950			0.950				0.900		
	Range			0.70–1.22			0.71–1.21				0.64–1.14		
Coventry[f]	N	133	242	243	216	216	205	162	141	136	56		
	Mean	1.165	1.115	1.115	1.105	1.095	1.050	1.065	1.035	1.025	1.035		
	Range	0.84–1.50	0.74–1.50	0.82–1.42	0.82–1.40	0.81–1.39	0.70–1.40	0.74–1.40	0.74–1.34	0.75–1.42	0.66–1.42		

a   All methods based on reduction of phosphomolybdate.
b   298 Caucasian men in good health.
c   Subjects from well-persons' clinic.
d   Blood donors.
e   Fasting. Excluded if over- or underweight.
f   Healthy hospital staff, as described in Chapter 2.

TABLE 31.
Serum Inorganic Phosphate in Healthy Females[a] (in mmol/L)

Reference		<20	21–25	26–30	31–35	36–40	41–45	46–50	51–55	56–60	61–65	66–70	>70
140	Mean		1.140		1.095		1.100		1.140		1.200		1.250
	Range		0.92–1.37		0.82–1.37		0.82–1.37		0.86–1.43		0.90–1.50		0.94–1.56
141	N		72		193		283		278		229		
	Range		0.83–1.53		0.84–1.50		0.77–1.55		0.88–1.59		0.89–1.60		
	Mean		1.180		1.170		1.160		1.230		1.240		
142	Mean	1.090	1.020		1.020		1.020		1.100		1.140		
321	N		956				2042				95		
	Mean		1000				0.990				1.020		
	Range		0.72–1.27				0.990				0.82–1.25		
Coventry	N Mean	1.080	1.100	1.095	1.105	1.065	1.075	1.105	1.165	1.125			
	Range	0.72–1.38	0.81–1.29	0.96–1.24	0.79–1.43	0.82–1.31	0.84–1.32	0.73–1.44	0.90–1.43	0.87–1.39			

a   Details as in Table 30.

TABLE 32.
Reference Intervals Derived from Hospital Records for Serum or Plasma Inorganic Phosphate in Males (in mmol/L)

Reference		<20	20–25	26–30	31–35	36–40	41–45	46–50	51–55	56–60	61–65	66–70	>70
								Age (Years)					
144	Mean		1.19	1.19	1.19	1.19	1.10	1.10	1.10	1.10	1.10	1.10	1.10
	Range		0.79–1.59	0.79–1.59	0.79–1.59	0.79–1.59	074–1.46	074–1.46	074–1.46	074–1.46	0.74–1.48	0.74–1.48	0.74–1.48
145	Mean		1.10	1.10	1.13	1.13	1.06	1.06	1.03	1.03	1.00	1.00	
	Range		0.77–1.61	0.77–1.61	0.77–1.52	0.77–1.52	0.74–1.42	0.74–1.42	0.65–1.65	0.65–1.65	0.65–1.42	0.65–1.42	
146	Mean	1.36	1.12	1.12	1.05	1.05	1.01	1.01	1.02	1.02	0.99	0.99	1.03
	Range	0.99–1.72	0.61–1.63	0.61–1.63	0.57–1.53	0.57–1.53	0.58–1.44	0.58–1.44	0.75–1.29	0.75–1.29	0.62–1.38	0.62–1.38	0.69–1.37
147	Mean		0.99	0.99	0.96	0.96	0.95	0.95	0.94	0.94	0.93	0.93	0.94
	Range		0.62–1.36	0.62–1.36	0.61–1.31	0.61–1.31	0.60–1.3	0.60–1.30	0.60–1.28	0.60–1.28	0.61–1.25	0.61–1.25	0.60–1.28

TABLE 33.
Reference Intervals Derived from Hospital Records for Serum or Plasma Inorganic Phosphate in Females (in mmol/L)

Reference		<20	21–25	26–30	31–35	36–40	41–45	46–50	51–55	56–60	61–65	66–70	>70
								Age (years)					
144	Mean		1.19	1.19	1.19	1.19	1.19	1.19	1.19	1.19	1.16	1.16	1.16
	Range		0.83–1.56	0.83–1.56	0.83–1.56	0.83–1.56	0.80–1.59	0.80–1.59	0.80–1.59	0.80–1.59	0.77–1.55	0.77–1.55	0.77–1.55
145	Mean		1.10	1.10	1.10	1.10	1.10	1.10	1.10	1.10	1.10	1.10	1.16
	Range		0.74–1.48	0.74–1.48	0.77–1.61	0.77–1.61	0.81–1.65	0.81–1.65	0.84–1.52	0.84–1.52	0.74–1.48	0.74–1.48	0.74–1.48
146	Mean	1.18	1.07	1.07	1.06	1.06	1.08	1.08	1.08	1.08	1.09	1.09	1.07
	Range	0.85–1.52	0.70–1.45	0.70–1.45	0.67–1.45	0.67–1.45	0.68–1.47	0.68–1.47	0.73–1.44	0.73–1.44	0.72–1.46	0.72–1.46	0.74–1.40
147	Mean		1.02	1.02	1.08	1.08	1.03	1.03	1.09	1.09	1.07	1.07	1.06
	Range		0.67–1.35	0.67–1.35	0.67–1.49	0.67–1.49	0.65–1.39	0.65–1.39	0.75–1.43	0.75–1.43	0.72–1.41	0.72–1.41	0.71–1.40

TABLE 34.
Effect of Menopause and Hysterectomy on Mean Levels
of Serum Inorganic Phosphate (in mmol/L)

Reference	Subjects	Time	Mean	Comment		
169	Nine patients; analysis using continuous-flow analyzer	Before oophorectomy 3 months after	0.97 1.05	Change not considered statistically significant, but rise in seven of nine		
		Before hysterectomy After	0.99 1.00			
142	Blood donors; analysis using continuous-flow analyzer	**Age (years)** Premenopause Post-natural menopause hysterectomy	**36–45** 1.031 0.995 0.967	**46–55** 1.017 1.145 1.075	**56–65** 1.137 1.156	

TABLE 35.
Variation of Serum Inorganic Phosphate within Individuals

Reference	Subjects	Method	N	Variation
163	Healthy subjects	Samples weekly for 10–12 weeks in morning from fasting subjects	68	Average personal variation when analytic variation excluded had SD of 0.259 in mmol/L
164	Healthy male Caucasian physicians	Samples weekly for 10 weeks from fasting subjects. All analyzed on same day to reduce analytical variation	10	Average personal variation when analytic variation excluded, 0.365 with range of 0.20–0.57 in mmol/L

TABLE 36.
Diurnal Variation of Serum Inorganic Phosphate

Reference	Subjects	Changes	
319	One subject	After 5 h of sleep On waking in morning	1.32 mmol/L 1.06 mmol/L
322	Three healthy adults	Highest level about 23.00 h Lowest level about 9.00 h	Highest mean about 0.25 mmol/L above lowest mean
323	8 men, 5 women	Highest level about 4.00 h Lowest level about 10.00 h	Highest mean about 0.28 mmol/L above lowest mean
324	9 men, 4 women	Maximum at about 3.00 h Minimum at about 11.00 h	Mean about 1.35 mmol/L Mean about 0.95 mmol/L

Most textbooks published in the past 30 to 40 years suggest a range in healthy persons for serum inorganic phosphate of about 0.80 to 1.40 mmol/L. This is probably a reasonable range for young adults of both sexes. Variation with age and time of collection are rarely mentioned, and these factors should be considered when interpreting results.

There is large variation within individuals over time, even when samples are collected under standardized conditions (Table 35). This has not been explained, but may be related to changes in phosphate in the diet and to changes in exercise patterns. If this is so, the variation is unlikely to be as great in hospitalized patients.

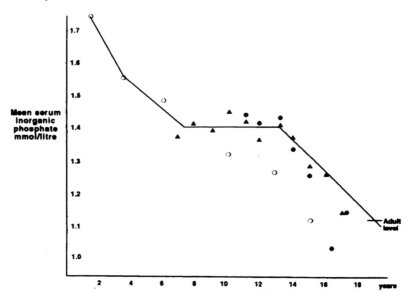

FIGURE 1. Change in mean serum inorganic phosphate with age in boys, reported by several groups. ○ from Cheng et al.,[171] ■ from Round,[325] ▲ from Widholm and Hötzel.[172]

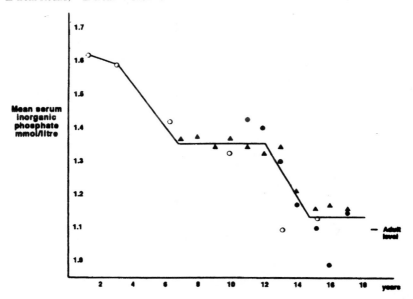

FIGURE 2. Change in mean serum inorganic phosphate with age in girls, reported by several groups. ○ from Cheng et al.,[171] ■ from Round,[325] ▲ from Widholm and Hötzel.[172]

Diurnal Variation

There is a well-defined diurnal variation, with the highest levels of serum inorganic phosphate during the night, and minimum levels in the midmorning (Table 36). Some of the changes are due to the effects of meals and exercise.

CHILDREN

The mean level of serum inorganic phosphate in children falls until the age of approximately 5 years and remains constant until the age of approximately 13 years, when there is a further decrease. Adult levels are reached at approximately 17 years of age in boys and at approximately 15 years of age in girls (Figures 1 and 2). Tables 37 and 38 show the ranges found by various workers. Mean values compare well, although Haas,[173] using fasting samples, found higher levels than other workers did.

TABLE 37.
Serum Inorganic Phosphate in Boys[a] (in mmol/L)

References		Age (Years)																
		0–2	2–5	6	7	8	9	10	11	12	13	14	15	16	17	18	19	20
325[a]	Mean				1.37	1.41	1.39	1.43	1.41	1.35	1.40	1.36	1.27	1.25	1.16			
	Range				1.19–1.55	1.16–1.68	1.13–1.71	1.13–1.71	1.13–1.71	1.10–1.61	1.16–1.68	1.03–1.74	0.94–1.58	0.94–1.58	0.83–1.48			
326[b]	Range			1.23–1.75	1.23–1.75	1.23–1.75		1.10–1.71	1.10–1.71	1.10–1.71	1.10–1.71	1.10–1.71	1.10–1.71	0.81–1.43	0.81–1.43	0.81–1.43	0.81–1.43	0.81–1.43
171[c]	Mean	1.74	1.55	1.48	1.48	1.48	1.32	1.32	1.32	1.26	1.26	1.26	1.13	1.13	1.13			
172[d]	Mean								1.42	1.41	1.42	1.33	1.24	1.04	1.16			
327[e]	Mean			1.6	1.6	1.6	1.6	1.5	1.6	1.6	1.6	1.5	1.4	1.4	1.3			
	Range			1.4–1.9	1.4–1.8	1.3–1.8	1.4–1.7	1.3–1.7	1.3–1.8	1.3–1.8	1.3–1.8	1.2–1.8	1.1–1.8	1.1–1.7	1.0–1.6			

a   All methods used were based on reduction of molybdate.

b   624 healthy children from six schools in London and Hertfordshire.

c   1062 healthy children from Toronto. Specimens collected in the morning.

d   837 healthy children. Finger puncture specimens.

e   111 healthy children from two schools near Vienna. Longitudinal study.

f   About 3600 children from a screening program in Marshfield, U.S. Mainly Caucasian. Fasting specimens analyzed same day.

TABLE 38.
Serum Inorganic Phosphate in Girls[a] (in mmol/L)

Reference		0-2	2-5	6	7	8	9	10	11	12	13	14	15	16	17	18	19	20
325	Mean				1.37	1.38	1.35	1.37	1.35	1.33	1.35	1.20	1.15	1.16	1.16			
	Range				1.16-1.61	1.16-1.61	1.16-1.61	1.16-1.61	1.13-1.68	1.10-1.55	1.10-1.61	0.94-1.45	0.90-1.39	0.94-1.35	0.94-1.35			
326	Range		1.28-1.74	1.28-1.74	1.28-1.74	1.28-1.74	1.28-1.74	1.13-1.64	1.13-1.64	1.13-1.64	1.13-1.64	1.13-1.64	1.13-1.64	0.90-1.39	0.90-1.39	0.90-1.39	0.90-1.39	0.90-1.39
171	Mean	1.61	1.58	1.42	1.42	1.42	1.32	1.32	1.32	1.10	1.10	1.10	1.13	1.13				
172	Mean								1.42	1.39	1.30	1.16	1.10	0.80	1.14			
327	Mean			1.6	1.6	1.6	1.6	1.6	1.6	1.5	1.4	1.4	1.3	1.3	1.3			
	Range			1.4-1.8	1.4-1.8	1.4-1.8	1.3-1.8	1.4-1.8	1.3-1.8	1.2-1.8	1.2-1.7	1.4-1.6	1.0-1.6	1.0-1.6	1.1-1.5			

[a] Details as in Table 37.

TABLE 39.
Serum Inorganic Phosphate in Pre- and Postpubescent Girls[a]

Subjects	Level (mmol/L)	
	Mean	2.5–97.5 percentile
Prepubertal girls 12–14 years of age	1.33	1.06–1.65
Postpubertal girls 12–14 years of age	1.26	0.96–1.46

[a] From Hitz, J., in *Interpretations of Clinical Laboratory Tests*, Siest, G., et al., Eds., Foster City, CA, Biomedical Publications, 1985, 346.

Widhalm and Hötzel, in a longitudinal study,[172] found a fall to a mean below that for adults, at the age of 16 years in both boys and girls. Other workers have not demonstrated this change. Hitz showed the relationship of the fall in the level of serum inorganic phosphate in girls aged 12 to 14 years to puberty (Table 39).[321] The level in postpubescent girls was found to be about 8% less than in prepubescent girls of the same age.

NEONATES

The level of serum inorganic phosphate in neonates depends on the type of feed being taken. Cow milk has a higher phosphate content than does human milk, so infants given artificial feed will have higher levels than will breast-fed infants. The results of several studies are shown in Table 40.

Racial differences have been reported (Table 41). The studies give no details, and it is possible that the proportion of breast-fed and artificially fed babies differed between the groups.

RANGE DURING PREGNANCY

Several studies suggest that there are small changes in serum inorganic phosphate during pregnancy, with a fall in mean values and a rise at term (Table 42). Studies by Moniz et al. differed[187] and showed little change from the fifteenth to the thirty-eighth week of pregnancy. The differences are difficult to explain. The higher levels obtained by Pitkin and co-workers may be due to the use of fasting samples. Different levels obtained by Tan et al., who used Malaysian subjects, could be due to racial differences that have been reported (Table 43).

OTHER CHANGES

BLOOD PRESSURE

An inverse relationship has been demonstrated between levels of serum inorganic phosphate and blood pressure (Table 44).

BODY WEIGHT

Serum inorganic phosphate is reported to be higher in thin subjects than in those of ideal weight.[321] The mean difference is said to be 6% in males and 3% in females. Obese men and women are stated to have lower levels, but no other quantitation is given.

BLINDNESS

Lower levels of serum inorganic phosphate are reported in blind subjects and those with impaired vision than in individuals with normal sight[329] (Table 45). Two weeks after an operation to remove cataracts, the patient's levels increased to approach levels in subjects with normal vision.

TABLE 40.
Serum Inorganic Phosphate in Neonates (in mmol/L)

		Reported values for method of feeding									
		Breast-fed		Adapted cow milk feed[a]				Unadapted cow milk feed[b]			
				SMA		S.26		Half cream		Full cream	
Reference	Subjects	Mean	Range	Mean	Range	Mean	Range	Mean	Range	Mean	Range
176	Babies on sixth day of life	1.97	1.48–2.71	2.58	2.00–3.26	2.52	2.13–2.90	2.74	2.29–3.19	2.74	2.29–3.52
177	Full-term babies with normal weight on sixth day of life	2.20	1.32–3.16				2.66	1.48–6.77[c]			
178	Sample taken 2.5–3 h after a feed on 5th–7th day of life	2.10	1.55–3.03					Babies with no convulsions		2.55	2.03–4.35[d]
								Babies had convulsions		2.94	2.03–4.35

[a] Cow milk modified to phosphorus content nearer to human milk.
[b] Evaporated or dried milk.
[c] Type of artificial feed not stated.
[d] Evaporated cow milk.

TABLE 41.
Serum Inorganic Phosphate in Neonates of Different Racial Groups (in mmol/L)

			Reported values		
Reference	Subjects	N	Day	Mean	SD
180	Caucasian	11	6	2.70	0.67
	Black	11	6	2.39	0.28
	Asian	11	6	2.64	0.75
181	Full-term babies	166			
	Caucasian				
	Male		1	1.70	
			2	2.20	
			3	2.35	
			4	2.17	
	Female		1	1.93	
			2	2.27	
			3	2.38	
			4	2.41	
	Black				
	Male		1	1.70	
			2	2.04	
			3	2.15	
			4	2.22	
	Female		1	2.35	
			2	2.63	
			3	2.99	
			4	2.60	

TABLE 42.
Serum Inorganic Phosphate During Pregnancy (in mmol/L)

Reference		1st trimester	2nd trimester	3rd trimester	Term	6 weeks postpartum
183	Mean	1.08	0.99	1.01	1.07	
	Range	0.80–1.44	0.67–1.28	0.72–1.44	0.72–1.28	
185	Mean	1.24	1.26	1.15		
186	Mean ± SD	1.42 ± 0.22	1.35 ± 0.23	1.33 ± 0.31		1.50 ± 0.24

TABLE 43.
Racial Differences in Serum Inorganic Phosphate During Pregnancy (in mmol/L)

		Race							
		Caucasian		Black		Asian			
Reference	Gestation weeks	N	Mean ± SD	N	Mean ± SD	N	Mean ± SD		
180	10–20	11	1.04 ± 0.15	11	1.14 ± 0.13	12	1.09 ± 0.23		
	29		1.01 ± 0.13		1.11 ± 0.13	12	0.95 ± 0.22		
	36		1.00 ± 0.14		1.11 ± 0.17		0.97 ± 0.24		
	Postnatal		1.20 ± 0.14		1.22 ± 0.15		1.22 ± 0.18		
190	10–20		1.21				1.16		
	21–30		1.13				1.09		
	31–40		1.12				1.07		

TABLE 44.
Relationship Between Serum Inorganic
Phosphate and Blood Pressure, Taken from a
Study of 2000 Men 45–50 Years of Age[a]

Serum inorganic phosphate (mmol/L)	Mean systolic b.p. (mm Hg)	Mean diastolic b.p. (mm Hg)
<0.6	137	86
0.61–0.70	135	85
0.71–0.80	132	83
0.81–0.90	132	82
0.91–1.00	129	79
1.01–1.10	127	80
>1.10	125	80

[a] From Ljundhall, S. and Medstrand, H., *Br. Med. J.*, i, 553, 1977. With permission.

TABLE 45.
Serum Inorganic Phosphate in Blind
and Partially Sighted Subjects[a]

Subjects	N	Mean ± SD (mmol/L)
Normal vision	50	1.08 ± 0.46
Impaired	140	1.03 ± 0.50
Blind	220	0.97 ± 0.40

[a] From Hollwich, F. and Dieckhues, B., *German Med.*, 1, 122, 1971. Analysis using a continuous-flow automatic analyzer. Specimens collected at 8 a.m. No details given of control group or ratio of males to females in each group.

DRUGS AFFECTING SERUM INORGANIC PHOSPHATE LEVELS

ALUMINUM SALTS

Aluminum used in antacids taken to buffer gastric acid combines with phosphate in the gut and is excreted as insoluble aluminum phosphate. This property is used to treat patients with hyperphosphatemia secondary to renal failure.

There are reports of patients found to have marked hypophosphatemia following antacid therapy.[330,331] Lotz et al.[332] gave a healthy volunteer 120 mL/day of aluminum hydroxide and 240 mL/day of aluminum and magnesium hydroxide, for over 70 days. Urine phosphate fell to undetectable levels by the 6th day, and at the end of the study, serum inorganic phosphate had fallen to 0.35 mmol/L. Spencer and Lender reviewed the adverse effects of aluminum-containing antacids[333] and found that it is believed that phosphate depletion will not occur if urinary phosphate can be maintained at 300 mg/day or higher.

Adrenalin

Administration of adrenalin lowers serum inorganic phosphate.[334] This is probably due to the rise in glucose,[335] and the effect may be analogous to that of intravenous glucose.

Body and co-workers infused epinephrine to maintain levels that spanned the physiologic range[336] and found a dose-dependent fall in serum inorganic phosphate of 0.2 mmol/L, with plasma epinephrine levels of 427 to 945 pg/mL. A plateau was reached after 20 to 30 min, and levels returned to the baseline on discontinuing the infusion.

Anticonvulsants

Reports of changes in serum inorganic phosphate in subjects taking anticonvulsants are confusing. Some have found no significant change.[213,337] Others have found a small increase of about 0.10 mmol/L in mean levels,[338] and others have found a mean decrease of about 7%.[218,339] Collection conditions have not always been standardized, and it can only be concluded that if there is any effect, it is small.

Cadmium

Scott et al. found that mean serum inorganic phosphate in 27 coppersmiths exposed to cadmium fumes was 0.78 ± 0.18 mmol/L compared with a mean of 0.93 ± 0.36 in 19 assembly workers in the same factory,[340] with a similar average length of service. Blood cadmium was high in both groups, compared with a control group. Details of the collection procedure were not given.

Calcitonin

There is a small fall in serum inorganic phosphate following administration of calcitonin. Cochran et al. found a fall of between 0.13 and 0.32 mmol/L in patients with Paget's disease and breast cancer,[202] but no fall in those with hyperparathyroidism, after giving porcine calcitonin intramuscularly. Wisneski et al. found a mean fall of 0.13 mmol/L 24 h after giving calcitonin.[341]

Cimetidine

Sherwood et al.,[219] who claimed that cimetidine reduces the PTH level in the blood of patients with hyperparathyroidism, described a patient with initial hypophosphatemia who had normal phosphate levels after 3 weeks of treatment with cimetidine.

Diphosphonates

Etidronate increases, and clodronate decreases, serum inorganic phosphate. Different effects reported (Table 46) may be related to different doses given.

Estrogen

Decreases in serum inorganic phosphate are found in subjects taking estrogen in milligram quantities, for treatment of osteoporosis, for instance, or in microgram quantities, as is done for oral contraception and for postmenopausal hormone treatment (Table 48).

Fluoride

Low levels of serum inorganic phosphate are found in people poisoned with sodium fluoride.[227]

Fructose

After intravenous administration of fructose, serum inorganic phosphate levels fall after 30 min by about 0.15 mmol/L, returning to the pretest level after 60 min. This is in contrast to the fall by about the same amount during the intravenous glucose tolerance test, with the level remaining this low for several hours.[343]

Glucocorticoids

High circulating levels of corticosteroids reduce renal tubular reabsorption of phosphate and depress serum inorganic phosphate.[344]

TABLE 46.
Effect of Diphosphonates on Serum Inorganic Phosphate[a]

Reference	Subjects	Dose	Effect
342	25 healthy adults	EHDP for 11–12 days	
		10 mg/kg/day	No significant change
		20	No significant change
		30	Mean increase from 1.21 to 1.64 mmol/L
210		EHDP in combination with calcitonin	No change
206	Patients with hypercalcemia associated with osteolytic metastases	500–100 mg/day EDHP intravenously	Increase of 0.1–0.2 mmol/L in 8 of 10 patients
		Cl_2HDP 500–1000 mg/day intravenously	Fall of 0.1–1.2 mmol/L in 16 of 21 patients
211	Patients with Paget's disease	800–3200 mg/day Cl_2HDP orally	Mean fall from 1.08 to 0.88 mmol/L after treatment

[a] EHDP = etidronate = ethane hydroxyphosphonate.
Cl_2MDP = clodronate = dichloromethylene diphosphonate.

TABLE 47.
Serum Inorganic Phosphate Before and After
Intramuscular HGH for 7 days[a]

Subject	Methods	Dose (mg/kg)	Mean (mmol/L)	
			Before	After
12 women and 6 men over 60 years of age	Recombinant HGH i.m. for 7 days. Patients randomly assigned to one of three dose groups	0.03	1.10	1.36
		0.06	0.95	1.16
		0.09	1.15	1.43

[a] Marcus, R., et al., *J. Clin. Endocrinol. Metab.*, 70, 519, 1990.

Growth Hormone
There is an increase in serum inorganic phosphate after administration of human growth hormone (Table 47). A reduction in phosphaturia has been noted.[345]

Insulin
Administration of insulin gives a fall in serum inorganic phosphate, which has been ascribed to increased phosphorylation of glucose.[346] Christian says, "the delicate interaction between insulin and growth hormone may provide some clue to the reported interaction."[347]

Iron Saccharate
After daily intravenous administration of iron saccharate, serum inorganic phosphate levels fall apparently due to increased renal loss of phosphate. Okada et al. gave nine iron-deficient patients doses intravenously for 14 to 42 days.[348] The level of serum inorganic phosphate fell from 1.18 ± 0.20 mmol/L to 0.82 ± 0.17 after 7 days and 0.67 ± 0.26 after 14 days.

Isoniazid
A reduction in serum inorganic phosphate is found in subjects taking isoniazid, this is thought to be due to the drug's inhibition of production of metabolites of vitamin D. Brodie et al. gave eight healthy subjects 300 mg daily for 14 days[349] and found that the mean serum

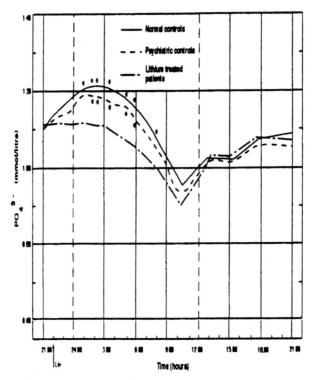

FIGURE 3. Diurnal variation in plasma phosphate during long-term lithium administration. Mean plasma phosphate in normal control persons, psychiatric control patients, and lithium-treated patients. Lithium tablets were taken at 10 p.m. (From Mellerup, E.T., et al., *Acta Psychiat. Scand.,* 53, 360, 1976. With permission of Munksgaard International Publishers Ltd., Copenhagen.)

inorganic phosphate level fell from 1.26 to 1.05 mmol/L after the last dose. The mean level was still 1.05 2 weeks after discontinuing the drug.

Lithium

Mellerup et al. found lower levels of serum inorganic phosphate for 14 h after giving subjects lithium,[252] compared with control subjects (Figure 3). Levels were compared for 24 h in 34 patients taking lithium at 10:00 pm, in 42 other psychiatric patients, and in 47 healthy persons. Mean levels can be seen to rise to a peak in those not taking lithium, at 2:00 am to 3:00 am, and to fall, as expected, to the lowest level at 10:00 am. In the lithium-treated group, the mean shows no rise, and there is a small fall to the lowest level at 10:00 am.

Mithramycin

Although some workers have reported no fall in serum inorganic phosphate levels in hypercalcemic patients treated with mithramycin,[233,350] Slayton et al.[351] found a mean fall of 0.21 mmol/L by the third day of treatment of 69 adequately hydrated patients given 25 µg/kg ideal body weight of mithramycin per day.

Paracetamol

Low levels of serum inorganic phosphate have been found after overdosage with paracetamol, in those with and those without liver damage (Table 49). Hypophosphatemia is a recognized feature of acute liver failure, but since low levels are also found in the absence of liver damage, it is considered possible that paracetamol causes renal loss of phosphate.

Phosphate

The level of phosphate in blood is dependent on the amount of phosphate in the diet. Smith and Nordin added 1.5 g of phosphate daily to the diet of volunteers and found that mean serum phosphate increased from 1.13 to 1.26 mmol/L.[356] Administration of drug

TABLE 48.
Effect of Estrogen on Serum Inorganic Phosphate (in mmol/L)

Reference	Administration	Effect			
352	Estradiol and stilbestrol given for osteoporosis	Small fall			
353	Stilbestrol given for osteoporosis	Mean fall of 0.2 mmol/L			
318	25 women not taking oral contraceptives	Mean 1.71			
	27 women on various oral contraceptives	1.06			
	"Estrogenic"	1.00			
	"Progesterogenic"	1.23			
354	Nonpregnant controls	Mean 1.41 (0.87–1.85)			
	Over 35 weeks pregnant	1.47 (1.15–1.97)			
	Oral contraception (mestranol/e thynodiol acetate)	1.27 (0.87–1.77)			
	Depot contraception (depomedroxy progesterone acetate)	1.53 (1.10–1.87)			
142	Female blood donors	Age (years)	18–25	26–35	36–45
	No oral contraception	Mean	0.915	0.880	0.968
	Oral contraception	Mean	1.088	1.023	1.031
237	Women less than 2 years after onset of menopause	Before	During	After treatment	
	Percutaneous estradiol cream	1.09	0.96	0.98	
	Oral estradiol	1.06	0.94	1.01	
238	Control group	Mean 1.18			
	32 women age 44–58 — previous hysterectomy 3 years earlier	1.17			
	16 given 20–40 μg mestranol daily for 1 year	0.96			
	Given placebo daily for 1 year	1.18			

TABLE 49.
Serum Inorganic Phosphate (in mmol/L)
on 273 Successive Admissions with Paracetamol Overdose[a]

Paracetamol taken	N	Mean	Male/female ratio
Insufficient to warrant treatment	63	1.05	1:1
Amount requiring acetyl cysteine	62	0.89	1:1.95
Amount causing liver damage; no encephalopathy	131	0.69	1:1.42
Amount causing liver damage and encephalopathy	17	0.45	1:1.50

[a] From Jones, A. F., et al., *Lancet*, ii, 608, 1989. With permission.

preparations containing phosphate might be expected to increase the level, although the quantity given would usually be small. Increased levels when drugs buffered with phosphate are given intravenously might be thought to be due to the drug when, in fact, the change is due to the buffer.

TABLE 50.
Serum Inorganic Phosphate in Subjects Taking Thiazides (in mmol/L)

Reference	Treatment	Effect
362	Healthy volunteers given 500 mg of chlorthiazide every 12 h for 15 days	No change found
363	5 mg/day of bendrofluazide to patients with idiopathic hypercalciuria	7 of 14 patients showed fall of 0.3 immediately following start of therapy
364	Prolonged treatment with hydrochlorothiazide	Increase in some cases, but no figures given
	36 hypertensive patients given thiazides at least 3 months	Mean increase 0.08
365	Control group:	Mean 1.09 (0.75–1.54)
	11 patients taking thiazides for 1–11 years given 100 mg hydrochlorthiazide daily for 3 months	Mean 0.90 (0.38–1.54)

Administration of purgatives containing phosphate will increase serum inorganic phosphate. Carrera found that the level increased two- or threefold over 3 h after purgation, prior to paracytic evaluation.[357] The patients had been given almost 25 g of phosphate in a single dose.

Conversely, any therapy that excludes phosphate from the diet, such as intravenous feeding with solutions containing little phosphate, can be expected to reduce levels. Travis et al. reported levels in the range of 0.4 to 0.7 mmol/L in five of eight patients given intravenous solutions lacking phosphate.[358] The effect varied. In two patients studied retrospectively, there was no fall after 19 days in one patient, and in the other there was a fall for 4 days and then no further change.

Propranolol and Metoprolol

Administration of the beta adrenoreceptor-blocking drugs propranolol and metoprolol gives a small increase in serum inorganic phosphate. Murchison et al. gave the drugs to 24 hyperthyroid patients.[359] After administration of propranolol, serum inorganic phosphate levels increased from a mean of 1.21 mmol/L to 1.35 after 2 weeks and 1.36 after 6 weeks. The level increased after administration of metoprolol, from a mean of 1.10 mmol/L to 1.33 at 2 weeks and 1.34 at 4 weeks. The increase was linked to a rise in renal tubular phosphate reabsorption and a rise in urine phosphate.

Rimiterol and Salbutamol

The selective B_2-adrenoreceptor stimulants rimiterol and salbutamol, given for reversible airway obstruction, cause a small fall in serum inorganic phosphate levels. Intravenous infusions were given to four healthy subjects by Phillips et al.[360] Rimiterol (0.44 μg/kg/min) was given over 60 min and reduced serum inorganic phosphate by a mean of 0.30 mmol/L, and salbutamol (0.70 μg/kg/min) was given over 90 min and reduced the level by a mean of 0.25 mmol/L.

Tetracycline

Treatment with tetracycline is associated with hyperphosphatemia. Christian considered that this was due to renal damage.[347] However, this seems unlikely, as Betro and Pain gave three instances of an increase within a day of administration.[335]

Theophylline

A small fall in serum inorganic phosphate levels has been found in patients given theophylline. Zantvoort et al.[361] gave theophylline (6 to 7 mg/kg body weight) intravenously over 20 min to seven patients with chronic obstructive lung disease. The mean level fell from 0.89 to 0.80 mmol/L after 2 h and returned to the baseline within 4 h.

Thiazides

There are different reports of the effect of thiazides on serum inorganic phosphate (Table 50). Prolonged treatment appears to result in an increase, whereas immediately after treatment, there is either no change or a small fall.

Chapter 5

SODIUM AND POTASSIUM

Sodium and potassium are closely related electrolytes, but have different roles in the body. Sodium maintains osmotic pressure and acid/base equilibrium and is implicated in maintaining tissue hydration. Potassium acts to maintain cellular hydration and is involved in transmission of nerve impulses.

Most analyses required for clinical purposes are made using serum or plasma, although some attempts have been made to obtain an estimate of intracellular fluid composition, by estimating red cell concentrations. Results do not always reflect intracellular composition as derived from analysis of a muscle biopsy.

Originally, estimation of sodium and potassium was slow. The author recalls that the first analysis allocated to him in a clinical laboratory was for sodium and potassium and took almost two days to complete. Introduction of relatively cheap commercial flame photometers in the 1950s enabled rapid analyses to be undertaken. Sodium and potassium are now probably the most frequently analyzed constituents of blood in most hospital laboratories except for hemoglobin, with nearly half of all requests for blood specimens including an analysis for sodium and potassium among the investigations.

ANALYTIC CONSIDERATIONS

The earliest method for the estimation of serum sodium was based on formation of a salt with zinc uranyl acetate, followed by gravimetric, titrimetric, or colorimetric quantitation. Potassium was estimated by precipitation as chloroplatinate or cobaltinitrite, followed by titrimetric or colorimetric quantitation. Henry has reviewed a number of analytic methods.[366]

Later, use of flame photometry made results available more quickly, and these instruments were adapted for use in continuous-flow and discrete automatic analyzers, in which sodium and potassium were estimated simultaneously using an internal standard of lithium or cesium.

ION-SELECTIVE ELECTRODES
Electrodes for estimating sodium and potassium have now been developed. Their advantage is that whole blood can be used, avoiding the need to separate serum. A disadvantage is that this can mask hemolysis, giving a false potassium level.

A greater problem is that ion-selective electrodes (ISEs) measure ionic activity, whereas flame photometric and other methods measure mass per unit volume. Indirect ISE methods involving the dilution of serum may give results close to those obtained by flame photometry,[367,368] but there are significant differences using direct-reacting electrodes, due to the volume displacement effect of protein and lipid. Instruments using blood or undiluted serum may give results for serum sodium from 0 to 11 mmol/L lower by ISE methods than by flame photometry.[369] Ladenson et al. found differences of up to 17 mmol/L in myeloma cases.[370]

Levy feels that there is no unambiguous theoretical basis with which to choose among various direct-reacting ISE techniques and instruments[371] and, as an alternative, suggests the use of indirect methods, with a numerical correction if required, with a table to correct values to 75 g/L of total protein and 7.5 g/L of lipid. It is necessary to decide whether activity or concentration should be reported by laboratories. Maas et al. considered that activity was more important than concentration,[372] as tissue cells "see" activity, thus, physiologically, ISE values will be the relevant ones. Nevertheless, they suggested that concentration should continue to be reported using a conversion factor, as large differences will only occur when there are substantial changes in plasma water, such as in hypo- or hyperproteinemia.

67

Broughton et al. found that the relationship between serum total protein and the difference between the serum sodium result obtained using ISEs and flame photometry was linear,[373] and they also suggested that the water content of serum also affects serum potassium levels obtained by ISE methods.

International committees have considered the problem. The IFCC Expert Panel on pH blood gases and electrolytes proposed that ISEs should be set to give results similar to those obtained with flame photometric methods, for sera with normal protein and lipid levels.[374] Later, Russell et al. said that the panel was considering making this a recommendation.[375] The IFCC Working Group on Ion Selective Electrodes has discussed the convention to be used for reporting measurements made by ISEs.[376] The choice was not easy; the possibilities include:

- Relative modal activity (essentially the quantity sensed by ISEs)
- Molality (the amount of substance per kilogram of water)
- Molarity (the amount of substance per liter of serum)

Physiologic activity of potassium ion is best expressed by modal activity, whereas the major physiologic role of sodium in maintaining osmolality is best expressed by the molality. The view of both users and manufacturers was said to be overwhelmingly that the results with specimens with normal protein and lipid concentrations should agree with those obtained by flame photometry, to avoid a number of practical problems. Most instruments incorporate a correction factor so that the readout is converted to molarity by an unspecified algorithm that is, in part, based on the specific volume of protein and lipid.

An attempt to decrease differences in method group means revealed by proficiency testing for sodium or potassium, has been made by the development of a reference material of ultrafiltered frozen serum requiring no reconstitution for the standardization of ISEs.[377]

OTHER METHODS

A color method for potassium, using dry chemistry reagents, has been described by Ng et al.,[378] using the indicator change caused by hydrogen ions liberated in the binding of potassium to valinomycin.

ACCURACY AND PRECISION

Accuracy of serum or plasma sodium and potassium estimation is concerned with problems of standardization and with the differences between the flame photometric and ISE methods already discussed. Differences have been found between flame photometric methods using serum standards and those using aqueous standards,[379] which were attributed to the higher viscosity of diluted serum standards. It was concluded that the procedure should either use a serum standard or should include an addition, such as polyvinyl pyrollidone, to correct for viscosity differences.

Several groups have given between-batch precision for the estimation of serum sodium and potassium (Table 51). There is considerable variation between laboratories, as shown in data from quality-assurance schemes. Fraser quoted figures from the Wellcome Scheme to indicate that there was a small improvement in analytic precision in the participating laboratories from 1977 to 1981.[383]

Between-batch precision for estimations using ISEs appears to be similar to that using flame photometric methods. Hawks says that it is about 1.6 mmol/L for the estimation of serum sodium.[382] This compares with 1.8 for discrete or manual flame photometric methods and 1.5 for continuous-flow methods.

SI UNITS

In early work, serum sodium and potassium were usually reported in mass units as

TABLE 51.
Between-Batch Precision for Serum Sodium and Potassium Estimation

Reference	Method		Between-batch precision	
			Sodium	Potassium
380	Flame photometer		1.5%	2.5%
381	Data from Wellcome quality control scheme	50% of labs	1.3 or less	0.08 mmol/L or less
		20%	0.7 or less	0.04 mmol/L or less
382	Discrete or manual flame photometer with int. standard		1.8	0.10 mmol/L
	Continuous-flow analyzer		1.5	0.09 mmol/L

milligrams per 100 mL. Later milliequivalent per liter was used. The SI recommendation is to use millimeters per liter (mmol/L), which, for univalent ions, is the same numerically as milliequivalent per liter (mEq/L).

$$\text{serum sodium mmol/L} = \text{mEq/L} = \frac{\text{mg/100 mL}}{2.3}$$

$$\text{serum potassium mmol/L} = \text{mEq/L} = \frac{\text{mg/100 mL}}{4.0}$$

INTERFERENCE WITH ANALYSIS

HEMOLYSIS

Potassium is found at higher levels in cells than in serum; this gives rise to an increase in serum or plasma in hemolyzed specimens. It is generally agreed that hemolysis giving 1 g/L of serum hemoglobin leads to an increase in serum potassium of about 0.3 mmol/L.[367] Mather and Mackie[384] suggest correcting by subtracting 0.33 g/L of serum hemoglobin from the serum potassium of hemolyzed specimens.

The presence of hemolysis has only a small effect on serum or plasma sodium. Brydon and Roberts added hemolyzed blood to plasma[282] and found a fall of about 4 mmol/L of sodium per 10 g/L of plasma hemoglobin. In practice few workers use corrections except in special cases, and most prefer to reject hemolyzed specimens.

HEPARIN

Mann and Green found that when commercial collection tubes were used,[385] plasma sodium was, on average, 0.9 mmol/L (range of −6 to +3) lower than the corresponding serum level, when estimated using ISEs. They calculated that if 1 mL of blood was placed in a tube with heparin required for 10 mL of blood, the sodium level could be depressed by 5 mmol/L. Variable results were also observed when specimens for blood gas analysis were subsequently used for sodium estimations, due to heparin being used as an anticoagulant. In conclusion, heparin in excess may affect the analysis for serum sodium, using ISEs.

OTHER INTERFERING SUBSTANCES
Tobacco Smoke

Tobacco smoke interferes with flame photometry, giving an increase in apparent serum potassium. In the early days of the author's career, this was a potential problem, but smoking in laboratories is now infrequent and is usually forbidden. Smoking must not be allowed in any area where flame photometry is used for potassium estimation.

TABLE 52.
Change in Serum Sodium and Potassium with Addition of Cefatoxime
and Its Metabolite des Acetyl Cefatoxime to Pooled Serum[a]

	Na (% change)		K (mmol/L)	
Serum pool	Cefatoxine	Metabolite	Cefatoxine	Metabolite
Normal female	+3.1	+2.4	+0.11	+0.10
Pregnant females	+3.0	+2.7	+0.13	+0.16
Patients on gentamicin	+5.8	+3.0	+0.26	+0.18
Patients on tobramicin	+1.6	+5.8	+0.09	+0.17

[a]   From Baer, D. M., et al., *Clin. Chem.*, 29, 1736, 1983. Analysis with American "Parallel" analyzer.

TABLE 53.
Potassium in Serum with Fluosol D. A. Added to Correspond to
Various Percentage Replacements of Plasma Volume[a]

	Replacement of plasma volume by 20% emulsion			
Method	0%	10%	25%	50%
SMA IIC	2.1	2.2	2.4	2.8
Astra 8	2.2	2.2	2.4	2.7
Ectochem 400	4.4	4.2	4.3	4.2
ACA		No change reported		

[a]   From Mullins, R. E., et al., *Am. J. Clin. Pathol.*, 80, 478, 1983.

Cefatoxime

The third-generation cephalosporin cefatoxime and its major metabolite in serum, des acetyl cefatoxime, have been reported to apparently increase serum sodium and potassium, when added to pools of serum[386] (Table 52).

Fluosol D. A.

A 20% emulsion of perfluorocarbons, which serves as a blood substitute, an oxygen transport medium, and a plasma volume expander, has been evaluated in the United States. Mullins et al. investigated the effect on an analysis,[387] by adding amounts of the emulsion to serum corresponding to a replacement of plasma volume. Serum sodium was not affected, but there were changes in potassium, which varied with the instrument used for the analysis (Table 53).

Liposol

The commercially available lipid-clarifying agent Liposol affects both serum sodium and potassium. Lacher and Elsea,[83] using the Beckman Astra Ideal analyzer, found that mean serum sodium of 26 randomly selected sera fell from 138.8 to 131.6 mmol/L after treatment with Liposol and mean serum potassium increased from 4.45 to 6.89 mmol/L.

Hyoscine-*N*-Butyl Bromide

Sonntag reported that hyoscine-*N*-butyl bromide above 20 mg/L affects estimations by ISEs, without predilution.[388]

PREANALYTIC ERROR

COLLECTION OF THE SPECIMEN

Potassium levels in serum are higher than the levels found in the plasma from correspond-

TABLE 54.
Potassium in Serum and Heparinized Plasma

Reference	Method	Observation
389	Dog's blood	Serum 0.1–0.6 mmol/L higher than heparinized plasma
390	Serum from 106 healthy subjects and plasma from 22 healthy subjects	Serum mean 0.7 mmol/L higher than heparinized plasma mean
391	Analysis using SMA 12/60 and IL Flame Photometer	Serum mean 0.23 mmol/L higher than heparinized plasma mean
392	203 subjects. Analysis with SMA 12/60	Serum mean 0.37 mmol/L higher than heparinized plasma mean
393	8 healthy subjects. Serum separated after 30 min. Plasma separated immediately.	Serum mean 0.19 mmol/L higher than heparinized plasma mean

ing specimens (Table 54). The smaller difference found by Kalsheker and Jones[393] was considered to be due to previous workers not taking into account the fall in potassium during the first hours after collection.[384] The higher level in serum is usually attributed to potassium derived from platelets on clotting. Despite this, many laboratories continue to use serum from clotted blood for electrolyte estimations, for reasons of either convenience or economy.

Small errors are introduced when polyester gel separators are used. Bailey compared the analysis of heparinized plasma separated within 2 h of collection, and of plasma from a container with polyester gel separator stored at 4°C overnight.[394] Plasma sodium from the gel separator tube was a mean of 0.53 mmol/L (range of 0.0 to 3.0) lower than in plasma from the other tube. Plasma potassium was a mean of 0.10 mmol/L higher (range of 0.0 to 0.5). The difference in sodium was thought to be due to an exchange with the red cells, and the higher potassium, due to leakage from cells. Mean differences were not considered to be clinically significant.

CONTAMINATION

Care must be taken to ensure that all glassware is clean and free from contamination with sodium and potassium. Unused glassware should be checked, as it is liable to have surface contamination with alkali. McCormick et al. found that soft glass pipettes, widely used to transfer sera, were contaminated.[395] Pipettes from different suppliers gave levels of 0.15 to 0.32 μmol of sodium per pipette and 0.02 to 0.04 μmol of potassium per pipette, after 1 minute contact time at room temperature. Errors on the order of 1 mmol/L of sodium and 0.1 mmol/L of potassium could be introduced.

Wooden applicator sticks used to remove fibrin have also been shown to produce contamination with potassium after a few minutes of contact with serum.[94] After 30 min an increase of 0.4 mmol/L was observed.

Specimens from indwelling catheter lines have been shown to be contaminated with benzalkalonium salts used as cationic surfactants, and this leads to erroneous results, using ISEs.[396]

SAMPLE STABILITY

The level of serum sodium remains constant after collection. However, serum potassium levels change if cells are not separated from the serum, decreasing a little over several hours before rising (Table 55). The initial fall is related to continuing glycolysis, and later increases are related to diffusion of potassium from cells. The diffusion is quicker at lower temperatures, as the sodium/potassium pump is less active. Samples should not be kept cold, as this results in greater error. Serum specimens are stable when frozen, but care must be taken to ensure thorough mixing after thawing. Omang and Vellar showed that a concentration gradient arises

TABLE 55.
Potassium Changes in Serum in Contact With Red Cells at Various Temperatures

Reference	Method	Temperature	Observation
397	Defibrinated blood from seven subjects	7°C	Increase at constant rate of 0.100–0.279 mmol/L/h for up to 48 h
	Defibrinated blood from two subjects	37°C	Decrease in first 4–5 h of about 1 mmol/L
			Increase in next 20 h of 0.1–0.2 mmol/L/h
398		25°C	Small fall after 2–8 h
399		4°C	Increase in 6 h 1.2 mmol/L
			Increase in 24 h 6 mmol/L
399		25°C	Increase in 24 h. 0.8 mmol/L
392	Lithium heparin samples		
	18 nonfasting	Room temp.	Mean decrease in 2 h 0.22 mmol/L
	10 fasting subjects	Room temp.	Mean decrease in 2 h 0.14 mmol/L
			Decrease continued for up to 8 h

TABLE 56.
Change in Serum and Plasma Sodium and Potassium
after Heating to 56°C for 30 min

Reference	Medium	Mean change	
		Na	K
101	Serum	+0.3%	No change
301	Plasma	–0.08%	
108	Plasma	+0.6%	
		(max. difference 3 mmol/L)	
302	Plasma	–0.3%	

in specimens frozen and thawed without mixing.[98] Serum sodium varied from 26 mmol/L in the top layer to 270 mmol/L in the bottom layer, compared with a concentration of 142 mmol/L in a well-mixed sample.

Salzmann and Male noted artifactual hypernatremia after centrifuging small amounts of blood (about 0.51 mL) from pediatric patients, in uncapped tubes.[400] Three minutes of centrifugation increased plasma sodium by about 10 mmol/L, due to evaporation of water.

Heating to 56°C

Studies of the effect of heating serum sodium to 56°C for 30 min to minimize the risk from HIV-positive specimens have shown small, but clinically insignificant, changes in serum or plasma sodium and no apparent change in serum potassium, if evaporation is avoided (Table 56).

Addition of B-propriolactone as an alternative has been found to affect sodium and potassium levels if added to whole blood, but causes no error when added to serum or plasma[401] (Table 57).

PHYSIOLOGIC CHANGES

EXERCISE

There are conflicting reports on the effect of severe exercise on serum sodium and potassium (Table 58). Some have found little change, and other have found increases, particularly in potassium. Differences may be related to the degree of exercise, although it is difficult to accept the large increase in potassium found by McKechnies' group.[402] Priest et al.

TABLE 57.
Effect of Treating Whole Blood and Separated Plasma
with B-Propiolactone[a]

	N	Na (mmol/L)	K (mmol/L)
Plasma from untreated whole blood	25	142.9 ± 5.2	4.05 ± 0.56
Plasma from treated whole blood	25	150.1 ± 5.6	4.74 ± 0.56
Untreated plasma	21	140.4 ± 1	4.08 ± 1
Treated plasma	21	139.9 ± 4	4.09 ± 1

[a] From Ball, M. J. and Griffiths, D., *Lancet*, i, 1160, 1985.

TABLE 58.
Effect of Severe Exercise on Serum Sodium and Potassium (in mmol/L)

			Effect			
			Na		K	
Reference	Exercise		Mean	Range	Mean	Range
402	20 men after a 50-km run	After			7.46	6.7–9.5
		3 weeks later			3.7	
403	9 men running same 50 km	Before				3.9–5.0
		After				3.1–4.5
404	Boston marathon	Before	139	137–141	4.20	3.8–4.6
		After	145	144–147	4.75	4.4–5.5
405	20 min of strenuous exercise		No change		Fall greater during morning than on previous day without exercise	
406	13-mile run	Before	140.8	SD 2.2	4.40	SD 0.60
		After	141.6	SD 2.8	4.90	SD 0.50

reported animal experiments[406] suggesting that there is an efflux of potassium from skeletal muscle during exercise. The modest amount of exercise by patients attending a clinic would not be expected to change serum sodium or potassium.

It has been shown that forearm exercise, as in the common practice of opening and closing the fist before venipuncture, can result in an increase in serum potassium (Table 59). The change can be great enough to affect the interpretation of results, and this should be borne in mind.

MENSTRUAL CYCLE

Small changes in serum sodium and potassium have been noted during the menstrual cycle.[409] The mean serum sodium level increased from 140.8 (SD 1.9) during the luteal phase to 142.5 (SD 2.1) during the follicular phase, and serum potassium fell from 4.0 (SD 0.36) to a mean of 3.8 (SD 0.29) mmol/L. The change in serum sodium was not found to be associated with a change in weight or an alteration in serum creatinine or albumin, suggesting that total body water and intravascular volume remained constant.

BLOOD DONATION

There is an alteration in plasma potassium in some individuals as a result of blood donation. Changes in serum sodium are infrequent. Flynn et al.[30] collected samples before and after donation of 420 mL of blood from each of 100 volunteers. Plasma potassium was found to change by more than 0.2 mmol/L in 38% of the subjects and by at least 0.8 mmol/L in 15% of the subjects. Care must be taken when using samples from blood donors to establish ranges in healthy people, and it should not be assumed that samples taken at the end of a donation are suitable.

TABLE 59.
Effect of Forearm Exercise on Serum Potassium

Reference	Exercise	Effect
407	Opening and closing fist 10 times with tourniquet on	Increase in potassium 10–20% persisting for about 2 min
408	Cuff pressure 10 mm below systolic b.p. 10–15 contractions of forearm muscles	During contractions potassium increase 0–2.7 mmol/L 15–30 s after potassium increase 0–2.0 mmol/L

TABLE 60.
Variation of Early Reports of Serum Sodium in Healthy Subjects

Reference	Method	Level (mmol/L)
149	Textbook range	141–152 (325–350 mg/100 mL)
7	Textbook range	141–152 (325–350 mg/100 mL)
410	Zinc uranyl acetate method	80% of the population had level in range of 137–148
125	Flame emission photometry. 111 healthy subjects	Male mean 143 Female mean 144
411	79 healthy staff. Plasma analyzed by flame emission photometry	Male mean 135 Female mean 133.8

RANGE IN HEALTHY SUBJECTS

WITHIN- AND BETWEEN-PERSON VARIATION
Serum Sodium

There are wide variations in the early reports of the level of serum sodium in healthy subjects (Table 60). It was not until the introduction of the continuous-flow analyzer that there was reasonable agreement in published ranges. The ranges found in some large surveys are shown in Table 61. The mean serum sodium level is approximately 140 mmol/L in males, with the mean level in young females about 1 mmol/L less. The difference disappears after menopause. There seems to be little variation with age in adults. Baadenhiutsen et al. obtained similar ranges by extracting data from hospital records,[146] but was not able to detect a sex-related difference.

Almost all workers think that the distribution is gaussian or near gaussian. The author has found a unimodal distribution that is leptokurtic.

Serum Potassium

Estimations of the range of serum potassium in healthy persons using chemical methods showed significant differences; with the introduction of flame photometric methods, better agreement was obtained about the level. Ranges found in some large surveys are given in Table 62. The mean serum potassium level is about 4.4 mmol/L, with a range of 3.7 to 5.1. Baadenhuitsen et al. obtained similar ranges by extracting data from hospital records.[146] As already discussed, the level in heparinized plasma is about 0.2 to 0.3 mmol/L lower than in serum.

There is no general agreement about the distribution that has been reported as "normal" by Roberts,[412] "lognormal" by Mohun and Cook[413] and Owen and Campbell,[414] or "positively skewed" by Li et al.[415] Studies in the author's laboratory (Figure 4) do not suggest that the distribution is skewed, and that it is approximately gaussian.

Following reports on Chinese subjects taking gossypol (a possible oral contraceptive for men), which showed hypokalemia in both controls and those taking the drug, Reidenberg et al.[416] studied serum potassium in subjects from six centers in different parts of the world (Table

TABLE 61.
Serum and Plasma Sodium in Healthy Subjects (in mmol/L)

Reference		≤20	21–25	26–30	31–35	36–40	41–45	46–50	51–55	56–60	61–65
Male											
141[a]	Mean		140.52	140.52	140.59	140.59	140.45	140.45	140.56	140.56	
	SD		2.96	2.96	2.67	2.67	2.64	2.64	2.71	2.71	
142[b]	Mean	141.1	141.1	141.1	141.1	140.7	140.7	140.7	140.7	140.7	140.7
Coventry[c]	N	95	232	145	139	82	90	61	77	54	33
	Mean	140.25	140.34	140.29	140.22	140.18	140.26	140.18	140.31	140.24	140.33
	SD	2.02	2.15	1.94	2.30	2.06	2.06	2.51	2.37	2.43	2.67
	2.5–97.5 percentile	136–144	136–144	136–144	136–145	136–143	135–143	133–146	135–146	136–145	
Female											
141[a]	Mean		139.80	139.80	139.89	139.89	140.02	140.02	140.76	140.76	
	SD		2.67	2.67	2.74	2.74	2.70	2.70	2.60	2.60	
142[b]	Mean	140.3	140.3	139.9	139.9	140.0	140.0	141.0	141.0	141.7	141.7
Coventry[c]	N	659	678	314	317	261	236	165	111	78	27
	Mean	139.21	139.32	138.97	139.02	139.33	138.89	139.43	140.02	140.27	140.13
	SD	2.06	2.22	2.15	1.90	1.93	2.50	2.29	2.23	2.29	2.63
	2.5–97.5 percentile	135–143	135–144	135–143	135–143	136–143	134–143	135–144	135–144	135–144	

[a] 3600 men and 1100 women from a well-persons' clinic.
[b] 1000 blood donors. Heparinized plasma.
[c] Coventry Healthy hospital staff, as described in Chapter 2.

62a). Mean levels in Shanghai were lower than those found elsewhere. For other Chinese populations, references are given to serum potassium levels within the usually accepted range. Although possible regional differences in dietary potassium were considered as a possible explanation, the protocol described did not record a standardized time for the separation of cells from the serum. Further studies are required to confirm this finding.

Diurnal Variation

A fall in serum potassium during the day has been reported. In a study of 7735 men ages 40 to 49 and selected randomly by Pocock et al.,[409] the time of venipuncture was noted. Mean serum potassium for samples collected between 9:00 am and 1:00 pm was 4.40 mmol/L and for samples collected between 1:00 pm and 6:00 pm, 4.26 mmol/L. The small change is unlikely to have any significant implication for the interpretation of serum potassium.

Meals are said to give a small increase in serum sodium and potassium. Hitz gives references showing that after a 700-cal meal, serum sodium and potassium increase by 0.42%,[410] a change that does not affect interpretation. A diet rich in sodium or potassium has no effect on the plasma levels.

CHILDREN

Levels of serum sodium and potassium in healthy children appear to be similar to those found in adults (Table 63), although Hitz claimed that sodium was slightly lower in children.[410] He reported that mean levels were about 140 mEq/L, compared with 141 in adults.

NEONATES

Serum sodium in the neonatal period is lower than that found later in life (Table 64), whereas potassium is higher[423] (Table 65). There may be a relationship between serum sodium and the amount of sodium taken in, particularly in very-low-birth-weight babies, in whom levels of less than 130 mmol/L are often found in the 1st week of life.[420]

RANGE DURING PREGNANCY

There is a small fall in the levels of serum sodium and potassium during pregnancy, with a rise to nonpregnant levels soon after delivery (Table 66).

OTHER CHANGES

SMOKING

Vasopressin levels in serum have been shown to increase fourfold after smoking two cigarettes within 15 min,[426] and this might be expected to give a hyponatremic effect. Little work has been reported on this, but Blum described a schizophrenic patient[427] who drank 6 to 8 L of water daily for at least 8 years and, on two occasions, suffered tonoclonic seizures and had a serum sodium level of 107 mmol/L. These were related to increased water and cigarette consumption, and it was thought that there was inappropriate antidiuretic hormone (ADH) secretion due to the ADH-releasing effect of nicotine. This was supported by a demonstration showing that serum sodium was lower when smoking was unrestricted than when it was confined to 18 cigarettes per day.

BLINDNESS

There is a report of significant differences in serum sodium and potassium in subjects either blind or with impaired vision (Table 67). The mean levels and ranges in subjects with normal vision differ from most other reports, suggesting that this finding requires further study.

TABLE 62.
Serum and Plasma Potassium in Healthy Subjects (in mmol/L)

Reference		20	21–25	26–30	31–35	36–40	41–45	46–50	51–55	56–60	61–65
Male											
141[a]	Mean		4.34	4.34	4.38	4.38	4.39	4.39	4.44	4.44	
	SD		0.34	0.34	0.37	0.37	0.37	0.37	0.38	0.38	
142[b]	Mean	3.99	3.99	3.99	3.99	4.06	4.06	4.13	4.13	4.13	4.13
	N	93	231	144	139	81	88	61	76	54	33
Coventry[c]	Mean	4.24	4.30	4.26	4.33	4.26	4.26	4.24	4.24	4.27	4.28
	SD	0.40	0.34	0.35	0.34	0.35	0.30	0.35	0.35	0.32	0.33
	2.5–97.5 percentile	3.7–5.0	3.7–5.1	3.6–5.0	3.8–5.1	3.7–5.0	3.9–5.0	3.7–4.9	3.6–5.0	3.8–5.0	3.7–5.1
Female											
141[a]	Mean		4.31	4.31	4.29	4.29	4.30	4.30	4.37	4.37	
	SD										
142[b]	Mean	3.80	3.80	3.85	3.85	3.90	3.90	3.98	3.98	4.02	4.02
	N	656	674	311	313	256	234	164	110	76	
Coventry[c]	Mean	4.26	4.24	4.25	4.23	4.26	4.21	4.26	4.32	4.26	
	SD	0.32	0.34	0.34	0.40	0.31	0.32	0.32	0.31	0.26	
	2.5–97.5 percentile	3.8–5.1	3.7–5.1	3.6–5.0	3.6–5.1	3.6–5.2	3.6–5.0	3.6–5.0	3.6–5.0		

a 3600 men and 1100 women from a well-persons' clinic.
b 1000 blood donors. Heparinized plasma.
c Coventry healthy hospital staff, as described in Chapter 2.

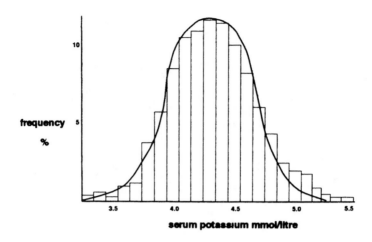

FIGURE 4. Distribution of serum potassium in 2794 healthy men and women 17–65 years old (from the author's laboratory). Curve shows gaussian distribution derived from the mean and SD.

TABLE 62A.
Serum Potassium in Men Living in Different Cities[a] (in mmol/L)

City	N	Mean	SD
Shanghai, China	53	3.82	0.27
Salvador, Brazil	100	4.06	0.29
Salzburg, Austria	30	4.14	0.44
Philadelphia, United States	51	4.31	0.32
Newark, United States	52	4.45	0.41
Santo Domingo, Dominican Republic	38	4.37	0.33

[a] From Reidenberg, M. M., et al., *Clin. Chem.*, 39, 72, 1993.

ALCOHOL

Small amounts of alcohol have some effect on serum sodium and potassium[428] (Table 68). Although the effect of social drinking can probably be ignored in clinical work when determining reference intervals, alcohol should not be taken for at least a day before samples are taken.

ANESTHESIA

Hypo- or hypercapnea may occur during anesthesia, depending on the degree of CO_2 retention allowed. There may also be a metabolic acidosis associated with increased lactate and pyruvate during deep anesthesia. These effects give rise to changes in serum potassium. Robertson and Fraser suggest[429] that there is a decrease of about 0.5 mmol/L for each 1.3-kPa (10 mm Hg) decrease in p_aCO_2. There is a corresponding rise in serum potassium if CO_2 retention is allowed. They also state that there is little change in serum sodium, although Grey, Nunn, and Utting found that a decrease of up to 5 mmol/L was not unusual.[430]

SPURIOUS HYPOKALEMIA IN MYELOPROLIFERATIVE DISORDERS

An increased uptake of potassium by abnormal white cells, causing a spurious hypokalemia in patients with myeloproliferative disorders, has been reported. Naparstek and Gutman described three cases of myeloid leukemia and one of undetermined myeloproliferative disease with apparent serum potassium levels of 2.2, 2.5, 2.5, and 3.4 mmol/L.[431] There was no hypokalemia if the sample was separated and analyzed immediately after venipuncture or

TABLE 63.
Serum and Plasma Sodium and Potassium in Children (in mmol/L)

Reference	Subjects and method	Sex	Age (years)	Na				K			
				N	Mean	SD	Range	N	Mean	SD	Range
317	Canadian children Analysis by flame emission photometry	M	4–20	500	139	2.1		500	4.3	0.36	3.3–4.7
		F	4–20	500	139	1.8		500	4.4	0.44	3.4–4.5
418	Heparinized plasma	M	7–16				135–144				
		F	7–16				136–144				
419	Children with morphologic disease and no medication or history of serious disease. Adult hospital staff	M + F	0					12	4.4		3.7–5.1
			1					24	4.4		3.7–5.1
			2					14	4.3		3.7–5.1
			3					27	4.3		3.7–5.1
			4					27	4.3		3.7–5.0
			5					34	4.3		3.7–5.0
			6	476	141		137–145	37	4.3		3.6–5.0
			7					22	4.3		3.6–5.0
			8					19	4.2		3.6–5.0
			9					29	4.2		3.6–4.9
			10					14	4.2		3.6–4.9
			11					14	4.2		3.6–4.9
			12					25	4.2		3.5–4.9
			13–19					178	4.1		3.5–4.8
			Adults 20–49		141		138–144		4.1		3.5–4.7

[a] From Meites, S., in *Paediatric Clinical Chemistry. A Survey of Normal, Method, and Instrumentation with Commentary*, Meites, S., Ed., Washington, DC, AACC Press, 1977, 93.

TABLE 64.
Serum Sodium in Neonates (in mmol/L)

Reference	Subject	Age	Mean	SD	N	Range
420	Full-term infants receiving	6 days	133	7	28	
	breast milk	3 weeks	137	9	17	
		6 weeks	137	11	16	
		3 months	136	9	15	
		6 months	137	9	11	
421	Low-birth-weight infants	7 days				131–140
	receiving SMA Goldcap-S26	11 days				133–142
		21 days				135–140
422	Very-low-birth weight infants					
	(less than 1.3 kg)					
	Sodium intake 2 mmol/kg/24 h	About 18 days	131			30% < 130
		25	129			41
		32	130			41
		39	130			39
		46	132			19
	Sodium intake 3 mmol/kg/24 h	About 18 days	131			32% < 130
		25	134			6
		32	135			0
		39	136			0
		46	137			0

TABLE 65.
Serum Potassium in First Weeks of Life[a]
(in mmol/L)

Age	Range
Premature	4.5–7.2
Full-term	5.0–7.7
2 days to 2 weeks	4.0–6.4
2 weeks to 3 months	4.0–6.2
3 months to 1 year	3.7–5.6

[a]   From Meites, S., in *Paediatric Clinical Chemistry. A Survey of Normal, Method, and Instrumentation with Commentary*, Meites, S., Ed., Washington, DC, AACC Press, 1977, 93.

if the sample was kept at 4°C. The findings were considered to be due to the abnormally increased sodium/potassium pump activity of the white cells, which was abolished at 4°C.

DRUGS AFFECTING SERUM SODIUM AND POTASSIUM

AMINO ACIDS

Some preparations, such as 10% aminosol prepared by the enzymic hydrolysis of casein, have a high sodium content and, in cases of cardiac or renal disease, can lead to sodium overload. Other preparations contain less sodium.[432] Arginine monohydrochloride, which has been used to treat metabolic alkalosis associated with hepatic encephalopathy, increases serum potassium. A dose of 30 to 60 g given to healthy subjects over 30 min increases serum potassium by 0.6 to 1.0 mmol/L.[433]

TABLE 66.
Serum Sodium and Potassium During Pregnancy (in mmol/L)

Reference		Gestation weeks	N	Na Mean	SD	K Mean	SD
424	200 subjects for diagnostic	20–30	43	139.0	4.9		
	amniocentesis. Analysis	31–32	38	138.0	6.4		
	using atomic absorption	33–34	32	138.0	4.5		
	flame photometry	35–36	43	138.0	5.3		
		37–38	15	136.0	5.9		
		39+	17	136.0	5.9		
425		10 ± 4	205	135.5		3.83	
		28 ± 4	198	134.6		3.78	
		37 ± 3	210	134.8		4.00	
		2–6 days after delivery	148	136.8		4.35	

TABLE 67.
Serum Sodium and Potassium in Blind Subjects, Subjects with Impaired Vision, and Controls[a] (in mmol/L)

Subject	N	Na	K
Blind	220	140.24	4.69
Impaired vision (less than 1/10)	140	141.47	
Controls	50	145.6	4.25

[a] From Hollwich, F. and Dieckhues, B., Endocrine systems and blindness. *Germ. Med.*, 1, 122, 1971.

TABLE 68.
Serum Sodium and Potassium after Alcohol[a] (in mmol/L)

	Na change mean	K change mean
1 h after 3rd dose	+2.14	–0.24
3 h after 3rd dose	+1	–0.24
15 h after 3rd dose		+0.26
38 h after 3rd dose	0	0

[a] From Leppänen, E. A., and Gräsbeck, R., *Scand. J. Clin. Lab. Invest.*, 47, 337, 1987.

Baseline samples taken on two successive evenings followed by 0.75 g/kg body weight ethanol given on three consecutive evenings.

TABLE 69.
Increase in Serum Potassium in Patients Given Captopril

Reference	Subjects	Effect
435	23 hypertensive patients given 150–800 mg daily for 10 days.	Increase up to 1 mmol/L
436	Five hypertensive patients given up to 450 mg daily with digoxin and frusemide	Mean increase 0.7 mmol/L
437	Men 20–69 years old with diastolic b.p. 72–109 mm given 37.5–150 mg daily for 12 weeks	Mean increase 0.11 mmol/L No significant increase in percentage with serum potassium above 5 mmol/L

Amphotericin B

About 25% of patients given Amphotericin B intravenously develop hypokalemia, which is not permanent if 4 g or less is given over 6 weeks.[434]

Angiotensin-Converting Enzyme Inhibitors

There is a small increase in serum potassium in patients taking angiotensin-converting enzyme inhibitors, related to the fall in serum and urine aldosterone. Table 69 shows increases found by several groups in patients given captopril. Ponce et al. found a mean increase of 0.3 mmol/L in patients given enalopril.[438]

Antibiotics

Changes in serum sodium and potassium have been reported after treatment with several antibiotics. Of 67 patients given 1 g of capreomicin daily for some months, three had serum sodium of from 125 to 130 mmol/L and serum potassium of from 1.6 to 2.5 mmol/L.[231] Ethambutol and isoniazid were also given, but were not considered responsible for the changes, which were considered to be due to capreomicin-induced secondary aldosteronism.

Hypokalemia due to the effect of carbenicillin on the renal tubules in patients with leukemia, lymphoma, and malignant neoplasms, who are given antibiotics, has been reported.[439,440] Hypokalemia and hypomagnesemia, attributed to drug-induced secondary aldosteronism, were reported in four patients on antitubercular therapy, by Holmes et al.[230] Serum potassium was from 2.2 to 3.4 mmol/L, and although the patients were taking several drugs, it was concluded that the effect was due to gentamycin.

There is an increase in serum potassium in patients given the potassium salt of penicillin intravenously and a decrease in patients given the sodium salt.[441] Brunner and Frick reported on three patients given large amounts of penicillin G;[442] two had high serum sodium (159 and 161 mmol/L), and all three had low serum potassium (2.0 to 3.2 mmol/L).

Polymyxin B, an antibiotic effective against Gram-negative organisms, affects serum sodium and potassium levels. Rodriguez et al. reported on 64 patients with 107 febrile episodes treated with polymyxin B.[443] Of 107 patients, 44 had serum sodium of less than 132 mmol/L.

Young found mithramycin, viomycin, and tetracycline to affect serum sodium and potassium,[56] but no primary reference is given, and Martin said methicillin gives an increase in serum potassium,[444] but again, no primary reference is given.

Beta Adrenoreceptor Blockers

Administration of nonselective beta blockers results in a small rise in serum potassium.

Propranolol

A dose of 40 to 450 mg of propranolol was given for 1 week to 47 hypertensive patients, by

Bühler et al.[445] There was an increase in serum potassium in 19 patients (0.37 ± 0.10 mmol/L), a decrease in 8 (0.30 ± 0.09), and no change in 5.

Drayer et al. gave patients 160 to 640 mg/day[446] and found a mean increase of 0.3 mmol/L in serum potassium and a mean fall of 3 mmol/L in sodium, whereas in 85 hypertensive patients given 85 mg/day by Bergland et al.,[447] mean serum potassium rose by 0.4 mmol/L after 2 months and remained at the same level for up to a year.

Timolol

In a study of 106 myocardial infarction patients given timolol by Nordrehaug et al.,[448] mean serum potassium increased by 0.5 mmol/L compared with little change in those given a placebo. A patient with serum potassium of 6.0 mmol/L, thought to be due to timolol maleate eye drops given for glaucoma, was described by Swenson.[449]

Alprenol, Oxprenol, and Pindolol

References suggesting that other beta blockers, including alprenol, oxprenol, and pindolol, increase serum potassium, are given by Ponce et al.[438]

Beta Adrenoreceptor Stimulants

Serum potassium falls after giving these drugs.

Fenoterol

Haalboom et al., in an experiment on healthy medical students,[450] found that after 12 puffs of fenoterol (each puff 0.2 mg), there was a mean fall in serum potassium of 1.0 mmol/L after 60 min. The decrease was shown to be dose-related, and no change was found using a placebo.

Ramiterol

Intravenous ramiterol was given in doses used in clinical practice (up to 0.44 μg/kg/min) to four healthy male subjects age 21 to 31, by Phillips et al.[451] A dose-related fall in serum potassium of up to 1.2 mmol/L was found.

Salbutamol

Güngoğdu et al. gave 5 μg/min of salbutamol intravenously for 1 h, followed by 20 μg/min for the next hour.[452] Mean serum potassium fell by 0.55 mmol/L in the first hour and a further 0.64 mmol/L in the next hour. An hour later the level had risen by a mean of 0.34 mmol/L.

O'Brian et al. reported a single case of a 76-year-old woman who had taken an overdose of 40×4 mg of salbutamol with distalgesic tablets.[453] Serum potassium was 2.3 mmol/L, with serum sodium of 140 mmol/L. Standard doses of salbutamol taken orally were said to have no effect on serum potassium.

Salmeterol

Ind found that the decrease in serum potassium, in healthy subjects and asthmatics after taking 25 to 200 μg of salmeterol, is similar to that produced by salbutamol.[454]

Terbutaline

Bengtssen found that both intravenous and oral terbutaline reduced serum potassium.[455] Mean serum potassium fell from 4.3 to 3.4 mmol/L in 11 healthy men 27 to 38 years old, who were given 0.25 mg intravenously. When 15 mg/day was given orally for 13 days, serum potassium fell from 4.4 to 3.5 mmol/L in 2 h on the first day, but by the thirteenth day, the mean had returned to the baseline level.

TABLE 70.
Serum Sodium Levels in Patients Taking Carbamazepine (in mmol/L)

Reference	Subject	N	Effect	
456	Patient with epileptiform attacks	1	Fall from 135 to 120	
457	Patients 14–65 years old	16	Five of 16 less than 135	
			Strong correlation between dose, steady state drug level, and serum sodium	
458	Patients on carbamazepine	13	Five of 13 had hyponatremia	
	Patients on other anticonvulsants with carbamazepine	67	Five of 80 had hyponatremia Range of serum sodium 125–134	
	Control patients	50	None with hyponatremia	
459	Children 6–18 years old			
	Carbamazepine alone	11	Mean 143	None with hyponatremia
	Carbamazepine with other anticonvulsants	17	Mean 142	None with hyponatremia
	Other anticonvulsants		Mean 142	None with hyponatremia

TABLE 71.
Reports of Hyponatremia in Patients on Chlorpromamide

Reference	Subjects	Level of serum sodium (mmol/L)	
460	Five diabetic patients taking chlorpromamide three also taking thiazides	On admission	113–132
		Lowest level	103–120
		Despite hyponatremia, sodium excretion continued	
461	Single case on 250 mg of chlorpromamide daily		118
	Also taking prednisolone and phenylbutazone		Potassium not abnormal
462	221 patients taking chlorpromamide	0 of 221	<120
		2 of 221	<130
463	Diabetic patients		
	64 on chlorpromamide		138.8 ± 3.7
	20 Moduretic		138.7 ± 3.0
	189 neither		139.7

Carbamazepine

Low serum sodium has been found in some patients taking carbamazepine (Table 70), although this appears to be less frequent in children.[459]

Chlorpropamide

Some workers have suggested that diabetic patients treated with chlorpropamide may show hyponatremia.[460,461] Other groups have disputed the incidence[462,463] and claim that it is very low (Table 71).

Cholestyramine

Cases of hypernatremia have been reported in babies treated with cholestyramine for liver disease. Primak et al.[464] described a case with serum sodium of 175 mmol/L and potassium of 4.7 mmol/L, in a baby with neonatal hepatitis, given 4 g with every feed for 8 weeks, instead of the 2 g intended. Another baby with biliary atresia had serum sodium of 155 mmol/L and serum potassium of 5.0 mmol/L, after taking 1 g with each feed. Care must be taken when treating babies with this drug, as they need extra water to compensate for the extra fecal loss and to deal with the increased urine solute load.

Cisplatin

A single case with serum potassium of less than 2.0 mmol/L during cisplatin treatment was described by Hill et al.[465] Serum calcium and magnesium were also low.

Corticosteroids

The main physiologic action of mineralosteroids such as aldosterone is on the kidney, decreasing sodium and water excretion and increasing potassium loss, resulting in increased serum sodium and decreased serum potassium. Some glucocorticoids have a mild mineralocorticoid effect, although this may be very small with some synthetic compounds. Bethone lists mineralocorticoid activity relative to that of cortisol:[466]

Drug	Relative mineralocorticoid activity
Cortisol	1.0
Cortisone	0.8
Aldosterone	300
Corticosterone	1.5
Deoxycorticosterone	20
Prednisone	0.3
Prednisolone	0.3
Methyl prednisolone	0
Dexamethazone	0
Fluorocortisone	250

Other Steroids and Related Drugs

Young described a number of drugs as affecting serum sodium or potassium,[56] but no primary references were given:

- Androgens[467]
- Anabolic steroids[444]
- Angiotensin;[468] due to salt-retaining action of aldosterone
- Beta metazone[467]
- Corticotrophin[444]
- Estrogen[468]
- Progesterone;[469] sodium diuresis at first, followed by retention. At higher levels, diuretic effect predominates.
- Testosterone[469] high dose causes salt and water retention.

Cyclophosphamide

Impairment of water excretion in normally hydrated cancer patients treated with more than 50 mg/kg body weight/day of cyclophosphamide was found in 17 of 19 patients, by DeFronzo et al.[470] The mechanism is not clear.

Some tumors (Burkitt's lymphoma and some leukemias) are very sensitive to chemotherapy, and rapid dissolution of malignant cells can cause the release of a large amount of potassium. Arseneau et al.[471] reported that 4 of 13 cases treated with chemotherapy had increased serum potassium (range of 5.2 to 8.9 mmol/L), with two deaths.

Cyclosporin

Renal allograft patients receiving cyclosporin have been found to have higher serum potassium levels than similar patients receiving other drugs (Table 72).

Diuretics

It can be anticipated that treatment with diuretics that inhibit sodium reabsorption in the kidney

TABLE 72.
Serum Potassium (in mmol/L) in Renal Allograft Patients Receiving Cyclosporin, Compared with the Level in Patients Given Other Drugs

Reference	Time	Cyclosporin		Prednisone and azothiaprine	
		N	Mean	N	Mean
472	3 months after transplant	40	5.0	25	4.2
	9 months after transplant	20	4.8	17	4.1
473	1 month	13 of 50 > 5.0			
	6 month	5 of 50 > 5.0			
				1 of 13 > 5.0	

TABLE 73.
Serum Sodium and Potassium in Patients on Thiazides

Reference	Subjects	Na (mmol/L) mean	K (mmol/L)	
474	Ten hypertensives given methylclothiazide for 12 weeks	Fall 2.2	Fall in mean 0.4	
475	Usual doses of thiazides		Fall in mean 0.6	
476	50 mg of hydrochlorthiazide daily		20–30%	<3.5
			5%	<3.0
	50 mg of chlorthalidone daily		40–60%	<3.5
	100 mg of chlorthalidone daily		80%	<3.5

will be associated with low serum sodium. Treatment with diuretics that increase renal clearance of potassium may, in some cases, lead to hypokalemia if potassium supplements are insufficient. Potassium-sparing diuretics can be used to avoid the need for potassium supplementation.

Thiazides
Although thiazides and related drugs inhibit sodium reabsorption in the kidney tubule and also increase renal clearance of potassium, only small changes in serum sodium and potassium are usually found after treatment (Table 73).

Severe hyponatremia in nonedematous patients taking thiazides is unusual, but a number of cases have been reported. Fishman et al. gave details of 25 cases taking a variety of thiazides, with serum sodium between 91 and 120 mmol/L.[477]

Carbonic Anhydrase Inhibitors
The carbonic anhydrase inhibitors acetazolamide and dichlorphenamide are little used for their weak diuretic action, but are used in reducing intraocular pressure. Hypokalemia is likely to be caused, in particular, in the elderly.[347]

Loop Diuretics
Powerful diuretics, such as frusemide, butmetamide, pitetanide, azosemide, and ethacrynic acid, act by inhibiting resorption from the ascending Loop of Henle in the renal tubule. Some reported changes are given in Table 74.

Potassium-Sparing Diuretics
Amiloride and triampterine are examples of potassium-sparing diuretics. Serum sodium is likely to fall, and serum potassium to rise, in patients given these drugs. Table 75 shows the findings of some workers.

TABLE 74.
Serum Sodium and Potassium Levels (mmol/L) after Loop Diuretics

Reference	Subjects	Na	K
478	122 men and 82 women mean age 69.8 on frusemide	50 of 204 hyponatremia	56 of 204 <3.9 5 of 204 <3.0 50 of 204 >5.0
475	Usual dose of frusemide		Mean fall 0.3
479	On frusemide		Mean fall 0.28 ± 0.11
	On bumetamide		Mean fall 0.24 ± 0.10
480	On azosemide	Mean fall 2	Fall 0.2–0.5

TABLE 75.
Serum Sodium and Potassium Levels (mmol/L) after Potassium-Sparing Diuretics

Reference	Subject and dose	Na		K	
481	Five healthy males given 75 mg of amiloride daily for 7 days	Mean fall from	141 to 131	Mean fall from	4.0 to 4.9
482	Thirteen male hypertensives given 5–10 mg of amiloride daily	Before After 3 weeks After 8 weeks	140 ± 0.5 138 ± 0.9 141 ± 0.9	4.2 ± 0.1 4.5 ± 0.1 4.4 ± 0.1	
483	Three cases admitted with epigastric pain being treated with 5 mg of amiloride and 50 mg of hydrochlorthiazide	107, 111, and 120		Low potassium in one case thought to be due to vomiting	

Hyperkalemia is a potential hazard of treatment with the aldosterone antagonist spironolactone. Two fatal cases from the early literature are quoted by Forland and Pullmin.[484] Greenblatt reported clinically important hyperkalemia in 68 of 788 (8.6%) patients taking spironolactone.[485] It was found in 20.3% of those with blood urea of more than 17 mmol/L and in 42.1% of those taking potassium supplements. Five healthy males ages 23 to 44 were given 300 mg daily for 7 days by Millar et al.,[486] who found that mean serum sodium fell from 138 to 134 mmol/L in the first 5 days and rose to 136 by the sixth day, and mean serum potassium increased from 4.0 to 4.4 mmol/L.

Other Diuretics

Clopamide acts similarly to thiazides, but does not have the diazine chemical structure. Wise et al. gave 22 patients 60 mg/day for 5 to 7 days[487] and found that mean serum potassium fell from 4.2 to 2.8 mmol/L if no potassium supplement was given, and from 4.3 to 3.8 mmol/L, with a potassium supplement. Jensen et al. described a single case with serum sodium of 150 mmol/L and serum potassium of 1.2 mmol/L, after 6 weeks of treatment.[488]

Indapamide is chemically related to chlorthalidone and is claimed to give less aggravation of diabetes than do other diuretics. Osei et al. reported a small fall in mean serum potassium from 4.1 to 3.8 mmol/L after giving 13 hypertensive diabetics up to 7.5 mg daily for 8 weeks.[489]

Metolazone is chemically a derivative of quinethazone and has diuretic properties similar to the thiazides. Pilewski et al.[490] found a mean serum sodium level of 137.2 and a mean serum potassium level of 3.26 mmol/L, in 21 hypertensive subjects given 5 mg daily for 4 weeks, compared with means of 140.2 and 3.93 for inpatients given a placebo.

Combination Diuretics

Diuretics containing both a thiazide and a potassium-sparing diuretic are used to aid

TABLE 76.

Serum Sodium and Potassium Levels in Patients Taking Combination Diuretics[a]

Subjects	Therapy	N	Na		K	
			<130 mmol/L	Mean	<3.0 mmol/L	Mean
197 consecutive new admissions (79 male, 118 female) taking diuretics as long term maintenance therapy for heart failure or hypertension	Thiazide alone	27	9 of 68	136 ± 4.2	2 of 27	Stated to be similar in all groups
	Thiazide and potassium supplement	41			4 of 41	
	Amiloride and hydrochlorthiazide	36	11 of 36	133.3 ± 5.1	3 of 36	
	Triampterene and hydrochlorthiazide	93	9 of 93	136.7 ± 4.8	4 of 93	

[a] From Bayer, A. J., et al., *Postgrad. Med. J.*, 62, 159, 1986.

compliance and to reduce the risk of hyperkalemia. Some patients taking the drugs have been found to develop hyponatremia or hypokalemia. Table 76 shows results of a study by Bayer et al.,[491] who concluded that a fixed-dose combination did not reduce the incidence of hypokalemia and that the combination amiloride-hydrochlorthiazide was associated with a higher proportion of cases of hyponatremia.

Danazol

Carlström et al.[492] reported a very small rise in mean serum potassium from 3.9 to 4.1 mmol/L in 18 women given 600 mg of danazol per day for 6 months as a treatment for endometriosis.

Dapsone

Single cases of patients with hyponatremia considered to be due to hypersensitivity to dapsone have been reported.[493,494] Serum sodium was 117 to 123 mmol/L.

Diazoxide

An antihypertensive agent with no diuretic action, diazoxide is a salt- and water-retaining thiazide. Changes in urine sodium and potassium were reported by Bartorelli[495] and Johnson,[496] but serum levels were not recorded.

Digitalis

Normal doses of digitalis do not produce changes, but doses of 20 (or more) times the therapeutic amount may produce hyperkalemia. Smith et al. found that 11 of 26 patients with digitalis poisoning (usually with a dose of 10 mg or more or caused by a long-term dosage error) had serum potassium in the range of 5.6 to 8.7 mmol/L.[497]

Heparin

Administration of heparin is known to interfere with aldosterone production and, potentially, could affect sodium and potassium levels in serum. Bailey and Ford found that these levels remained within "normal limits," after giving heparin to healthy subjects.[498] Single cases of hyperkalemia after heparin have been reported with potassium above 6 mmol/L.[499-501]

Heroin

Cases of hyperkalemia in patients unconscious following heroin abuse have been reported.[502,503] It is likely in these cases that hyperkalemia was due either to ischemic muscle injury or to contamination of street heroin with ergot.

Epinephrine

Early experiments by Silva, reported in 1934,[504] showed a transient rise in serum potassium, followed by a sustained decrease. Ponce et al. later stated that serum potassium increases by a maximum of 2 mmol/L within 1 min of an intravenous administration of epinephrine.[438] It falls to original levels within 4 min and then falls further.

Hypertonic Sodium Chloride

Both serum sodium and potassium increase when hypertonic sodium chloride is given intravenously. Moreno et al. gave healthy volunteers 1 L of 2.25% sodium chloride at a rate of 10 mL/min.[505] Mean serum sodium increased from 139 to 145 mmol/L, and mean potassium increased from 3.9 to 4.4 mmol/L.

Ketoconazole

The imidazole ketoconazole, used to treat fungal infections and given for advanced cancer of the prostate, inhibits adrenal steroidogenesis. Tractenburg and Pont found hypoadrenalism in 2 of 15 patients treated for prostatic carcinoma,[506] and White and Kendall-Taylor[507] found a blunted synacthen response and reduced urine free cortisol. Pillans et al. reported a serum sodium level of 121 mmol/L in a patient taking 600 mg for 2 1/2 months,[508] which returned to normal after 4 days of treatment.

Licorice and Carbenoxolone

Both carbenoxolone and its parent substance, licorice, have an aldosterone-like effect, and there are a number of reports of the production of severe hypokalemia.

The earliest reports[236,237] involve long-term treatment of tuberculosis with *p*-amino salicylic acid flavored with licorice to mask the unpleasant taste. Later cases had gastric ulcers treated with carbenoxolone.[238,239] There are some reports of hypokalemia in subjects eating large amounts of licorice for long periods.[240,241]

Lithium

Small changes in serum sodium and potassium levels have been found in patients given lithium salts. Murphy et al. found that sodium fell by a mean of 2 mmol/L on the 1st day of treatment with 1.2 to 1.8 g of lithium carbonate daily and then returned to predrug levels.[509] Coggins noted a significant increase in serum potassium during the first 3 months of treatment,[510] but levels remained within physiologic limits. A single case with potassium increasing from 4.6 to 5.7 mmol/L by the 4th week, and later with a level of 6.2, was reported.

Lactulose

The synthetic disaccharide lactulose, which is not absorbed from the gastrointestinal tract, is used in the treatment of hepatic encephalopathy. An osmotic diuresis is produced, and more water is lost from the bowel than sodium, which may lead to high serum sodium levels. Nelson et al.,[511] in a study of 75 admissions of 33 patients with hepatic failure treated with lactulose, found sodium of more than 145 mmol/L on 20 occasions. No correlation was found between serum sodium and the dose of lactulose.

Lorcainamide

Oral treatment with the antiarrhythmic drug lorcainamide causes a temporary decrease in serum sodium. Somani et al. gave oral treatments to 33 patients showing a good response to an intravenous dose.[512] The day after intravenous administration of 200 mg of lorcainamide, mean serum sodium was 138.5 mmol/L. After 6 days of oral treatment, mean sodium was 133.4, and after 6 months, it was 138.2 mmol/L. Sixteen patients developed significant hyponatremia during oral treatment, and in 14, serum sodium returned to normal within 3 to 12 months of continued therapy.

Mannitol

Serum sodium decreases, and potassium increases, in subjects given intravenous mannitol. Bucknell gave 500 mL of 10% mannitol, over a short period, to neurologic patients.[513] There was an increase in mean serum potassium after 1 h, and levels returned to normal after another hour. Six healthy volunteers were given 1 L of 12.5% mannitol at a rate of 10 mL/min, by Moreno et al.[505] Mean serum sodium fell from 140 to 127 mmol/L, and mean serum potassium increased from 4.0 to 4.7 mmol/L.

Methylfluorane

Crandell et al. found that a toxic nephropathy developed in 16 of 94 cases given methylfluorane,[514] with serum sodium in the range of 150 to 165 mmol/L.

Miconazole

Hyponatremia has been found in 40% of cases of the antifungal drug miconazole, with a mean decrease of 10 mmol/L.[515]

Nonsteroidal anti-inflammatory drugs (NSAIDs)

Over 20 NSAIDs are listed in the British National Formulary, and the most universal side effect is water and salt retention as a result of reduced renal plasma flow and enhanced tubular reabsorption of sodium. A decrease of the glomerular filtration rate and inhibition of the renin–angiotensin system may lead to hyperkalemia.

Ibuprofen

Clive et al. reported that sodium retention causes edema in 25% of arthritis patients taking ibuprofen.[516] A single case of lupus erythromatosis given 2.4 g of ibuprofen per day was described by Kimberley et al.[517] By the third day, serum potassium had increased from 4.7 to 6.1 mmol/L, and sodium had fallen from 142 to 130 mmol/L.

Indomethacin

There is an increase in serum potassium during treatment with indomethacin. Kutyrina et al.[518] found that the mean level of serum potassium in 30 patients with glomerulonephritis increased from 4.57 to 5.82 mmol/L (range of 5.3 to 6.7) during treatment. The mean level fell to 4.60 after treatment, Zimram et al.[519] investigated the increase in serum potassium in 50 patients, defined as the difference between the highest level found before and after indomethacin treatment had started. Levels in twenty patients increased less than 0.5 mmol/L, in seventeen levels increased between 0.5 and 0.9, and in thirteen levels increased 1.0 or more.

Preexisting azotemia and old age were associated with an increased risk of hyperkalemia. In six patients treatment was stopped, as potassium was above 6.0 mmol/L.

Only small increases in serum potassium were found in eight healthy volunteers given 150 mg of indomethacin daily for 4 days, by DeJong.[520] Mean serum potassium increased from 4.15 to 4.40 mmol/L on the 1st day and fell to 4.26 mmol/L by the final day.

Naproxen and Fenoprofen

A single case of lupus erythromatosis treated with naproxen, showing an increase in serum potassium from 3.8 to 4.3 mmol/L and a decrease in sodium from 137 to 129 mmol/L by the 10th day, was described by Kimberley et al.[517] Another case treated with fenoprofen showed an increase in potassium of from 3.7 to 4.2 mmol/L after 6 days, with no change in serum sodium.

TABLE 77.
Serum Sodium (mmol/L) Following Intravenous Oxytocin[a]

	Control group no i.v. treatment		Intravenous oxytocin		Intravenous glucose	
	N	Mean	N	Mean	N	Mean
Cord blood serum	52	135.0	45	131.4	43	132.6
Mothers' blood serum	52	135.4	45	132.5	43	133.3

[a] From Singhi, S., et al., *Br. J. Obstet. Gynaecol.*, 92, 356, 1985.

Piroxican

Several cases of hyperkalemia following piroxican therapy have been reported. Some[521,522] were also given other drugs that could have contributed to the findings, but Miller et al. described a case given 20 mg of piroxican daily, with no other drugs.[486] Serum potassium was 8.0 mmol/L after 7 months and 9.3 after 9 months, with serum sodium 135 mmol/L.

Oxytocin

A small decrease in the serum sodium of mother and of cord blood has been noted in subjects given an intravenous administration of oxytocin[523] (Table 77). The antidiuretic effect of oxytocin was considered to cause a dilutional effect.

Phenoxybenzamine

A single case of hyponatremia following administration of the alpha adrenogenic blocker phenoxybenzamine was described by Aron et al.[524] A dose of 10 mg was given daily for 5 days, and on the sixth day 2 L of water were given as part of a urodynamic study. Serum sodium was 95 mmol/L 24 h later. After discontinuing the drug and treatment, this increased to 132 mmol/L.

Potassium Salts

There is little change in serum potassium in subjects with good renal function, when small amounts of potassium are given orally,[525] but administration of single doses larger than 0.5 mEq/kg body weight usually produces a rise.[526] A dose of 1 mEq/kg of potassium increases serum potassium by up to 1 mEq/L, and 2 to 2.5 mEq/kg may give serum potassium levels of 6 to 8 mEq/L. Larger changes may occur in patients having difficulty with excretion. Shapiro et al. found five cases, among 6199 consecutive hospital admissions,[527] in whom taking potassium salts was considered to contribute to death. Causes were taking potassium citrate, taking a salt substitute, or taking potassium in a nutritional supplement.

Collins solution

Preservation of cadaver kidneys for transplantation uses Collins' solution, whose composition resembles that of intracellular fluid. After transplantation and release of vascular clamps, a bolus of Collins' solution may move to the right atrium. Soulillou et al.[528] found that seven of nine patients showed ECG changes indicative of hyperkalemia after renal transplantation, with a mean rise of serum potassium of 2.6 mmol/L (range of 0.4 to 5.1). Slower removal of vascular clamps resulted in a rise of only 1.2 to 1.6 mmol/L. It was pointed out that this was not the only possible cause of hyperkalemia after renal transplantation.

Transfusion of Stored Blood

Blood to be used for transfusions that has been stored for more than 10 days will have a plasma potassium level of 7 to 13 mmol/L. On transfusing the blood, the patient's serum potassium may increase by a mean of 1 mmol/L.[438] Problems with hyperkalemia following blood transfusion are uncommon, but there is some risk when large amounts are given.

Prolactin

Intramuscular administration of prolactin increases serum sodium, but has no effect on serum potassium. Horrobin et al. gave 8 mg of sheep prolactin intramuscularly to five fully hydrated adult males[529] and noted an increase in mean serum sodium of from 140.2 to 147.06 mmol/L. Injecting 1 mL water on a control day gave no change.

Sodium Sulfate

Occasionally, patients given sodium sulfate to treat hypercalcemia have increased serum sodium. Chakmakjian and Bethune found high levels in 2 of 13 patients, with a maximum of 160 mmol/L.[529a] Sherwood reported a case with serum sodium of 158 mmol/L,[530] and Heckman and Walsh reported a case with maximum serum sodium of 179 mmol/L.[531]

Somatostatin

Two cases developing water retention and hyponatremia after being given intravenous administration of somatostatin (250 μg/h) were reported by Halma et al.[532] In one patient, serum sodium was 113 mmol/L and potassium 3.4 mmol/L, and in the other, sodium was 127 mmol/L and potassium 5.0 mmol/L. The cause was considered to be inappropriate ADH secretion.

Streptozotocin

Murray-Lyon et al. described a patient with a malignant islet cell tumor and intractable hypoglycemia, who developed hypokalemia with serum potassium of 2.8 mmol/L, after treatment with streptozotocin.[533] They considered that a renal tubular defect was responsible for the loss of potassium.

Succinyl Choline

There are several reports of an increase in serum potassium a few minutes after giving succinyl choline as a muscle relaxant (Table 78). Greater increases have been found in patients with various traumatic conditions. Ponce et al. stated that dramatic hyperkalemic response can occur in patients with

1.   Spinal cord injury
2.   Head injury
3.   Peripheral and central nervous system disease
4.   Increased intracranial pressure
5.   Cerebral vascular accident
6.   Severe burns
7.   Encephalitis
8.   Severe intraabdominal infection
9.   Tetanus

Theophylline

There is a small fall in serum sodium and potassium levels in patients given intravenous theophylline. Zantvoort et al. gave 6 to 7 mg/kg body weight intravenously for 20 min to seven patients with severe chronic obstructive lung disease.[538] Mean serum sodium fell by 1.9 mmol/L in 8 h, and mean potassium fell by 0.3 mmol/L in the first hour and then rose.

TABLE 78.
Change in Serum Potassium After Succinyl Choline

Reference	Subjects	Effect (mmol/L)
534	6 patients given 40 mg of succinyl choline	Highest serum potassium after 3 min; mean increase 0.408
	11 patients given 100 mg of succinyl choline	Highest serum potassium after 7 min; mean increase 0.551
	27 patients 3 min after anesthesia; no succinyl choline	Mean increase 0.102
535	10 renal transplant patients; presurgery 5 min after succinyl choline	Mean increase 5.0 ± 0.71 Mean increase 5.2 ± 0.76
	10 other patients; presurgery 5 min after succinyl choline	Mean increase 3.7 ± 0.42 Mean increase 4.0 ± 0.42
536	Renal transplant patients after succinyl choline	Mean increase 0.45
	Other patients after succinyl choline	Mean increase 0.46
537	20 patients anesthetized; no succinyl choline	Little change in serum potassium
	63 patients with no trauma anesthetized + succinyl choline	Increase <1.0 in 63 of 63
	59 traumatized patients (burns, multiple fractures, etc.) anesthetized + succinyl choline	Increase >1.0 in 43 of 59 Increase >2.0 in 13 of 59 Increase >4.0 in 1 of 59

Vinchristine

Cases of hyponatremia in patients given vinchristine have been reported. Rothanthal and Kayfman reviewed seven cases, in the literature, with serum sodium in the range of 96 to 125 mmol/L.[539] Hyponatremia was thought to be due to the syndrome of inappropriate ADH secretion. A case of hyperkalemia due to rapid dissolution of malignant cells in a patient on chemotherapy including vinchristine was reported by Arseneau et al.,[471] with serum potassium of 6.0 mmol/L.

Chapter 6

ALKALINE PHOSPHATASE ACTIVITY

Alkaline phosphatases are a group of nonspecific phosphatases that hydrolyze various phosphoric esters at an alkaline pH. Chemically, they are glycoproteins, and three types of activity are known: hydrolytic, phosphotransferase, and pyrophosphatase.

Most tissues show alkaline phosphatase activity. The richest sources are osteoclasts in bone, bile caniculi in liver, the intestinal epithelium, proximal tubules in kidney, breast tissue during lactation, and placenta. Each tissue is associated with a different isoenzyme, with a different optimal pH. Alkaline phosphatase activity has been measured by many different methods that differ in substrate, buffer type, buffer concentration, temperature of incubation, and unit of measurement.[540] Magnesium, zinc, manganese, and cobalt are required for maximum activity, and an optimal Mg^{3+}/Zn^{2+} ratio is required, as zinc is essential for catalysis, but by binding to the magnesium site, zinc can also inhibit enzyme activity. Activity is inhibited by copper, mercury, and EDTA and by some amino acids such as phenyl alanine.

Activity of alkaline phosphatase in blood was first described by Martland et al.[541] and Lawaczeck[542] in 1924. Martland and Robison reported that the bone enzyme was inhibited by liberated phosphate,[543] but later Bodansky showed that inhibition by blood levels is negligible even when the patient is uremic.[544]

Kay demonstrated in 1930 that the enzyme is most active at an alkaline pH,[545] and although finding that the optimum pH in a glycine buffer was between 8.8 and 9.1, described a method using glycerophosphate as substrate at a pH of 7.5 to 7.6. Kay also noted that magnesium ions had a stimulating effect and that higher levels were found in children.

ANALYTIC CONSIDERATIONS

Methods of estimating serum alkaline phosphatase activity are reviewed in the monograph by McComb, Bowers, and Posen[546] and by McLaughlan.[540] A number of substrates have been used. Much of the early work in the United States used B-glycerophosphate as the substrate in a method introduced by Bodansky.[544] The procedure measured phosphate produced and had an additional advantage — the blank could be used to estimate inorganic phosphate. In the method of King and Armstrong,[547] disodium phenyl phosphate was used as a substrate for measuring phenol produced. This was widely used, particularly in the United Kingdom. A later variation using amino antipyrin as a color reagent[548] had the advantage that protein was not precipitated; it was later adapted for use on continuous-flow analyzers.

Many other substrates have been used, including naphthyl phosphate,[549] phenolphthalein diphosphate,[550] phenolphthalein monophosphate,[551] thymolphthalein phosphate,[552] and the phosphates of fluorescent compounds such as eosin and fluorescein.[553] A method using dinitrophenyl phosphate, which had a colored reaction product, was described in 1946 by Bessey, Lowry, and Brock.[554] The method was little used at first, as pure substrate was not readily available, but it is now almost universally recommended, as it has the advantage of being suitable for continuous monitoring of the reaction.

COMPARISON OF METHODS

A number of factors make comparison of the estimation of alkaline phosphatase activity by different methods difficult:

1. The nonspecificity leads to different activities with different substrates.

TABLE 79.
Range of Serum Alkaline Phosphatase Activity in Healthy Persons,
Using Different Methods[a]

Reference	Substrate	Unit/dL	IU/L
Bodansky	B-glycerophosphate	1.5–4.0	8–32
King–Armstrong	Diphenyl phosphate	3.5–13.0	21–92
Bessey–Lowry–Brock	Dinitrophenyl phosphate	0.3–2.7	14–50
German Soc. recomm.	Dinitrophenyl phosphate		30–170
Scand. Soc. recomm.	Dinitrophenyl phosphate		70–390
Am. Assoc. recomm.	Dinitrophenyl phosphate		6–110

[a] From Posen, S. and Doherty, E., *Adv. Clin. Chem.*, 22, 163, 1981. With permission.

2. Optimal pH is usually in the range of 10.0 to 10.5, but it may vary with the buffer, substrate concentration, incubation temperature, and the tissue source of the enzyme.
3. The activity of different isoenzymes may vary.
4. The reaction products may have different color intensities.
5. The reaction rate is increased by transphosphorylation buffers.

As a result, the use of conversion factors for comparison is not usually appropriate. In an attempt to compare results from different workers, recommended methods have been suggested. One group proposed a method based on the King–Armstrong procedure[555] that reflected the practice in the majority of laboratories in the United Kingdom at the time.

Most recommendations have been based on the use of dinitrophenyl phosphate as substrate.[556-562] The conditions are suitable for continuous monitoring of the reaction, and as the substrate is less affected by intestinal enzymes, the results are more sensitive to changes in the clinically significant bone and liver isoenzymes. Differences remain,[562] as shown in Table 79. These are expected in methods using different substrates, but are present even in methods using the same substrate. The different reaction conditions for recommended methods that use dinitrophenyl phosphate as substrate are shown in Table 80, and differences can be seen to be due to the use of varying buffers and reaction temperatures.

COMPARISON OF RESULTS BY DIFFERENT METHODS

It is difficult to compare results of serum alkaline phosphatase activity from different studies. Several groups have attempted to obtain factors to convert the results, but the general view is that the use of such factors is unreliable. Tietz et al. compared analyses by the Bodansky and the Bessey–Lowry–Brock methods and concluded that it was not permissible to use a conversion factor,[563] as 15 of 135 sera (70 considered to have normal activity) gave normal results with one method and abnormal results with the other.

Penittilä et al.[564] found that, on average, 4.73 × Bessey–Lowry–Brock unit/L gave the level by the recommended Scandinavian method, but that the range for the conversion factor was 4.1 to 6.0, depending on the isoenzyme composition.

Use of the upper range limit (URL), discussed earlier, is probably the procedure to use, despite its imperfections, if comparisons are required.

ACCURACY AND PRECISION

The mean between-batch cv for estimation by manual methods is reported to be about 5% by several groups.[546,559,565] Precision for automatic methods is probably about the same. Sterling et al.[566] reported a between-batch cv of 6% for a King and Kind method adapted for use on a continuous-flow analyzer, and Lohff et al.[567] reported a cv of less than 5% for within-laboratory precision at three different levels of accuracy.

TABLE 80.

Reaction Conditions for Various Recommended Methods of Estimation of Serum Alkaline Phosphatase Activity

	AACC[605] 1975	AACC[607] 1982	Scand. Soc.[604] 1974	Germ. Soc.[603] 1972	IFCC[606] 1983
Temperature	30°C	30°C	37°C	25°C	30°C
pH	10.30	10.5	9.80	9.80	10.40
Buffer molarity	2A 2M 1P[a]	2A 2M 1P	Diethanolamine	Diethanolamine	2A 2M 1P
	0.80	1	1	1	0.35
Magnesium molarity	0.100	1	0.5	0.5	2
Zinc molarity					1
					HEDTA[c] 2 mmol/L
DNP[b] molarity	15	16	10	10	16
Wavelength	402.5	402	405	405	405

[a] 2A 2M 1P = 2-amino 2-methyl 1-propanol.
[b] DNP = dinitrophenyl phosphate.
[c] HEDTA = *N*-(2hydroxyethyl) ethylene diamine triacetic acid.

Between-laboratory comparisons are much greater due to method differences. Cvs of 17 to 20% have been suggested for manual methods,[568,569] but use of standardized methods could improve this figure.

INTERFERENCE WITH ANALYSIS

HEMOLYSIS

The effect of hemolysis on the estimation of alkaline phosphatase activity varies according to the method used. Sterling et al.[566] and Brydon and Roberts[292] found no significant interference with up to 10 g/L of hemoglobin in serum, using a continuous-flow method. Proksch et al. found only a minimal increase caused by hemolysis, using a thymolphthalein phosphate method.[568] Methods using spectrophotometric measurements may have problems caused by high absorbance blanks.

Hemolysates were found to give an apparent reduction in alkaline phosphatase activity using dinitrophenyl phosphate as substrate, which varied according to the buffer used.[569a] The fall was shown not to be due to dialyzable substances and was probably due to hemoglobin. Using ethanolamine buffer, a sample blank almost compensated for the apparent reduction in enzyme activity, whereas using amino methyl propanol, amino methyl propanediol, or a tris/carbonate buffer, a serum blank had a minimal compensating effect. The fall in alkaline phosphatase activity caused by hemolysis was 2 to 30%, depending on the buffer and the enzyme level, with higher enzyme levels giving a lower-percentage reduction.

THEOPHYLLINE

A dose of 20 mg/L of theophylline added to serum has been found to decrease alkaline phosphatase activity by almost 10% when estimated using a dinitrophenyl phosphate method on a Technicon SMAC analyzer,[570] This concentration of the drug was considered to be within the therapeutic range. Caffeine did not affect the enzyme activity. The effect of theophylline varied with the isoenzyme and was much less with placental enzyme. It was suggested that theophylline might be acting as an enzyme inhibitor.

PENICILLAMINE

D-Penicillamine added to serum (in the concentration range found in patients under treatment with 2 to 6 g/day) reduces the apparent alkaline phosphatase activity by more than 50%.[571] It is possible that activators, particularly metals, are bound.

PREANALYTIC ERROR

COLLECTION OF THE SPECIMEN

Most laboratories estimate alkaline phosphatase activity, using serum. Heparinized plasma is probably satisfactory, but other anticoagulants affect the assay.

The use of heparinized tubes containing a polyester gel separator was investigated by Bailey,[572] who found a small difference compared with serum (difference between means of 1.14 IU/L), but poor correlation, with a range from 24 IU/L lower to 19 IU/L higher. The author states that the mechanism for poor correlation remains to be proven, but does not comment on any possible contribution by the increase on storage.

ANTICOAGULANTS

Heparin

Although Lum and Gambino found that alkaline phosphatase activity in heparinized plasma was a little less than in serum,[391] a number of other groups have not confirmed this.[544,573,574] Tietz et al.,[575] proposing an official AACC reference method, concluded that there was no significant difference between the results obtained using serum and heparinized plasma.

EDTA

A concentration of 50 mmol of EDTA completely inhibits alkaline phosphatase activity in serum.[556]

Citrate

In the absence of magnesium, citrate inhibits alkaline phosphatase activity. A dose of 25 mmol of citrate inhibits activity by 50%.[556] Using enzyme from rat intestine, Evered and Stevenson found that relatively high concentrations of magnesium eliminate the inhibition,[576] they considered that this was due to chelation of magnesium and citrate.

Oxalate

Bodansky, in 1933,[544] found that alkaline phosphatase activity in plasma from oxalated specimens was about 90% of that in the corresponding serum. He considered that this was due to dilution by a shift of water from cells, by an osmotic effect. This was confirmed by Belfanti et al.[577] using tissue extracts, and it was noted that as phosphate was produced, inhibition was reduced, and that inhibition of activity was prevented by addition of phosphate before analysis.

VENOUS STASIS

Because enzymes are proteins, venous stasis would be expected to increase serum protein. Although Henny and Schiele stated that there is no such effect,[578] Statland et al. found a mean increase in serum alkaline phosphatase activity of 3.4% when applying pressure with a tourniquet on healthy subjects for 3 min.[38] It is desirable to use minimum restriction of the veins when collecting blood samples.

CONTAMINATION

Some substrates have been reported to be contaminated with impurities that inhibit the enzyme reaction. Disodium phenyl phosphate has been found to be contaminated with orthophosphate, which inhibits the enzyme.[546,579] Some preparations of dinitrophenyl phosphate have been found to contain impurities affecting the assay. Bowers et al. found that of 16 lots from 10 suppliers, only 6 met acceptable specifications;[574] the same group later described the specification for high-purity dinitrophenyl phosphate.[580] Some lots obtained commercially that did not meet the specification could be purified by crystallization or sublimation. Detergent left as a

TABLE 81.
Stability of Alkaline Phosphatase in Serum and Reconstituted Lyophilized Serum

Reference	Sample	Stability
582	Serum	Increase up to 20% after 24 h of refrigeration
583	Serum	4% increase after 96 h of refrigeration
584	Serum	3–10% increase after several hours at room temp.
585	Serum	6% increase after 96 h at 25°C
586	Serum	8% increase in 24 h of standing on clot
587	Serum deep frozen and thawed	Alkaline phosphatase extracted from liver added to pooled serum frozen and thawed. After 24 h at 25°C, 20–30% increase. After 48 h at 25°C, further 5% increase
585	Pooled serum frozen and thawed	Increase of 1%
588	Reconstituted lyophilized serum	Increase of up to 60% in 7 h with commercial sera
589, 590	12 commercial reference sera from six manufacturers	After reconstitution kept at 25°C, 130–200% increase within 24 h. Kept at 4°C, less than 15% increase within 24 h. Frozen no change. Lyophilization caused a reduction in activity; restored by 98 h after reconstitution

contaminant on washed glassware can affect the estimation of alkaline phosphatase activity. The activity is inhibited 17 to 24% by 0.6 to 0.8 mg/mL of detergent.[581]

SAMPLE STABILITY

Bodansky, in 1932, reported a rise in serum alkaline phosphatase activity of up to 20% following refrigeration for 24 h.[582] However, little notice was taken of this and other similar reports until the introduction of analyzers requiring calibration by serum-based standards caused renewed interest in the matter. Table 81 shows the findings in various reports. A greater increase was found in serum thawed after deep freezing and in reconstituted serum.

Bowers and McComb,[559] suggesting a reference procedure, concluded that the increase in alkaline phosphatase activity in freshly drawn blood kept at room temperature for less than 4 h was probably a maximum of 1 to 2%.

Szaaz considered that the changes in reconstituted lyophilized control sera depended on the pH after reconstitution,[589,590] and he found that the activity on reconstitution was not increased if the pH was decreased to less than 5.8.

Deep freezing sera for long periods can lead to a loss in activity. Henny and Schiele found a loss of activity of 5.5% in serum frozen at −30°C for 1 month,[578] and a further 20% decrease after 1 year. The changes in sample and standard must be considered when assaying alkaline phosphatase, and appropriate procedures must be adopted to minimize the errors.

Heating to 56°C

Several groups have shown that heating serum or plasma to 56°C for 30 min to minimize the risk from HIV samples decreases alkaline phosphatase activity. Goldie found a mean fall of 38.5%, using serum,[101] and Ball, a mean fall of 88.5%, using plasma.[312] Ball suggested treating with B-propionolactone as an alternative,[312] as this gave no significant change in alkaline phosphatase activity.

PHYSIOLOGIC CHANGES

POSTURE

There is a decrease in serum alkaline phosphatase activity of about 10% in supine subjects compared with upright subjects, as would be expected. Statland et al. found a mean 6.1% increase in serum from healthy subjects lying down for 30 min compared with the level after patients sat for 30 min,[405] and a mean increase of 4.6% after patients stood for 30 min, giving a mean difference between lying down and standing of almost 11%. This was confirmed in experiments on healthy medical students by Dixon and Paterson,[591] who found an average difference of over 10% between lying down and standing subjects.

MEALS

No change in serum alkaline phosphatase activity after meals was found by Statland et al.,[592] but other groups have reported increases after a fatty meal. Table 82 shows changes found by workers using diphenyl phosphate as a substrate, with different increases according to blood group. Increases are not found when dinitrophenyl phosphate is used as a substrate, as it is less readily hydrolyzed by intestinal enzymes. These findings support the use of dinitrophenyl phosphate as a substrate, as it is less affected by changes in alkaline phosphatase after meals.

DIET

Alkaline phosphatase activity in serum is higher if dietary carbohydrate is taken as sucrose than if it is taken as starch. Irwin and Staton studied ten healthy young men and nine healthy young women taking a normal diet,[596] except that in one group, 84% of the carbohydrate was taken as sucrose, and in the other, the same proportion was taken as wheat starch. Using a method similar to that of Bessey–Lowry–Brock, mean serum alkaline phosphatase activity was 1.57 units per milliliter for men and 0.77 units per 100 mL for women on the sucrose diet, and 1.37 units per 100 mL for men and 0.69 units per 100 mL for women on the wheat starch diet. No explanation was offered for the difference found.

IMMOBILIZATION AND BED REST

Prolonged bed rest has little effect on serum alkaline phosphatase activity, but there may be increased levels during the post bed rest period. Hully et al. subjected five healthy male volunteers to continuous bed rest for 24 to 30 weeks, preceded by a 5-week baseline period, and followed by an 8-week post bed rest period.[117] There was no change using an "automated Bodansky" procedure during the bed rest, but increased levels were found in four of the five subjects during the post bed rest period.

EXERCISE

Exercise can cause an increase in serum alkaline phosphatase activity. Riley found a mean rise of 25% after a marathon run.[317] Galteau and Siest found that moderate exercise increases activity by 2 to 5%,[120] but gave no further details.

King et al. found that normal sports activity did not affect the level,[597] and Statland et al. also reported that mild exertion had no effect.[404] It seems unlikely that the modest activity involved in traveling to a clinic would affect levels significantly.

RANGE IN HEALTHY SUBJECTS

WITHIN- AND BETWEEN-PERSON VARIATION

The difficulties of comparing results by different methods have been discussed. As it is unsatisfactory to use conversion factors, reports of the range given by various groups will be given as in the original publications.

The earliest reports of serum alkaline phosphatase activity in healthy subjects did not report differences between males and females,[547,598] although Bodansky and Jaffe gave the mean for 18 men of 2.7 Bodansky units per 100 mL, and for seven women, of 2.3 Bodansky units per 100 mL, without comment.[599] Later workers have consistently reported higher levels in males

TABLE 82.
Changes in Serum Alkaline Phosphatase Activity after a Fatty Meal, Showing Differences with Blood Group and Method

Reference	Method	Time of collection	Blood group	Mean increase (KA unit per 100 mL)	Mean different methods IU/L	
					Phenyl phosphate method	Dinitrophenol phosphate method
593	8.9 g cream per kg body weight given	5 h after		2.32		
	Skim milk or dextrose given	5 h after		Range up to 40% increase No increase		
594	Fatty breakfast given to healthy male students	Fasting	O and B	2.20		
		4.5 h after	AB	2.00		
		7.5 h after	A	0.80		
			nonsecretors	0.55		
595	Nonfat meal	4 h after	A nonsecretors	−0.15		
			A secretors	+0.16		
			O nonsecretors	+0.23		
			O secretors	−0.63		
	Fatty meal	4 h after	A nonsecretors	−0.07		
			A secretors	−0.16		
			O nonsecretors	+0.32		
			O secretors	+1.55		
592	Eleven healthy young men	Day 1				
		Fasting 11.00			49.5	143.0
		Fasting 14.00			48.9	141.8
		Day 2				
		Fasting 11.00			48.9	147.0
		Meal 12.00				
		Sample 14.00			54.4	143.0

than in females.[140,142,413,600] The distribution of values is skewed toward the lower levels[600] and is close to log normal.[413] Increases with age have been reported and can be summed up by the comments of Roberts,[412] who wrote, "examination of the alkaline phosphatase/age scattergram of our figures demonstrates no obvious regression between the ages of 20 and 50 years. After 50 years the alkaline phosphatase values increase progressively." These findings are confirmed in a number of large surveys, as shown in Tables 83 and 84. The work of McPherson et al.[142] confirmed by results from the author's laboratory, suggests that the higher levels found in adolescence do not fall to adult levels until the age of almost 25 years in males. Levels begin to rise at the age of about 55 in both men and women.

In most studies the highest level observed in a group of healthy subjects exceeds the lowest by at least three times, but in individuals, remarkable consistency has been found over long periods. McComb et al. reported analyses over a period of 8 years on samples taken from one of the authors.[546] Thirty observations were made with specimens taken under standard conditions. The subject was fasting, in good health, and had sat for 15 min prior to venipuncture. A range of 41 to 51 units per liter was found, with a mean of 45.8 and a SD of 2.7. Another subject had 20 observations over a year, with little attention paid to standardizing the conditions, and again, low variability was found, with a mean level of 27.6 units per liter and a SD of 2.4.

THE ELDERLY

Most studies suggest that there is an increase in serum alkaline phosphatase activity from the age of 50 or 55 years (Tables 83 and 84). The extent that the changes are due to the presence of occult disease, rather than to genuine change with age, is not clear. Several groups have found that levels are from 50 to 100% higher in the elderly than in younger subjects (Table 85). However, when Hodkinson and McPherson excluded diagnostic categories expected to give higher-than-average levels,[604] including bone trauma within 6 months, malignant secondaries, Paget's disease, rheumatoid arthritis, liver disease, osteomalacia, skin ulceration over bone, gastric surgery, and osteoarthritis; the range in the remaining patients was only a little higher than in those in younger age groups, at 3.8 to 13.8 KA units per 100 mL in 97 males and 3.5 to 14.9 in 162 females. A lack of correlation with serum calcium, urea, phosphate, albumin, or globulin was considered to support the view that patients with osteomalacia had been successfully eliminated.

EFFECT OF MENOPAUSE

Serum alkaline phosphatase activity increases in women from about age 45 (Table 86). This is due to menopause, as shown by Henny and Schiele,[578] who found a range of 25 to 95 IU/L (mean 48) in menstruating women 40 to 55 years old, compared with a range of 31 to 126 IU/L (mean 62) in women of the same age who had ceased to menstruate. McPherson et al. found that the difference between males and females ceased after menopause.[142]

CHILDHOOD

Levels of serum alkaline phosphatase activity remain higher than those in adults, from the age of 1 year until after puberty. Tables 89 and 90 show the ranges found at different ages by various workers. Pubertal changes are less apparent in girls and occur several years earlier than in boys. Levels in girls fall to approximately adult levels at the age of approximately 16 to 17 years, whereas in boys, adult levels are not reached until over the age of 20 (Tables 87 and 88). Better correlation may be shown with a sexual maturity rating than with age.[605] Others have found a general parallel with growth rate[607] or with skeletal age[608] (Table 89).

In some healthy subjects there is a large rise in serum alkaline phosphatase activity during childhood, especially during the natural growth spurt. Levels of up to 7 × URL (adults) have been observed in some children, by McComb et al.[546] Stevens and Stevenson reported several

TABLE 83.
Serum Alkaline Phosphatase Activity in Healthy Men

Reference		<20	21–25	26–30	31–35	36–40	41–45	46–50	51–55	56–60	61–65	66–70	71–79	Method and units
140	Range			18.51–73.99	19.18–75.34		19.87–76.70		20.58–78.08			21.29–79.47	22.02–80–87	IU/L
141	Mean			9.42	9.50		9.79		9.98			10.21	8.64	KA units per 100 mL
142	Mean	48.3		42.6		42.4		45.3		49.0				King–Kind method in IU/L
601	N	149	101		178		132	137		103		93	40	IU/L
	Mean	102	62		58		63	68		70		74	80	
	Range	48–182	33–102		35–109		36–122	39–139		37–159		36–161	52–227	
578	N	75			18		152	129		69				French Society-recommended method at 30°C
	Mean	80			60		60	65		65				
	Range	50–160			35–105		35–105	35–100		40–100				
Coventry	N	62	134	152	106	114	92	64	70	40	18			Scandinavian Society-recommended conditions
	Mean	210	190	165	158	157	155	152	155	166	188			
	Range	112–315	97–312	98–282	97–260	90–280	95–290	90–286	92–290	95–	100–325			

TABLE 84.
Serum Alkaline Phosphatase Activity in Healthy Women

Reference		Age (years)												Method and units
		<20	21–25	26–30	31–35	36–40	41–45	46–50	51–55	56–60	61–65	66–70	71–79	
140	Range		12.21–62.77		13.95–66.66		15.82–70.67		17.80–74.79		19.90–79.04		22.12–83.40	IU/L
141	Mean		7.28		7.11		7.75		9.87		10.66		10.51	KA units per 100 mL
142	Mean	37.5		35.9		37.2		43.3			50.4			King–Kind method in IU/L
601	N	156	119	211		164		188		129		105	43	IU/L
	Mean	60	47	48		49		60		72		78	79	
	Range	29–176	26–98	25–100		30–80		34–121		31–132		38–172	49–199	
578	N	99		148		104		130			78			French-recommended method at 30°C
	Mean	55		50		45		65			75			
	Range	35–85		30–90		30–80		45–105			45–145			
Coventry	N	242	209	188	158	176	172	128	84	38				Scandinavian Society-recommended conditions
	Mean	144	132	123	132	127	135	143	171	172				
	Range	80–220	70–220	70–200	70–220	80–210	80–220	70–270	100–250	120–270				

TABLE 85.
Serum Alkaline Phosphatase Activity in Elderly Subjects

Reference	Subjects	Age (years)	Male			Female		
			N	Mean	Range	N	Mean	Range
602	Subjects living in north London. Mobile and free from disease known to raise alkaline phosphatase. Phenolphthalein phosphate method expressed as King–Armstrong units.	65–99	65	9.2	4–30 Omitting highest 4–18	156	9.9	4–33 Omitting highest 4–22
166	Subjects living at home excluding those taking diazepines or diuretics. King–Armstrong method	64–74 74+	300	10.0 10.6	5–20 6–20		11.0 12.5	6–21 5–20
603	25 women aged 61–87 years					25	Mean 50% higher than mean of 34 healthy men aged 21–30 years; Increase considered due to liver isoenzyme	
591	91.5% of admissions to a geriatric unit over 15 months King–Armstrong method	Over 60	384	2.8–28.8		209	2.6–30.3	

TABLE 86.
Change in Mean Serum Alkaline Phosphatase Activity
with Natural and Artificial Menopause[a] (in IU/L)

Age (years)	Premenopause	Post-natural menopause	Posthysterectomy
18–25	37.5		
26–35	35.9		
36–45	36.4	39.2	41.4
46–55		45.5	43.4

[a] From McPherson, K., et al., *Clin. Chim. Acta,* 84, 373, 1978.

cases with levels of more than 100 KA units per deciliter.[609] A transient hyperphosphatasemia of infancy has also been reported.

Posen et al. reported five infants with levels more than $20 \times$ URL (adults)[610] and reviewed 11 previously reported cases. Heat-activation studies suggested a skeletal origin for the increase. Wieme described 11 similar children[611] and, by studies on agar and starch gel, showed that the increase in enzyme activity originated in both liver and bone, but noted an unexplained difference in mobility, on agar. Rosalki and Foo investigated four cases and found no evidence of bone or liver disease.[612] They postulated that the cause was a response to a viral infection of the alimentary tract, which might lead to Chrohn's disease, but they could not support this theory with animal experiments. The same authors later showed that the increase was due to an abnormally sialyated enzyme,[613] probably of hepatic origin and of unknown cause.

In most cases the abnormal levels return to normal for age, within about 2 months of diagnosis.

TABLE 87.
Serum Alkaline Phosphatase Activity in Boys

Reference		½–2	2–3	4–5	6	7	8	9	10	11	12	13	14	15	16	17	18	Adult	Method and units
325	Mean					16.8	15.9	16.6	16.1	16.4	18.1	19.3	18.5	14.1	11.8	9.1			KA units per 100 mL
	Range					11–26	10–25	11–30	16–25	12–29	11–31	12–32	10–33	7–27	5–27	4–21			
564	Mean	605.4	476.2	489.2	549.7	549.7	485.3	485.3	466.3	466.3	552.6	552.6	529.7	529.7	303.1	303.1	303.1	107.5	Scandinavian Society-recommended method
	Range	250–1000	250–1000	250–1000	250–1000	250–1000	250–750	250–750	200–730	200–730	275–875	275–875	170–970	170–970	125–720	125–270	125–270	50–200	
605	Mean								76	79	99	100	102	103	75	64	42		Phenolphthalein method
	Range								58–110	55–105	55–207	49–240	36–192	41–195	32–142	21–228	23–63		
606	Range				340–570	340–620	340–670	340–720	340–820	380–1100	380–1100	450–1100	480–1100	210–830	210–660	120–500	120–350		AACC-selected method
172	Mean									440	440	510	410	350	240	180			Scandinavian Society-recommended method

TABLE 88.
Serum Alkaline Phosphatase Activity in Girls

Reference		½–2	2–3	4–5	6	7	8	9	10	11	12	13	14	15	16	17	18	Adult	Method and units
325	Mean					18.1	15.5	17.0	17.1	17.1	17.9	14.6	9.1	7.4	6.3	6.3			KA units per 100 mL
	Range					12–27	11–23	11–26	10–28	10–27	11–30	7–29	5–16	3–18	4–10	4–10			
564	Mean	647.3	500.3	463.8	564.4	564.4	486.7	486.7	572.9	572.9	458.2	458.2	249.9	249.9	151.0	151.0	151.0	107.5	Scandinavian Society-recommended method
	Range	205–1000	250–850	250–850	250–1000	250–1000	250–750	250–750	250–950	250–950	200–730	200–730	170–460	170–460	75–270	75–270	75–270		
605	Mean						84	90	90	103	91	78	52	38	31	28	21		Phenolphthalein method
	Range						59–102	49–136	51–118	72–147	65–148	25–144	22–91	17–91	13–56	16–46	18–24		
606	Range				340–620	340–670	340–720	340–770	340–820	340–880	340–900	240–900	180–590	130–250	120–250	100–220	100–220		AACC-selected method
172	Mean									470	450	360	200	170	120	100			Scandinavian Society-recommended method

TABLE 89.
Serum Alkaline Phosphatase Activity in Children, According to Sexual Maturity Rating and Skeletal Age

Reference			Sexual maturity rating									
			1		**2**		**3**		**4**		**5 (adult)**		
			Mean	Range	Mean	Range	Mean	Range	Mean	Range	Mean	Range	
605	Boys	White	72	54–110	77	42–106	101	53–141	95	41–158	58	21–120	Babson method
		Black	77		94	53–204	122	46–240	116	32–228	75	23–228	
	Girls	White	70	51–90	89	49–134	76	36–108	33	16–60	38	23–76	
		Black	84	69–108	95	65–138	86	26–148	34	18–144	31	13–70	

Reference		Skeletal age (years)									
		8–9.9	10–10.9	11–11.9	12–12.9	13–13.9	14–14.9	15–15.9	16–16.9	Adult	
608	Girls										Bessey–Lowry–Brock method
	Mean	4.59	4.61	5.85	5.47	4.92	3.03	2.45	2.70	1.93	

Reference			Mean	Range	
578	Girls	Age 10–15 years			French-recommended method at 30°C
		Not menstruating	223	72–384	
		Menstruating	120	61–251	

TABLE 90.
Serum Alkaline Phosphatase Activity in First Year of Life

Age (days)	Mean[a] (Bodansky units per 100 mL)	Mean[b] (KA units per 100 mL)	Range (KA units per 100 mL)	Day	Male mean[c] (KA units per 100 mL)	Female mean (KA units per 100 mL)	Mean[d] (KA units per 100 mL)	Range (KA units per 100 mL)	Adult range
1	⎫	8.355							
2	⎬ 7.1	8.014							
3	⎭	7.426	⎫ 5–19				813	3.5–14	7–15
4		7.021	⎪						
5		6.945	⎪						
6		7.424	⎭						
3–15	8.9								
(months)									
0.5–1.5	10.4	17.58		28	22	19			
1.5–2.5	11.9	16.77	12–20	56	21	17			
2.5–3.5	12.1	13.95		84	21	17			
3.5–4.5	11.6	⎫		112	18	17			
4.5–5.5	13.0	⎬ 15.647							
5.5–6.5	11.4	⎭							
6.5–7.5	12.3								
7.5–8.5	9.9								
8.5–9.5	11.6								
9.5–10.5	10.8								
10.5–11.5	11.8								
11.5–12.5	11.5								

[a]   From Barnes, D. I. and Munks, B., *Proc. Soc. Exp. Biol. Med.*, 44, 327, 1940.
[b]   From van Sydow, G., *Acta Paediatr.*, 33 (Suppl. 2), 17, 1946.
[c]   From Fomen, S. Jr., et al., *Acta Paediatr.*, 202 (Suppl.), 1, 1970.
[d]   From Izquierdo, J. M., et al., *Clin. Chim. Acta*, 30, 343, 1970.

TABLE 91.
Mean Serum Alkaline Phosphatase Activity in Preterm Babies[a]
(in King–Armstrong units per 100 mL)

Age (days)	Human milk mean	Human milk + vit. D mean	Cow milk mean
1–3	12.5		12.6
4–6	12.0		13.4
7–15	17.7		22.7
16–45	32.4		24.8
46–75	33.0		
76–105	29.8		
31–105		29.4	

[a] From van Sydow, G. A., *Acta Paediatr.*, 33 (Suppl. 2), 17, 1946.

NEONATES AND INFANTS

Changes in serum alkaline phosphatase activity during the first months of life are described by the earliest workers on the subject. In 1933 Stearns and Warweg reported that levels increased from near-adult levels at birth to a maximum during the first month of life and that this peak was maintained for only a short time.[598] There was a fall during the second or third month of life, followed by a gradual decline during the remainder of the first year of life, although the level remained higher than that found in adults. This pattern was confirmed by a number of later workers[614,615,616,618] (Table 90). Sydow found higher levels in preterm babies than in full-term babies, and in babies fed on breast milk than in those taking cow milk (Table 91).[618] The supplementation of feeds with vitamin D did not significantly alter the enzyme activity.

DeBaare et al. found higher levels in black babies than in white babies, during the first days of life.[181] At 36 h after birth, the mean level in black babies was 66.2 μ/L compared with a mean level of 46.7 in white babies.

CORD BLOOD

Most reports of serum alkaline phosphatase activity in cord blood give levels about twice that in healthy adults. Similar levels have been found in cord blood from full-term and preterm babies.

Reference	Method	Range	Adult
617	Bodansky	2.9–7.9	1.4–4.0 μ/dL
619	King Armstrong	7–28	3–13 μ/dL
620	Scand. Soc. rec.	108–420	70–390 IU/L
621	AACC rec.	32–245	6–110 IU/L
622	King Armstrong		
	Full-term	Mean 12.3	
	Preterm	11.9	

The source of the increased level has not been identified, but may be derived from the high placental level.

RANGE DURING PREGNANCY

An increase in serum alkaline phosphatase during pregnancy was recognized by Coryn in 1934,[623] who investigated a single patient with a normal pregnancy. The increase is mainly during the third trimester, with maximum levels at term (Table 92). An enzyme fraction stable at 65°C, originating from the placenta and representing 40 to 60% of the alkaline phosphatase

TABLE 92.
Serum Alkaline Phosphatase Activity During Pregnancy

Reference	Method	N	Gestation (weeks)	Mean	Range
624	Analysis by	231	12	1.42	0.91–2.06
	Bessey–Lowry–Brock		16	1.51	0.94–2.55
	method		20	1.40	0.90–2.37
	(unit/100 mL)		24	1.66	1.00–3.40
			28	1.76	1.05–3.12
			32	2.30	1.04–3.58
			36	3.09	1.47–5.48
			40	3.67	1.65–5.75
			Post partum		
			4	2.31	1.22–4.78
			13	1.80	0.55–3.22
			26	1.69	1.07–2.40
			39	1.78	1.24–2.56
625	Analysis by		1st trimester	7.30	
	King–Armstrong		2nd	12.30	
	method		3rd	19.40	
			Female nonpreg.	7.10	
			Male	10.10	

activity, is responsible for the increase.[625,626] The apparent increase varies with the substrate and is greater with B-glycerophosphate than with *p*-nitrophenyl phosphate.

Fishman et al. claim[627] that the presence of the placental isoenzyme can be detected about 4 to 6 weeks after conception in mothers with blood group O, and 6 to 12 weeks after conception in other mothers. Later, in a discussion, Fishman said that enzyme activity is higher at term in mothers with blood group O than in other mothers,[628] that primipara showed higher levels at term than multipara, and that levels in the latter often fall immediately before delivery. The biologic half-life of the placental isoenzyme is about 7 days, and according to Vermehren,[629] levels return to the prepregnancy range about 3 to 4 weeks after delivery, in nonlactating subjects. However, the figures from Beck and Clark (Table 91) suggest that prepregnancy levels are not reached for several months,[624] and Young et al. found a mean level of 7.6 KA units per deciliter 12 months after delivery,[630] compared with a mean of 4.4 during the first 24 weeks of pregnancy. Some workers have found slightly higher levels in lactating women than in those not lactating;[618,630] this could explain some of the differences found.

Ebbs and Scott reported higher serum alkaline phosphatase activity in mothers carrying twins.[631] Although the level was usually within the range of 4 to 9 KA units per deciliter, four cases were quoted with levels in the range of 11.0 to 15.7 units per deciliter. The findings could be due to the larger placenta, as could the finding of Beck and Clark[676] of higher levels in mothers carrying boys than in those carrying girls.

OTHER CHANGES

ALBUMIN INFUSION

Very high serum alkaline phosphatase activity has been found in patients given some commercial albumin products. Neale et al. reported increases up to and over 500 KA units per deciliter in patients infused with one albumin preparation believed to be placental in origin.[632] Bark confirmed that albumin of placental origin gave this effect[633] and noted levels rising from pretreatment levels of 5 Bodansky units per deciliter to 160 units per deciliter on the thirteenth day.

BLOOD GROUPS

Subjects with different blood groups have been found to have different mean serum alkaline phosphatase activities. Bamford et al., using the Bessey–Lowry–Brock method,[634] found higher levels in blood group O and B subjects than in those with blood group A and in those that were Le(a⁻), mainly ABH secretors.

	Mean	unit/dL
Group	**Le(a⁻)**	**Le(a⁺)**
O	7.67	6.90
B	7.70	6.02
A	6.66	6.35
AB	6.69	5.89

Similar results were reported by McPherson et al.[142]

Group	IU/L above the mean
O	4.7
B	0.5
A	4.4
AB	6.1

The different levels are probably related to differences in the isoenzyme derived from the intestine.

BODY WEIGHT

Body weight does not appear to affect serum alkaline phosphatase activity in men, but Henny and Schiele found that women 15% overweight had a 20% greater median level than women not overweight.[578]

FLUORIDE

Serum alkaline phosphatase activity in groups living in areas with fluoride added to the water supply were studied by Ferguson.[635] In one study the mean level fell by 16% 4 weeks after fluoridation of the water supply, using a dinitrophenyl phosphate method of estimation. In another study of a group of women sampled weekly for a year, the mean level fell to 73% of the basal level 1 week after fluoridation, but slowly rose until, after 22 weeks, it was at the prefluoridation level.

Addition of fluoride at twice the level found in blood had no effect on the enzyme level, which was in line with a report in 1935 by Belfanti et al.[636] they found that fluoride *in vitro* inhibits serum acid phosphatase activity, but has no effect on alkaline phosphatase.

Ferguson discussed the changes in enzyme activity following fluoridation, but a satisfactory explanation was not found.

MACROALKALINE PHOSPHATASE

The presence of alkaline phosphatase in serum, in a high-molecular-mass form called a macroenzyme, has been reported. Nagamine and Ohkuma showed in a patient with skeletal abnormalities and serum alkaline phosphatase activity of 32 KA units per deciliter, that IgG was able to bind with liver and bone isoenzyme, but not with other isoenzymes.[637] Dingjan et al. found a macroenzyme in 7 of 2500 sera submitted for routine analysis,[638] Crofton and Smith reported eight patients with serum containing macroenzyme and either intestinal or lung disease, but no common clinical condition.[639]

Complexes of alkaline phosphatase with lipoprotein have been reported in patients with cholestasis.[640]

Patients reported as having a macroenzyme can have various clinical conditions, and it is possible that subjects appearing healthy, but having an unexplained persistent increase in serum alkaline phosphatase activity, may have a macroenzyme present.

DRUGS AFFECTING SERUM
ALKALINE PHOSPHATASE ACTIVITY

The toxic effects of a number of drugs on the liver give an increase in serum alkaline phosphatase activity.[55,56]

Some drugs increase the bone isoenzyme, for instance, the antithyroid drugs, reflecting the increase in bone turnover in hypothyroidism.[641] These drugs can also give rise to hepatitis or cholestasis when the liver isoenzyme is increased.[642] Lithium is also reported to increase bone alkaline phosphatase.[643]

Some drugs reduce serum alkaline phosphatase activity. Oral contraceptives decrease the mean by up to 20%, depending on the period taken and the estrogen content.[644] Clofibrate, used to treat hyperlipidemia, is also reported to reduce serum alkaline phosphatase activity. Schade et al.,[645] using a dinitrophenol method giving normal levels up to 120 units per liter, found that the mean level fell from 82.1 units per liter to 52.3 units per liter, during 2 years of treatment. Ferrari et al. found that much of this change was during the first weeks of treatment.[646] In 27 male patients given 2 g of clofibrate daily, and estimating using a "standard method," the mean fell from 114 units per liter to 98 after 1 week, and 72 units per liter after 2 weeks.

Chapter 7

AMINOTRANSFERASE (TRANSAMINASE) ACTIVITY

Transamination plays a key role in intermediary metabolism, as it provides a means for the synthesis and degradation of amino acids in living cells. The three amino acids, glutamic acid, aspartic acid, and alanine, can be converted by a transamination reaction into the corresponding keto acids, which are components of the citric acid cycle.[647] Enzymes catalyzing the interconversion between amino and keto acids, without the intermediate participation of ammonia, were first reported by Braunstein and Kritzsman in 1937.[648] The two of most interest in clinical work are aspartate aminotransferase (glutamic-oxalacetic transaminase, GOT) and alanine aminotransferase (glutamic-pyruvic transaminase, GPT).

Estimation has been by measuring the decrease in absorption at 340 nm resulting from the oxidation of NADH by oxalacetic or pyruvic acid under the influence of malic or lactic dehydrogenase[649,650] or by determining the keto acid produced as dinitrophenyl hydrazone,[651,652] or by coupling with a stabilized diazonium salt.[653] An account of both manual and automatic methods is given by Demetriou et al.[654]

ANALYTIC CONSIDERATIONS

PYRIDOXYL PHOSPHATE

Addition of pyridoxyl phosphate (a cofactor for aminotransferase activity) to serum has been found to give a variable effect. This may be due to the use of different buffers, as phosphate inhibits the association of the cofactor with apoenzyme.

Rej et al. found a mean increase of 16% in GOT activity,[655] after adding pyridoxyl phosphate to 125 sera with varying levels and estimating using a spectrophotometric method and a phosphate buffer, whereas Cheung and Briggs, adding pyridoxyl phosphate to 125 heparinized plasma samples from hospital patients,[656] found a mean increase of 37% (range of 0 to 389%), using an optimized method at 37°C with a tris buffer. The increase in GPT was usually less than 15%.

RECOMMENDED METHODS

A problem when attempting to standardize conditions of estimation is that optimal conditions vary for the two isoenzymes found in serum: one is of cytoplasmic origin, and the other is derived from mitochondria.

Proposals for reference methods have been made by the Scandinavian Committee on Enzymes[657] and by the IFCC Expert Panel on Enzymes.[658-660] Table 93 shows the recommended conditions; for full details the references given should be consulted. Apart from some differences in reagent concentration, the methods differ in the proposed reaction temperature and in the addition of pyridoxyl phosphate, which is obligatory in the IFCC method. In the Scandinavian Society proposal, it is suggested that pyridoxyl phosphate can be added if "of interest."

The IFCC Expert Panel explains that they selected optimal conditions, with reference to sera from patients with liver and myocardial disease, by studying both pools of sera and individual sera. In these studies there is an increase in GOT activity, mainly of mitochondrial origin. Reagent conditions are therefore a compromise based on the proportion of isoenzymes present in abnormal sera and biased to the mitochondrial enzyme.

Between-laboratory surveys in Scandinavia in 1975 and 1978 suggested that imprecision between laboratories is about 7%.[661] Vincent-Viry et al. found between-batch precision to be 2.3 to 5.1% for GPT and 1.8 to 4.3% for GOT, using the German Society-recommended methods.[662]

TABLE 93.
Recommendations for Conditions for Estimation of Serum Amino Transferases

	Serum aspartate amino transferase (GOT)		Serum alanine amino transferase (GPT)	
	Scandinavian[657]	IFCC[658]	Scandinavian[657]	IFCC[659]
Temperature (°C)	37	30	37	30
pH	7.7	7.8	7.4	7.5
Buffer				
tris (mmol/L)	20	80	20	100
EDTA (mmol/L)	5		5	
Aspartate (mmol/L)	200	240	1 alanine 400	500
NADH (mmol/L)	0.15	0.18	0.15	0.18
MDH	600 unit/L	71 µkat/L		
LDH	200	10	2000 unit/L	20 µkat/L
Pyridoxyl phosphate (mmol/L)		0.10		0.10
2 oxo glutarate	12	12	12	12
Wavelength (nm)	340	339	340	339
Volume fraction of sample	1/8	1/12	1/16	1/8

INTERFERENCE WITH ANALYSIS

HEMOLYSIS

The average aminotransferase activity in whole-blood hemolysates is up to ten times that in serum. Slight hemolysis does not appreciably increase the level.[663] Henry, using published concentrations, calculated that the increase in aminotransferase activity with visible hemolysis (about 0.6 g/L of hemoglobin) was about 1.2%,[664] whereas Sax and Moore considered it to be about 10%.[665] Using a color method, they found that serum hemoglobin did not significantly increase GOT activity, but at 2.5 g/L, the apparent activity increased by up to 30%. As red cell GPT activity is only about four times that of serum, they noted that the effect of hemolysis was correspondingly smaller. The variation in findings may be due to method differences.

LIPEMIA

Color methods with serum still present in the final test mixture, but not in the blank, will show falsely high final optical densities, in the presence of lipemia.[305] Reaction rate methods would not be affected.

Changes due to the rate of clearing of lipemia, and its effect on the inverse colorimetry used in the Technicon SMAC analyzer, were found by Miyada et al.[666] They clarified 50 sera with varying amounts of lipemia by centrifuging for 10 min at 100,000 g. Serum GOT decreased in 35 of 50 sera, and the mean level fell from 33.5 to 22.6 µ/L (range of 1 to 350). Serum GPT decreased in 41 of 50 sera, with the mean level falling from 65.0 to 27.8 µ/L (range of 6 to 203).

OTHER INTERFERING SUBSTANCES

Procedures using the coupling of a keto acid produced with a stabilized diazonium salt, as are frequently used in continuous-flow analyzers, suffer from interference from any metabolite or drug with a labile hydrogen atom between two carboxyl groups.

Acetoacetate

False increases in aminotransferase activity have been found in sera from patients with ketoacidosis, when using procedures involving coupling with diazonium salts. Cryer and

Daughady reported an increase in 38 of 55 patients with ketoacidosis,[667] using the Technicon SMA 12/60 analyzer. They believed that the increase was hepatic in origin, but Moore and Sax showed that it was due to the reaction between acetoacetate and Fast Red PDC (Fast Panneau L),[668] used as a coupling agent, and recommended inclusion of a serum blank to correct for the interference. The findings have been confirmed by other workers.[669,670]

L-Dopa and Methyl Dopa

Apparent increases in serum GOT activity, using the Technicon 12/60 analyzer, have been found when L-dopa and methyl dopa were added to serum, at therapeutic levels.[82] A dose of 83.3 µg/mL, representing the maximum level after a single dose of 3000 mg of L-dopa, increased the apparent activity by 48 units. A dose of 20.8 µg/mL, representing the maximum level after a single dose of 250 mg, increased the apparent activity by 37 units. Methyl dopa at 62.5 µg/mL, representing the maximum level after a 750-mg dose, increased apparent GOT activity by 12 units.

Para-aminosalicylic Acid

Falsely high serum aminotransferase levels have been found in patients treated with para aminosalicylic acid (PAS), using methods coupled with stabilized diazonium salts. Apparent levels of up to ten times those before treatment or found using a spectrophotometric method were found by Glynn et al.,[671] using Azoene Fast Red PDC. This finding was confirmed by Singh et al.,[82] who, using the Technicon 12/60 analyzer, found an apparent increase of GOT activity of 245 units when PAS of 75.5 µg/mL was added.

Glutamic Dehydrogenase

Interference by glutamic dehydrogenase is potentially possible if high levels are present.[672] The glutamic dehydrogenase reaction cannot proceed with a minimal ammonia concentration. To avoid potential problems, the IFCC Expert Panel on Enzymes recommends that MDH and LDH in glycerol be used.

PREANALYTIC ERROR

ANTICOAGULANTS

It is usually stated that serum or plasma can be used for the estimation of aminotransferase activity,[391,673] although heparinized plasma has been reported to give rise to errors, with some methods.[674] Hakkensceid and Hectors, using the Scandinavian Society-recommended method,[675] found that plasma GOT was 95% of the serum level, and plasma GPT was only 70% of the serum level. No difference between serum and plasma was found using a phosphate buffer or using the method of Bergmeyer et al.,[676] which is similar to the IFCC-recommended method, but uses 25°C. The difference using the Scandinavian method was attributed to a lag phase.[677]

Heparinized plasma has also been reported to cause occasional turbidity, and the IFCC Expert Committee recommends that the use of plasma be avoided. It is said that plasma from EDTA specimens can be used, but that sodium citrate inhibits aminotransferase activity.[662] Fluoride affects methods using diazo reagents. Sax and Moore, using Fast Ponceau L as a coupling reagent,[665] found that 10 mg of fluoride enhanced the color obtained by 17%.

VENOUS STASIS

Venous stasis would be expected to increase serum aminotransferases. It was reported by Statland and Winkel660,[678] that mean GOT is 9.56% higher if a tourniquet is in place for 3 min, compared with the level if it is only on for 1 min. Mean GPT was only 1.56% higher.

TABLE 94.
Stability of Serum GOT and GPT at 25 and 4°C,
Measured as Mean Loss of Activity[681]

| | Mean loss of activity | | | |
| | GOT | | GPT | |
After	4°C	25°C	4°C	25°C
24 h	2%	2%	2%	8%
48 h	5%	6%	5%	12%
3 day	8%	10%	12%	17%
5 day	10%	11%	14%	19%
7 day	12%	13%	15%	20%

CONTAMINATION

Detergents inhibit aminotransferase activity, and care must be taken to avoid contamination of glassware. Bergmeyer studied the effect of detergents[581] and found that at a concentration of 0.8 mg/mL, one inhibited serum GOT activity by about 16%.

NADH solutions that have been frozen and thawed are liable to contain LDH inhibitors affecting the reduction of pyruvate.[679] The inhibitor is also formed in solid NADH exposed to a moist atmosphere. Some commercial preparations contain the inhibitor, and different products have been found to have up to threefold differences in activity. Unsatisfactory NADH preparations should be indicated by internal quality control procedures, and special attention should be given when changing reagents.

SAMPLE STABILITY

Although some workers say that serum aminotransferases are stable for 2 days at room temperature, and 2 weeks at 4°C,[581,680] Schmidt and Schmidt suggest that there is a small loss of activity (Table 94).[681] Serum GOT is said to be stable for at least 4 months if frozen.[682] Serum GPT is unstable when frozen, as the enzyme does not tolerate thawing well.

Hanok and Kuo found GOT in reconstituted commercial lyophilized serum to be stable for 8 days at 10°C, and for at least 20 days when frozen.[95]

PHYSIOLOGIC CHANGES

POSTURE

Both GOT and GPT in serum are reported to be higher in standing subjects than in sitting or supine subjects, as would be expected. Statland et al. found[38] the following:

Posture	Serum GOT	Serum GPT
Subject supine 30 min after sitting	−4.7%	−3.1%
Subject standing 30 min after sitting	+9.8%	+11.4%
Subject changes from standing to supine	−14.5%	−14.5%

MEALS

Serum GPT has been shown to increase by about 6% in healthy subjects after a 700-cal meal.[683] Serum GOT was also higher, but the increase was not considered statistically significant.

EXERCISE

A number of studies have shown that serum GOT increases with exercise (Table 95). There is less change in serum GPT. Levels after severe exercise, such as a long-distance run, show

TABLE 95.
Changes in Serum Aminotransferases Following Exercise

Reference	Method		N	GOT	GPT
684	Spectrophotometric	1 hour exercise		Doubled	Increased 20%
685	Reitman and Frankel	Moderate exercise such as ½-mile jog, 150-yd swim, etc.		Rise to 36–96 Fall to normal (less than 40 units) in 12–16 h	Smaller rise not outside normal range
686	Spectrophotometric	Healthy men using bicycle ergonometer for 90 min	12	Before mean 22, range 17–30 After mean 27, range 17–45	Before mean 20, range 14–24 After mean 21, range 11–29
687	Spectrophotometric	After completing a 50-km run	20	Immediately after mean 60, range 31–114 2 weeks after mean 39, range 5–93 Normal range 9–40	Immediately after mean 50, range 22–104 2 weeks after mean 35, range 10–57 Normal range 5–35
688	Reitman and Frankel	Officer cadets Five days of strenuous exercise followed by exercise at about 50% of previous level	18	Day 1 mean 25, range 10–42 Day 2 mean 262, range 42–1360 Day 4 mean 267, range 76–1580 Day 7 mean 113, range 44–298 Day 10 mean 44, range 28–124	

TABLE 96.
Changes Reported in Serum Aminotransferases During the Menstrual Cycle

Reference	Method	Phase of cycle	GOT mean	GPT mean
692	Reitman-Frankel	Preovulatory	17.80	8.20
		Ovulatory	14.50	6.80
		Postovulatory	12.80	6.10
693	Spectrophotometric	Day 1–14 of cycle	8.83	6.99
		Day 15–28 of cycle	9.34	8.69
		Postmenopausal	9.73	10.45

aminotransferase levels that would normally be diagnostic of severe tissue damage, which may mislead if used for diagnostic purposes. Preexercise levels may not be achieved for several weeks. Changes may reflect an increase in membrane permeability as a result of prolonged exertion. The small changes produced by relatively modest exercise need to be taken into account when taking specimens from outpatients and when standardizing conditions for establishing reference intervals.

SEASONAL VARIATION

Small changes in serum aminotransferase activity have been reported during the year. Röcker et al.[689] noted lower GPT levels in the summer, whereas Gidlow et al., in two studies of employees over a 5-year period, found consistent seasonal variations.[690,691] A statistically significant change in serum GPT, with a mean spring level of 27 units and a mean autumn level of 25 units, was shown, with greater change in those 25 to 45 years of age than in those below the age of 25. GOT activity showed similar changes, which were not considered statistically significant. The reasons for these differences were not discussed, and possible changes in exercise patterns were not investigated.

MENSTRUAL CYCLE

Different changes in serum aminotransferase activity during the menstrual cycle have been reported (Table 96), with one group finding an increase in the second half of the cycle, and another reporting lower levels in the postovulatory phase. Neither group suggested any explanation for the changes or the discrepancy.

RANGE IN HEALTHY SUBJECTS

WITHIN- AND BETWEEN-PERSON VARIATION

The level of serum aminotransferase activity is a little higher in men than in women (Table 97). There is a small change with age (Table 98), although in a study of 6036 blood donors, Hetland et al. found that serum GPT activity correlated with body mass and not with age.[697] McPherson et al. found a small increase in serum aminotransferase activity in females, due to menopause (Table 99).[142]

CHILDREN

Most reports suggest that there is a small fall in both serum GOT and GPT activity during childhood (Table 100), although a report from Emanuel et al. said that serum GPT levels from 1 month, the earliest age studied, were similar to adult levels.[698]

NEONATES

Activity of serum aminotransferases in the 1st week of life is about two or three times that found in adults (Table 101). The level in cord blood serum is similar to that found in

TABLE 97.
Serum Aminotransferase Activity in Healthy Adults

Reference	Subjects	N	Method	GOT Male Mean	GOT Male Range	GOT Female Mean	GOT Female Range	GPT Male Mean	GPT Male Range	GPT Female Mean	GPT Female Range
694	"Normal" adults	75	DPNH color IU/L	70.43	35–107	67.04	28–113	53.95	27–105	47.95	17–92
695	Subjects for routine health examination	12682	Spectrophotometric with phosphate buffer at 37°C	22.4 (Median)		18.5 (Median)		18.1 (Median)		16.3 (Median)	
696	Finns over 30 years old. Exclusion for disease, overweight, excessive alcohol consumption	8000	Scandinavian Society method		13.4–39.4		12.5–32.9				

TABLE 98.
Serum Aminotransferase Activity with Age in Healthy Adults

GOT

Reference	Subjects	Method		Male age (years) 18–25	26–35	36–45	46–55	56–65	Female age (years) 18–25	26–35	36–45	46–55	56–65
142	1000 healthy blood donors	Fluorimetric method on continuous-flow analyzer	Median	17.9	18.2	17.4	17.7	19.0	14.3	14.8	15.2	16.2	18.3
662	Healthy subjects	IFCC method at 30°C	N	320	879	400	172	95	314	736	320	157	50
			2.5 percentile	13.5	14.5	15.5	15.5	15.5	11.5	11.5	11.5	11.5	12.5
			50 percentile	23.0	25.5	26.5	26.5	25.5	19.5	19.0	19.0	19.5	21.5
			7.5 percentile	45.0	52.5	56.5	54.5	50.0	40.0	40.0	45.5	35.0	43.0

GPT

Reference	Subjects	Method		Male age (years) 18–25	26–35	36–45	46–55	56–65	Female age (years) 18–25	26–35	36–45	46–55	56–65
662	Healthy subjects	German Society-recommended method at 37°C	N	351	765	462	362	208	376	588	346	261	102
			2.5 percentile	8.5	9.5	10.0	10.0	8.8	6.5	6.5	7.0	7.0	9.0
			50 percentile	17.0	19.0	21.0	19.5	17.5	13.0	13.0	13.5	13.5	15.0
			97.5 percentile	33.0	45.0	45.0	45.5	33.5	26.0	26.0	28.0	26.0	28.0

TABLE 99.
Median Serum GOT in Groups of Female Blood Donors
Showing an Increase at Menopause[a] (units per liter at 25°C)

Age (years)	Premenopausal	Posthysterectomy	Postmenopausal
18–25	14.3	—	—
26–35	14.8	—	—
36–45	15.2	13.6	19.4
46–55	15.1	16.0	16.8
56–65	—	19.0	18.2

[a] From McPherson, K., et al., *Clin. Chim. Acta,* 84, 373, 1978.

the mother (Table 102). A study by Kristenson et al. found that addition of pyridoxyl phosphate increased mean GOT activity by about 30%,[705] but there was little increase in GPT activity.

RANGE DURING PREGNANCY

The mean level of aminotransferase activity during pregnancy is similar to that in nonpregnant subjects, but occasionally a high level is found. Knutson et al.,[706] using a spectrophotometric method at 25°C, found a mean serum GOT of 20 units (range of 7 to 33) compared with a mean of 16 units (range of 7 to 31) in 31 healthy nonpregnant women. Borglin, using a similar method,[707] found a mean GOT of 18.5 units (range of 5.8 to 72.4) in 34 pregnant women, gestation 36 to 40 weeks, compared with a mean of 28.9 units (range of 15.6 to 59.3) in eight subjects at term and a mean of 20.5 (range of 9.4 to 32.4) in ten nonpregnant women of similar ages.

Kristenson et al., using the Scandinavian Society-recommended method,[705] found similar levels in pregnant subjects at term and in nonpregnant women. Addition of pyridoxyl phosphate increased GOT activity by approximately 40% and GPT activity by approximately 25%.

OTHER CHANGES

BODY WEIGHT

Both serum GOT and GPT activity increase with body weight. Table 103 shows the findings of some workers.

ALCOHOL

Even moderate consumption of ethanol in healthy subjects affects blood levels of aminotransferase activity. In a study of the acute effect of alcohol, Freer and Statland[48] gave four men and five women alcohol, 0.75 g/kg body weight each evening for 3 days, in the form of "hard liquor" diluted with a mix. Sixty hours after the last drink, mean GPT had increased by 12% and mean GOT had decreased by 12%. GPT had increased in seven of the subjects by 10 to 40%, and GOT had decreased in 8 subjects (by more than 20% in 2).

Jarvisalo et al., in a study of 8000 Finns over 30 years of age, using the method recommended by the Scandinavian Society,[696] found higher levels of GOT in those taking more than 140 g/week of ethanol than in those taking less than this amount. For subjects taking more than

140 g/weeks, men had a mean of 25.7 units, and women, 21.7 units. For those taking less than 140 g/week of alcohol, men had a mean of 23.1 units, and women, 20.3 units.

Patients with a history of heavy alcohol abuse have a greater increase in serum GOT. Konttinen et al.[709] found that in 64 of 100 patients admitted to the hospital, with a history of a large intake of alcohol for several years, the level was more than the 99% limit for healthy controls. Alcohol intake must be considered when selecting subjects and standardizing conditions for the determination of reference intervals.

TRAUMA

An increase in serum GOT is found in a number of patients, following surgery and accidents involving surgery. Lieberman et al. found that 25 of 51 patients with accidents involving bodily trauma without evidence of cardiac injury had an increase.[710] In most cases the maximal level was within 2 days of the injury, and the return to normal took variable times, up to the ninth postoperative day. Blodgett et al. found an increase in only 2 of 33 patients subject to transurethral prostatic resection.[711] The increase was probably due to the cutting of muscle and to an anesthetic-induced spasm of the Sphincter of Oddi, causing regurgitation.

HEMODIALYSIS

Wolf et al. found that serum GOT activity decreased in patients undergoing long-term hemodialysis.[712] They considered that either a nondialyzable enzyme inhibitor was accumulating or that dialysis was causing a pyridoxyl phosphate deficiency.

MACROAMINOTRANSFERASES

High-molecular-mass forms of aminotransferases are found with the enzyme combined with immunoglobulin. There are reports of this in healthy subjects and in patients with liver disease. Kottinen et al.[713] reported two healthy young women, ages 20 and 23, with an unexplained increase in serum GOT when being checked after taking oral contraceptives. The level fluctuated from five to ten times the URL in one woman and from 7.5 to 15 times in the other. Kijita et al. found the high-molecular-mass form of GPT in 16 of 506 sera from patients with chronic liver disease when investigated by an electrophoretic technique.[714] Activity was from one to seven times the URL, although most had an increased level due to liver disease. Both groups showed that the enzyme was bound to IgG.

DRUGS AFFECTING AMINOTRANSFERASE LEVELS

The toxic effects of drugs on the liver and the induction of the enzymes both give rise to increases in aminotransferase activity in serum, as discussed in Chapter 6. The lists edited by Young,[55,56] Tryding and Linblad,[59] and Salway[60] should be consulted for information on the many drugs affecting levels of aminotransferase activity.

In the case of oral contraceptives taken by a proportion of healthy subjects, the increase is over 30% in those taking higher-dose preparations, and about 10% in those taking a lower-dose preparation. The greatest effect is in those treated for 1 to 2 years and is greater in those 20 years of age than in those 40 years of age.

Some drugs given intramuscularly are reported to result in an increase in serum GOT. Knirsch and Gralla reported levels of up to twice the mean normal after 3 days of treatment, but no increase in GPT.[715]

TABLE 100.
Serum Aminotransferase Activity in Healthy Children

GOT

Reference	N	Age	Male Mean / Median	Male Range 2.5–97.5 percentile	Female Mean / Median	Female Range 2.5–97.5 percentile	Comment
698	463	In young children, about 2× adult levels					Adult levels attained at about 3 years
699		6	47		35		Fall almost linear from age 6 to age 7
French children (units mU/L)		17	35		28		
700	About 3600		Median		Median		
Technicon SMAC (unit/L)		5	28	19–36	27	17–39	
		6	28	17–40	27	18–37	
		7	26	18–40	25	17–39	
		8	27	17–42	25	17–40	
		9	25	15–37	24	17–35	
		10	24	16–37	22	14–32	
		11	23	14–35	20	11–30	
		12	22	13–38	18	11–30	
		13	21	12–37	16	8–24	
		14	21	11–32	16	9–26	
		15	19	10–38	14	88–26	
		16	19	11–31	15	8–27	
		17	18	11–31	14	9–24	

GPT

698

701 Pediatric patients in Tokyo with morphological disease such as Burn scars, nevus Analysis with Technicon SMAC unit/l

	Median	Range	
0	19	8–46	Mean GPT activity similar to adult from about 1 month
1	19	8–45	Young adults 20–29 years old, median 13, range 6–32
2	18	7–44	
3	18	7–43	
4	17	7–41	
5	17	7–40	
6	16	7–39	
7	16	6–38	
8	15	6–37	
9	15	6–36	
10	15	6–35	
11	14	6–34	
12	14	6–33	
13	13	6–33	
14–19	13	6–32	

TABLE 101.
Serum Aminotransferase Activity in Neonates

Reference	Subjects		GOT Range	GOT Adult range	GPT Range	GPT Adult range
702	Infants in first week of life	Spectrophotometric method (unit/mL)	13–120	8–40	12–90	5–35
703	Infants 2–6 days old	Spectrophotometric method (unit/mL)		**Older children**		
			29–79	4–36		
			Mean	Mean		
			51	20		

TABLE 102.
Serum Aminotransferases in Cord Blood Serum

Reference	Method	Subjects	N	GOT Range	GOT 50 percentile	GPT Range	GPT 50 percentile
704	DPNH method	European mother					
		Serum at term		39–255		10–134	
		Cord serum	19	80–205		10–116	
		Bantu mother					
		Serum at term		40–150		10–118	
		Cord serum	26	70–190		15–78	
705	Scand. Soc. method	Cord serum		16–47	27	4–23	10
		Cord serum with pyridoxyl phosphate		22–58	36	4–24	12

TABLE 103.
Effect of Body Weight on Serum Aminotransferase Activity[a]

Reference	Subjects	GOT percentile			Mean	GPT percentile		
		2.5	50	97.5		2.5	50	97.5
708	12,682 subjects for routine health exam. Men 20–30 years old (unit/L)							
	Weight between 15th and 25th percentile	14.7	22.4	44.4		13.5	24.4	65.5
	Weight above 85th percentile	16.5	24.8	68.0				
696	8000 Finns over 30 years old (unit/L)							
	Body Mass Index below 29 kg/m²				23.1			
	Body Mass Index above 29 kg/m²				26.1			

[a] Body Mass Index = weight/height²

Chapter 8

TOTAL PROTEIN

Over 60 different proteins have been identified in blood plasma. All are synthesized in the liver, with the exception of those immunoglobulins formed in the reticuloendothelial system. The molecular size at which a substance is considered a protein has not been precisely defined, but commonly corresponds to about 10,000, the molecular size that does not pass through a dialysis membrane.

ANALYTIC CONSIDERATIONS

The number of different proteins present in serum give rise to problems that make accurate estimation of total protein difficult. It has been proposed that the polypeptide content should be used as the basis for determining total protein.[716] Nonprotein moieties, such as carbohydrate and lipid found in conjugated proteins, would then not be included in the protein weights estimated. The percentage of polypeptide varies from approximately 7% in alpha$_2$ lipoprotein and 20% in B-lipoprotein, to over 99% in albumin.

NITROGEN CONTENT

Analysis for protein has been based, since the earliest work, on determination of the nitrogen content. The Kjeldahl procedure has become the accepted reference method for protein estimation in biologic material. For serum, the nonprotein nitrogen level obtained by analysis of a protein-free filtrate is subtracted. An analytic precision of ±1% can be achieved. Calculation of protein content assumes that the various proteins in serum have the same nitrogen content. Multiplication of nitrogen by the factor 6.25 to give the protein level has been used since the late 19th century. This represents the nitrogen as 16% by weight of protein.

Investigation of serum fractions has shown that the factor varies. A number of different figures are given in the literature. Peters, in one study,[716] found that the factor varied from 5.69 to 6.52 for proteins in normal plasma when nonprotein moieties were disregarded. Earlier, Brand, who analyzed air-dried samples by the Dumas method and corrected for ash and moisture,[717] obtained factors of 6.27 for albumin and 6.24 for gamma globulin, whereas Sunderman et al.[718] and Chiaravigcio et al.[719] both suggested 6.54, Watson, reviewing the literature up to about 1960,[720] concluded that the most reliable figure for albumin was 6.40, and for total protein, 6.45. Despite these different proposals for the factor, 6.25 has continued to be used.

BIURET REACTION

The reaction of polypeptides with alkaline copper solutions, known as the biuret reaction, has been used to estimate protein at least since 1914.[721] Modifications of the reagent by reducing alkalinity and copper content to prevent precipitation of copper have been developed,[722,723] and now most clinical laboratories use a technique based on the biuret reaction, to measure serum total protein. An American Society of Clinical Pathology survey in 1963 found that 89% of laboratories in the United States were using the biuret method, and in 1990 over 97% of laboratories participating in the "Wellcome" quality-assurance scheme used a method based on the reaction. Accuracy of analysis is variable, as different proteins give varying amounts of color, with biuret reagents, from 97 to 116% of that given by serum albumin.[766] The precision obtained is good.

OTHER METHODS

In some early work the Folin–Lowry method was used.[724] This procedure measures mainly the tyrosine content of protein. Reaction of copper in alkaline solution is followed by reduction by the Folin and Ciocalteau phosphomolybdate phosphotungstate reagent. A number of substances are known to interfere, including tris and other buffers, sulfhydryl groups, carbohydrates, and chelating agents.[725] The tyrosine content of different proteins in plasma can vary by a factor of five; therefore the method is strongly influenced by the amino acid composition of the proteins present.

Both the specific gravity and refractive index of serum have been used as the basis of methods for estimating serum protein. Other procedures have used the absorption in the UV region. Measurement at 270 to 290 nm uses absorption mainly due to tyrosine, phenylalanine, and tryptophan, and at 200 nm, absorption due to the peptide bond is used.

STANDARDIZATION

Bovine serum albumin and human albumin are considered to consist of a single peptide chain without prosthetic groups, and are possible reference materials for the standardization of methods. Both are available in very pure forms, except for the presence of dimers and trimers. Primary preparation of standards can be based on dry weight, and the best estimation was obtained by heating *in vacuo* at 110°C.[726] At this temperature the weight remained constant for at least 10 days.

The Standards Committee of the AACC recommends standardization of biuret methods, based on bovine serum albumin.[716] Bovine serum albumin is cheaper than human albumin and is readily available, and the color follows Beer's law better.

ACCURACY AND PRECISION

Accuracy is difficult to assess with most methods, because a mixture of proteins with different properties is being assayed. Precision is good for most methods. When based on the between-batch coefficient of variation at normal levels of serum total protein, using the biuret reaction, precision is about 3.7% for manual methods and 2.6% for automatic methods.[727]

SI UNITS

As a mixture is being assayed, the relative molecular mass is not known, and so levels of serum total protein are expressed in mass units of gram per liter. Many earlier reports used grams per 100 mL and can easily be converted by multiplying by ten.

INTERFERENCE WITH ANALYSIS

HEMOLYSIS

As hemoglobin is a protein, its presence in serum will affect methods based on the measurement of nitrogen content.

Interference in the biuret method may also be due to optical interference. Henry et al. found that the biuret color produced by 1 mg of hemoglobin is equivalent to 1.9 mg of protein.[728] This figure was confirmed by Doumas et al.,[723] who found that interference was small and probably negligible by up to 3 g/L of hemoglobin in serum, using a blank in their proposed candidate reference method based on the biuret reaction.

BILIRUBIN

Interference by bilirubin with the biuret method can be corrected by using a suitable blank. Kingsley found that 85 μmol/L of bilirubin does not interfere appreciably,[729] and Doumas et al.[723] stated that 513 μmol/L of bilirubin increases serum total protein by about 2 g/L if no blank is applied in their proposed reference method. A blank corrects reasonably well.

LIPEMIA

Henry et al. found that many serum and biuret mixtures that appear clear exhibit a definite Tyndall effect that introduces significant error.[728] The most successful correction technique was considered to be ether extraction. The blank of reagent, without copper, that can be used to correct for interference by bilirubin or hemoglobin is not satisfactory for correction of lipemia.

Ulracentrifugation to remove lipemia may increase apparent serum protein. Miyada et al. centrifuged 50 sera with varying amounts of lipemia for 10 min at 100,000 g and found that mean total protein increased from 68.4 to 69.5 g/L when estimated on a Technicon SMAC analyzer.[666] The change was considered to be due to volume displacement.

BROMSULFOPHTHALEIN

The color given by bromsulfophthalein in an alkaline solution will interfere with protein estimation by the biuret method.[285]

GLUCOSE

Doumas reported that glucose interfered with the biuret reaction,[722] but the group proposing a candidate reference method[723] later concluded that glucose (as much as 55 mmol/L) did not interfere.

DEXTRANS

Dextrans, administered as plasma volume expanders, combine in serum with copper in a biuret reagent to form a precipitate.[730] A blank with copper omitted from the reagent is unsatisfactory, as no precipitate forms.[690] In manual assays the mixture can be centrifuged, and the optical density of the clear supernatant liquid can be measured. Interference in automatic systems can be detected by noting unusual blank readings or suspiciously high serum total-protein results. Hydroxyethyl starch, also used as a plasma volume expander, does not interfere.[690]

Specimens identified as containing dextrans should be estimated using a manual method, with centrifugation to remove the precipitate.

ANTIBIOTICS

Panek et al. reported that carbenicillin interfered with the estimation of serum total protein, using the Technicon SMAC analyzer,[731] and this was investigated by Doumas et al.,[690] who tested antibiotics that may be administered to patients in high doses. They considered

1. Ampicillin
2. Carbenicillin
3. Cephalothin
4. Chloramphenicol
5. Methicillin
6. Nuficillin
7. Oxacillin
8. Penicillin G

and found an apparent increase in serum total protein of 0.1 to 1.0 g/L at antibiotic concentrations of 0.5 g/L. Therapeutic concentrations are much less than this, and so no significant interference was expected.

SULFASALAZINE

Moriarity et al. found that 50 mg/L of sulfasalazine reduced apparent serum total protein from 66 to 49 g/L,[732] using a biuret method on the DuPont ACA analyzer. An increase in absorption at 510 nm after the biuret reaction is complete was shown to give rise to overblanking.

PREANALYTIC ERROR

COLLECTION OF THE SPECIMEN

Most laboratories use serum for estimating total protein. Analysis of plasma from anticoagulated specimens gives results 2 to 4 g/L higher due to the inclusion of fibrinogen.

Lacher and Elsea showed that the use of the commercially available product Liposol to decrease lipemia affected serum total protein.[83] The mean level of 26 randomly selected sera increased from 56.2 to 61.6 g/L after shaking with Liposol the analysis used the Beckman Astra Ideal analyzer.

ANTICOAGULANTS

When blood is taken into an anticoagulant such as oxalate there is a water shift from the erythrocytes within 15 min, which is proportional to the amount of anticoagulant used. This causes a reduction of total protein, which balances, to some extent, the higher level due to the presence of fibrinogen, giving an apparent content similar to that of the corresponding serum.

VENOUS STASIS

It has been known for many years that serum total protein increases following venous stasis, although the earliest reports exaggerated the effect. Böhme, in 1911,[733] reported that the level increased from 77 to 114 g/L after 16 min of stasis and that it returned within 5 min of releasing the restriction. In 1924 Peters et al. found that 5 min of stasis increased total protein from 63 to 93 g/L.[734]

In a controlled experiment, Husdan et al. later studied seven male staff and five female staff,[167] who were fasting and lying down throughout the experiment. After applying a tourniquet for 3 min with a pressure 10 mm Hg less than the systolic pressure, mean serum total protein was 73 ± 4 g/L compared with a mean of 69 ± 4 g/L when no tourniquet was used.

For reliable estimations of serum protein, particularly when serial estimations are being made, it is essential that a minimum of venous stasis be applied.

ARTERIAL AND VENOUS BLOOD

Young found that the protein content of venous blood was 2 to 5 g/L higher than in the corresponding arterial blood,[735] but no further details or references were given.

SAMPLE STABILITY

Little change is found in the level of serum total protein after long periods of storage if the container is tightly capped to avoid evaporation. Peters and Biamonte found that there is no change after 1 week or longer at room temperature, for up to a month at 2 to 4°C, and for up to 2 months at –20°C. Hanok and Kuo stored reconstituted lyophilized serum at –15°C and found an apparent increase after 10 days,[95] which was thought to be due to bacterial contamination.

Heating to 56°C

Several groups have investigated the effect of heating serum or plasma to 56°C to minimize the risk from HIV-positive samples (Table 104). The fall in the level of serum total protein in plasma is mainly due to the formation of a precipitate of fibrinogen. Different effects are reported on sera, which are probably not of significance in the interpretation.

TABLE 104.
Effect of Heating to 56°C for 30 min on Serum and Plasma
Total Protein Compared with the Effect of B-Propriolactone

Reference	Method	Serum or plasma	Mean change
311	Heat	Plasma	Fall 5.9%
102	Heat	Plasma	Fall 5.4%
		Serum	Fall 0.9%
101	Heat	Serum	Fall 0.6%
103	Heat	Serum	Rise 2.13%
312	Heat	Plasma	Fall 4.3%
	B-propriolactone	Plasma	Fall 0.3%

PHYSIOLOGIC CHANGES

POSTURE

There is a fall in serum total protein when a subject moves from the upright to a lying position. Thompson et al., in 1928,[736] found a mean change of 11%, and similar figures have since been reported by a number of workers (Table 105). It is said that 2 h in either position is required for the maximum change to take place.[741] It can be concluded that levels in outpatients will be about 8% (5g/L if not abnormal) higher than in bedridden patients. The posture and time in the position must be defined precisely when determining reference intervals. Seating the patient for a few minutes to collect a sample is unlikely to affect the level.

MEALS

Some workers reported a small increase in serum total protein after a meal, although one group suggested that there is a decrease. Statland et al. reported a mean increase of 1 to 3% after a meal,[38] and Steinmetz et al. reported a mean of 77.6 ± 3.70 g/L at 12 noon and a mean of 79.00 ± 3.70 2 h after a 700-cal meal. Annino and Relman noted a mean decrease of 1.1 g/L 45 min after a standard breakfast,[109] and a mean decrease of 0.3 g/L 2 h after, in a study of 32 subjects, mainly hospital personnel. Changes are small and may not be significant. Increases caused by the effect of turbidity on biuret methods are possible.

EXERCISE

An increase in serum protein after exercise was first reported in the early years of this century.[733] There is an increase of approximately 5% after strenuous exercise and of approximately 10% when exerting to the point of exhaustion (Table 106). It is unlikely that the mild exertion involved in traveling to a clinic would affect levels significantly, but previous exercise should be standardized when determining reference intervals. The effect may be due to dehydration, which can be shown to increase serum protein. Senay and Christensen subjected males to a hot room for up to 11 h to induce dehydration[744] and found that a decrease in plasma volume was accompanied by a corresponding increase in total protein.

STRESS

Severe stress has been shown to increase serum total protein. This is linked to hemoconcentration possibly related to muscular tension. Dugue et al. found little change with mild stress,[745] but in a group of young healthy subjects, mean serum total protein in blood taken immediately before the subjects first parachute jump was found to be more than 8% higher than the mean of samples taken some days previously.

TABLE 105.
Serum Proteins in Standing and Supine Subjects (in g/L)

Reference	Subjects	N	Change	Comment
737		10	Fall during night with lowest after 6 h rest	Fall reversed when subject rose and complete in about 2 h
738			Mean change standing to lying down 14.0%	Mean in men standing significantly higher than in women standing, but little difference lying down
739	Males	10	8 a.m. after lying down for about 9 h Mean serum protein 69.1 Mean serum albumin 39.1	Serum total protein and serum albumin alter by about same amount
	Females	5	4 p.m. after upright for about 8 h Mean serum protein 73.8 Mean serum albumin 43.2	
740	Male medical students	20	Before rising Mean serum protein 67.3 (59.8–75.1) Mean serum albumin 38.6 (38.1–42.3) 15–30 min after rising Mean serum protein 72.6 (67.8–76.3) Mean serum albumin 42.5 (39.6–47.3) Midmorning Mean serum protein 76.1 (67.3–84.6) Mean serum albumin 44.1 (40.7–48.5)	
37	Nonedematous	10	Maximum lying down to standing + 19.1%	
38	Edematous	10	Maximum lying down to standing + 28.7% Standing 2.15% higher than sitting Sitting 6.5% higher than lying down	

TABLE 106.
Effect of Exercise on Serum Total Protein

Reference	Exercise	Change	
		Mean	Range
733	After "work"		+3%–+10%
	After "severe exertion"		+8%–+14%
742	2.5 minutes "standing running"	+17.6%	
738	7–8 min "running up and down stairs and round the garden"	+8.86%	+6%–+12%
743	28 Olympic athletes 15–21 min on a bicycle ergometer until exhausted	+8.6% (2 min after)	Baseline level 30 min after

SEASONAL VARIATION

Several groups reported serum total protein to be approximately 10% lower in summer than in winter. Frank and Carr found levels highest in November and December and lowest in June.[125] Lellough and Claude, in a study of 4422 French civil servants, 46 to 52 years old, also found a decrease in summer.[746] Gitlow et al. found a consistent seasonal variation.[691] No explanation for the finding has been suggested.

RANGE IN HEALTHY SUBJECTS

WITHIN- AND BETWEEN-PERSON VARIATION

The level of total protein was given by Berzelius as 8.6% and by Marcett as 8.7%, as long ago as 1831,[738] although it is not clear if the figures referred to blood or serum. Most workers in this century have obtained similar figures for the range in serum, probably reflecting analysis by the Kjeldahl method or a standardization based on the nitrogen content.

The range found by Salveson in 1926,[747] of 65.3 to 79.6 g/L in 16 "normal" men and 63.4 to 79.6 in 16 "normal" women, compares well with that of 63.0 to 88.6 g/L for heparinized plasma in 60 men and 55 women, 18–59 years old, mainly students and doctors using a Kjeldahl method obtained by Lange in 1946.[738]

Levels found at different ages in some large studies using the biuret method are shown in Tables 107 and 108. A small fall with age is found up to about 50 years, with the level higher in men than women.

Unlike figures given for some other blood constituents, there is little difference between the range given in various textbooks over many years. A range of 60 to 80 g/L, given by King in 1946[7] and McMurry in 1988,[741] probably represents a reasonable overall range without taking posture into account.

BETWEEN-DAY VARIATION

Serum total protein remains reasonably constant over several weeks in an individual, with a coefficient of variation of 3 to 4% (Table 109).

RACIAL DIFFERENCES

Higher serum total-protein levels in non-Caucasian subjects compared with groups of Caucasians have been noted by a number of workers. Rawnsley gave references to studies in Africa, Jamaica, and the United States,[749] reporting higher globulins and lower albumin in blacks, and it was suggested that the differences could be due to tropical disease, liver disease, malnutrition, or genetic variation. Immunoglobulin levels are higher in blacks than in whites,[750] but it is difficult to distinguish genetic from socioeconomic factors.

Using an estimation by a micro-Kjeldahl method on oxalated plasma, Milam[751] found a

TABLE 107.
Serum and Plasma Total Protein Levels in Men by Biuret Methods (in g/L)

Reference		<20	21–25	26–30	31–35	36–40	41–45	46–50	51–55	56–60	61–65	66–70	71–75	76–80
140[a]			62.48–76.56	62.48–76.56	61.78–75.86	61.78–75.86	61.08–75.15	61.08–75.15	60.38–74.45	60.38–74.45	59.67–73.75	59.67–73.75	58.97–73.05	58.97–73.05
145[b]			68–83	68–83	68–82	68–82	66–83	66–83	66–81	66–81	66–84	66–84		
141[c]	Mean	72.6	72.6	72.0	72.0	71.0	71.0	69.5	69.5	69.5	69.7	69.7	69.7	
748[d]	50 percentile	72.2	70.6	70.6	71.7	71.7	71.3	71.3	71.7	71.7	69.5	69.5	70.3	70.3
	5–95 percentile	64.1–80.5	61.7–78.9	63.6–81.4	63.6–81.4	63.1–77.4	63.1–77.4	64.8–78.7	64.8–78.7	64.8–78.7	63.1–75.9	63.1–75.9	59.1–77.9	59.1–77.9
Coventry[e]	N	32	78	70	55	35	32	29	23	27	11			
	Mean	75.09	74.26	74.40	73.45	73.14	70.75	71.52	71.61	70.81	71.36			
	2.5–97.5 percentile	70–81	66–81	67–79	66–83	66–83	62–82	66–80	63–78	63–80	66–76			
	SD	3.33	3.46	3.39	3.73	3.44	4.83	3.10	3.87	4.78	3.44			

a　Caucasian employees and subjects, without complaints, undergoing routine check ups. Fasting and recumbent.

b　Patients from eight geographic areas of U.S., excluding those with active disease

c　Caucasian blood donors. Specimen taken into lithium heparin.

d　Subjects with no acute or chronic disease. No medication alcohol or smoking within 48 h

e　Healthy hospital staff. Specimen collected seated. Details in Chapter 2.

TABLE 108.
Serum and Plasma Total Protein Levels in Women by Biuret Methods[a] (in g/L)

Reference		Age (years)												
		<20	21–25	26–30	31–35	36–40	41–45	46–50	51–55	56–60	61–65	66–70	71–75	76–80
140			60.42-74-84	60.42-74-84	59.95-79.37	59.95-79.37	59.48-73.90	59.48-73.90	59.01-73.45	59.01-73.45	58.54-72.95	58.54-72.95	58.06-72.48	58.06-72.48
145			66-84	66-84	66-84	66-84	64-83	64-83	65-83	65-83	64-86	64-86		
141[b]	Mean	72.0	72.0	70.6	70.6	70.2	70.2	69.9	69.9	70.4	70.4			
748	50 percentile	70.5	72.5	71.6	71.6	70.5	70.5	71.7	71.7	70.5	70.5	70.5	70.5	
	5–95 percentile	64.1-80.1	63.7-80.6	64.1-79.4	64.1-79.4	62.4-77.9	62.4-77.9	65.0-80.0	65.0-80.0	59.0-78.1	59.0-78.1	62.8-77.5	62.8-77.5	
Coventry	N	239	194	84	102	81	82	53	38	22				
	Mean	73.10	74.12	73.45	72.11	72.15	71.90	72.49	72.03	70.59				
	2.5–97.5 percentile	67-81	67-81	64-86	63-80	64-79	63-85	64-80	64-83	64-78				
	SD	3.65	3.72	4.47	3.89	3.23	4.00	4.22	4.33	3.87				

a Details as in Table 107.
b Subjects taking oral contraceptives excluded.

TABLE 109.
Intraindividual Variation of Serum Total Protein

Reference	Subjects	Method	N	Individual variation (mean cv)	Comment
163	Male and female white and black subjects 20–59 years old	Fasting specimen taken at 9 a.m. weekly for 10–12 weeks. Analysis using a biuret method	68	3.9%	After allowing for analytical variation of 3.9%
164	White doctors	One fasting specimen taken weekly for 10 weeks. Stored frozen and all analyzed on same day	9	2.9%	After subtracting mean analytic variation
165	Male students 21–27 years old	Five fasting samples taken within 3 weeks. Analysis using "Autochemist" analyzer	18	2.9%	

mean 73.8 g/L (range of 64.6 to 83.0) in a group of blacks, compared with a mean of 71.3 g/L (range of 62.9 to 79.8) in a group of whites. Bronte-Stewart et al. found similar differences in different racial groups in Cape Town,[752] using a copper sulfate SG method calibrated by a Kjeldahl assay. (Those with ESR of more than 8 mm/h were excluded.)

Cape Town racial group	N	Serum total protein
Europeans	133	73.8 ± 4.8 g/L
Coloreds	68	75.2 ± 4.4
Bantu	117	75.9 ± 5.0

A curious finding was reported by Luzzio,[753] who found higher serum levels in Eskimos than in Caucasian Americans, in summer, but that the difference disappeared when outdoor activity was minimal.

CHILDREN

In the first years of life, levels of serum total protein slowly increase, and most workers report that adult ranges are reached by about the age of 5[754,755,326,756] (Table 110).

NEONATES

Levels in the newborn are low, and mean levels increase with gestational age. Levels slowly increase during the first months of life (Table 111).

CORD BLOOD

Cord blood serum has a lower total protein level than serum from the mother. Stürmer et al. found a mean of 58.7 g/L in 72 cord sera.[759] This was confirmed by Sternberg et al.,[760] who found a mean of 59.8 g/L in 126 cord sera, compared with a mean of 68.8 g/L in serum from the mothers.

RANGE DURING PREGNANCY

There is a fall during the first trimester of pregnancy to a level of serum total protein of about 10 g/L below the nonpregnant level. This level is maintained throughout the rest of the pregnancy (Table 112). Not all proteins are affected similarly. For instance, alpha globulins increase, whereas there is a small fall in gamma globulins.

OTHER CHANGES

BLINDNESS

Hollwich and Dieckhues[329] showed that blind and partially sighted subjects had lower serum total protein levels than those with normal vision.

N	Subjects	Serum total protein (g/L)
220	Blind persons	62.5 ± 3.8
140	Vision less than 1/10	65.0 ± 4.7
50	Normal vision	68.2 ± 4.4

DRUGS AFFECTING SERUM TOTAL PROTEIN

Drugs stimulating protein synthesis, including corticosteroids, anabolic steroids, corticotrophin, androgens, growth hormone, insulin, and thyroid hormones, can cause an increase in serum total protein.[764] An increase can also result due to drugs increasing hemoconcentration, such as angiotensin and epinephrine[765] and diuretics. Mohamdi et al., in a study of 11 patients taking 100

TABLE 110.
Serum Total Protein in Children (in g/L)

Age (years)	Mean[a]	N[b]	Mean	SD	Male[c] Mean	Male[c] SD	Female Mean	Female SD	Male[d] N	Male[d] Median	Male[d] 2.5–97.5 percentile	Female N	Female Median	Female 2.5–97.5 percentile
.25	70.8	21	68.6	7.4										
.5	70.8	51	70.8	7.4										
.75	70.8	33	70.8	6.6										
1	70.8	28	72.2	7.5										
1.5	70.8	16	71.6	5.4										
3		11	72.0	7.0										
4					72	3.6	73	4.2						
5					72	3.6	73	4.2	81	67	61–74	93	63	68–75
6		13	71.7	4.6	72	3.6	73	4.2	150	63	61–75	136	68	62–76
7					72	3.6	73	4.2	147	68	62–76	160	69	63–76
8					72	3.6	73	4.2	151	69	62–75	155	71	64–77
9					72	3.6	73	4.2	149	70	64–76	155	71	65–78
10					72	3.6	73	4.2	156	71	64–77	156	71	65–77
11									199	70	65–78	158	72	67–79
12									178	70	63–76	165	70	64–78
13									157	69	63–76	144	71	66–77
Adults		28	76.9	4.9										

a From Rennie, J. B., *Arch. Dis. Child.*, 10, 415,1935.
b From Josephson, B. and Gyllenswärd, C., *Scand. J. Clin. Lab. Invest.*, 9, 29, 1957.
c From Cherian, A. G. and Hill, J. G., *Am. J. Clin. Path.*, 69, 24, 1978.
d From Haas, R. G., in *Paediatric Clinical Chemistry. Reference (Normal Values)*, 3rd ed., Meites, S., Ed., Washington, AACC Press, 1989, 228.

TABLE 111.
Serum Total Protein in Neonates and Infants (in g/L)

Reference	Subjects and method	N	Age (days)														
			0–1 mean	SD	1–2 mean	SD	2–3 mean	SD	3–4 mean	SD	≤14 range	21 range	28 range	70 range	150–210 mean	SD	Adult mean	SD
757	Micro-Kjeldahl method								55.5	5.8					62.9	3.3		
758	Full-term babies	108									40–70	47–74	37–54	60–74				
	Premature babies	20																
755	Newborn	92	71.6	9.6														
	Adults	28															76.9	4.9
181	White male	11–18	67	8.7	67	8.1	65	6.1	63	6.9								
	White female	9–17	67	7.7	65	6.1	67	5.5	63	5.4								
	Black male	7–11	66	10.2	65	8.3	58	6.7	60	5.3								
	Black female	7–10	69	7.6	65	6.1	67	5.5	63	5.4								
	Analysis by biuret method																	

TABLE 112.
Serum Total Protein During Pregnancy

Weeks of pregnancy	Mean[a]	Mean[b]	Mean[c]	Mean[d]	Mean[e]	SD
6				69.9	72.70	1.84
8				69.9		
10				69.9		
12				69.9	66.12	5.66
14	73.17	73	66	69.9		
16				69.6	56.24	5.66
18				68.9		
20				68.7	55.92	8.67
22						
24				67.2		
26	68.28	68	62		55.59	6.35
28						
30						
32				66.7	60.13	6.78
34					57.36	8.91
36						
38	64.80	66		66.7	58.96	6.20
Delivery			65			
1–6 days postpartum			72			
6–7 weeks postpartum						
Nonpregnant	71.00					

a   Normal healthy pregnancies. Biuret method.[759a]
b   Micro-Kjeldhal method.[760]
c   Nine subjects followed throughout pregnancy. Biuret method.[761]
d   Micro-Kjeldahl method.[762]
e   Estimated through each pregnancy. Biuret method.[763]

mg of hydrochlorthiazide daily,[365] found a mean serum total protein of 78.6 g/L (range of 61.9 to 105.8) compared with a mean of 75.5 g/L (range of 62.4 to 83.7) in controls. Oleson et al. found that bumetamide increased mean serum total protein from 68.9 to 75.9 g/L, after 3 months of treatment,[766] in 100 patients with organic heart disease.

Dale and Spivey showed that progesterone, when given by injection (Table 113),[767] increased serum total protein. Stringer et al. showed that gemfibrozil given for hyperlipidemia increased the mean level of serum total protein from 73.1 to 76.3 g/L in patients given 600 mg daily for 12 weeks.[768]

Falls in serum total protein levels may be caused by drugs affecting liver synthesis and drugs causing loss through the kidney,[769] such as mercury compounds or trimethadine. Carbamazepine is reported to cause a small fall. Dellaportus et al. found a fall from a mean of 75 g/L to a mean of 72 g/L after 2 years of treatment.[770]

McPherson et al. showed that oral contraceptives in a study of blood donors[142] reduced serum protein, with the effect decreasing with increasing age.

	Mean (g/L) at Age		
	18–25	26–35	36–45
On oral contraceptives	68.8	70.6	70.0
Not on oral contraceptives	72.0	72.5	68.4

TABLE 113.
Effect of Long-Acting Injectable Medroxy
Progesterone Acetate on Serum Total Protein[a]

Contraception	Mean SD
150 mg of Depoprovera[b] Injected every 3 months	76 ± 4.1
Oral contraceptive (Ovulen 21)[c]	70 ± 4.8
Nonoral contraception (IUCD)	72 ± 4.9

[a] From Dale, E. and Spivey, S. H., *Contraception*, 4, 241, 1976. With permission.
[b] Depoprovera — medroxy progesterone acetate (UpJohn Co, CA)
[c] Ovulin 21 — ethynodiol acetate + estriol (G. D. Searle Co, IL)

Chapter 9

ALBUMIN

Human albumin is a protein containing a single peptide chain of 573 amino acids, with a molecular weight of about 67,000 and a biologic half-life of about 21 days. Albumin variants have been described, and are reviewed by Tarnky.[771] About 10 g of albumin per day is produced by the healthy adult, synthesized exclusively in the liver.

Serum albumin concentration is the net result of a number of factors, such as the rate of synthesis and degradation and the plasma volume, which can individually, or in combination, be altered by disease.[772] The function of serum albumin is to contribute to the colloidal osmotic pressure that regulates the distribution of extracellular fluid, and to transport a number of substances, such as bilirubin, fatty acids, calcium, hormones, and some drugs.

ANALYTIC CONSIDERATIONS

ESTIMATION BY SALTING-OUT METHODS

For many years serum albumin was estimated by estimating the protein remaining after precipitating globulins with various salts. The earliest workers mixed diluted serum with saturated ammonium sulfate so that the final concentration was 2.05 M, and removed the precipitated globulins.[773,774]

Howe introduced sodium sulfate in the early 1920s to avoid the interference of ammonium sulfate with the Kjeldahl reaction.[775,776] A concentration of 1.50 M sodium sulfate was used in the final solution. It has now been shown that this concentration does not completely remove alpha globulin and that a final concentration of 1.80 M gives a measure of albumin closer to that obtained by electrophoretic methods.

The different concentrations of precipitating agents must be taken into account when considering figures in the early literature.

ELECTROPHORETIC METHODS

Electrophoretic techniques using either the Tiselius techniques or electrophoresis on paper, cellulose acetate, or other media, followed by estimation of the stained strip, usually by scanning, were used by a number of workers in the 1950s and 1960s. A disadvantage was that the various protein fractions often did not take up dye in proportion to their concentration thus introducing errors.

DYE-BINDING METHODS

Currently, most clinical laboratories use methods involving dyes that bind with albumin, but not the globulins, as they are more suitable for automatic analytic equipment.

Originally, azo dyes such as methyl orange and 2-(4′-hydroxybenzene azo)-benzoic acid (Haba dye) were used, but several problems were found. The dye varied according to its source. The albumin–dye complex was thermolabile; bilirubin, salicylates, and some other drugs interfered. Now the phenolphthalein dyes bromcresol green (BCG) and bromcresol purple (BCP) are used.

BCG, introduced by Bartholomew and Delaney in 1966,[777] was found by Northam and Widdowson[778] to give a good correlation with salt fractionation methods and to be suitable for use in continuous-flow analyzers. Later, Webster et al. compared the BCG method with the estimation of serum albumin immunologically[779] and concluded that the BCG method gave high results at low albumin concentrations. They suggested that samples with low albumin should be reanalyzed by a more specific method, for accurate results. Globulins have been shown to react slowly with BCG, compared with the almost-immediate reaction with albumin.[780] Doumas et al. suggested that the best procedure is to mix and read the absorption after not more than 30 s.[781]

Estimation with BCP was described by Louderbeck et al.[782] Pinnell and Northam showed that BCP reacted immediately with albumin and not with globulins.[783] The analysis for serum albumin compared well with an electroimmunoassay. BCP reacts much less strongly with equivalent quantities of bovine and other animal albumins, limiting the use of nonhuman control sera.

Wells et al., in a study of sera from 100 patients,[784] found good agreement between a BCP method and an immunologic assay, and low results using BCG; but in 19 pediatric patients on hemodialysis, agreement was not as good. Results by a BCG method were a mean of 6.3 g/L higher than by an immunologic method, and a mean of 7.1 g/L lower than by a BCP method.

STANDARDIZATION

Human serum albumin (HSA) is preferred to bovine serum albumin (BSA) as the standard for dye-binding methods, as the absorptivity of the dye–BSA complex is 2 to 3% higher compared with the dye–HSA complex.[781] BSA is also unsuitable for standardizing BCP methods. A satisfactory product must be used for standardization, as commercial preparations of crystalline albumin may contain aggregates that can introduce a bias.

A specially selected calibration procedure has been used to assign an albumin value to human serum pool IFCC 74/1, by an Expert Panel.[785] Hill found this pool to be satisfactory for assays using BCG,[786] but interference from the preservative phenyl methyl sulfonyl fluoride altered the dye-binding characteristics, making the pool unsuitable for dyes using BCP.

ACCURACY AND PRECISION

The accuracy of serum albumin estimation depends on the method used. Differences have been discussed when considering different methods. McMurray found the between-batch precision[787] to have a cv of about 4.5%. The precision of automatic assays is probably better than this.

SI UNITS

It is recommended by the IFCC Education Division Expert Panel that specific protein concentrations should be expressed in molar units if the relative molecular mass is known.[788] Conversion from mass to molar units can be made using a relative molecular mass of 67,000 for albumin. This may be preferred when the concentration of albumin is being compared with those of compounds such as bilirubin, which bind with albumin or with other specific proteins. Mass units must be used when comparing with total protein, as no molecular mass can be assigned to the heterogeneous mixture of macromolecules included in total protein. In this work, mass units will be used, since molar units are not yet generally used for albumin. If necessary, conversion can be made easily.

$$\text{grams per liter of albumin} = 10 \times \text{g/100 mL of albumin}$$
$$\text{micromoles per liter} = 149 \times \text{g/L}$$

INTERFERENCE WITH ANALYSIS

HEMOLYSIS

Salting-out and electrophoretic methods are not affected by hemolysis. Dye binding methods may be altered. For every gram per liter of hemoglobin in serum, apparent serum

TABLE 114.

**Effect of Bilirubin (Serum Level in μmol/L) on Albumin Assay
by Haba Dye and BCG Methods with Apparent Albumin[a] (in g/L)**

	Bilirubin					
	30.8	**61.6**	**82.1**	**128.3**	**167.8**	**249.7**
HABA dye	38	37	34	32	29	30
BCG	38	38	37	37	36	36

[a] From Leonard, P. J., et al., *Clin. Chim. Acta*, 35, 409, 1975.

albumin increases by about 1 g/L.[781] As a guide, serum hemoglobin of about 0.5 g/L is just visible in most sera.

BILIRUBIN

An increase in serum bilirubin gives a significant reduction in apparent serum albumin estimated by the HABA dye method.[789] The same authors found that there was no interference with the BCG method, but inspection of their results suggests that there may be a small fall in apparent albumin, with increased serum bilirubin level (Table 114). Doumas and Biggs found no difference when up to 342 μmol/L of bilirubin was added to serum, when using their analytical procedure.[781]

LIPEMIA

Slight or moderate lipemia does not introduce an error into the assay of serum albumin by dye-binding methods. A triglyceride concentration of more than 10 mmol/L gives a blank of about 1 g/L of albumin.[781]

OTHER INTERFERENCE WITH DYE-BINDING METHODS

A number of drugs are reported to interfere with dye-binding methods. Methods using HABA dye are affected by substances that compete for binding sites. Caraway reported that sulfonamides and salicylate affect the method.[295]

Underestimation of serum albumin, using the BCG method, was reported by Calvo et al.[790] when amounts of phenyl butazone and clofibrate, considered therapeutically attainable, were added to serum.

	μg/mL	Mean (g/L)
Phenyl butazone	0	30.0
	50	27.8
	100	27.4
	150	26.7
Clofibrate	50	27.1
	100	27.5
	150	25.9

Beng and Lim noted a high result in a patient on intravenous ampicillin,[791] which was not found when the same patient was taking the drug orally. The addition of 1 mg/mL of ampicillin to serum increased serum albumin by 1 g/L.

PREANALYTIC ERROR

COLLECTION OF THE SPECIMEN

Albumin is usually estimated in serum, because the same specimen taken for total protein

TABLE 115.
Effect of Heating to 56°C for 30 min on
Serum and Plasma Albumin

Reference	Plasma or serum	Mean change
102	Plasma	+1.50%
	Serum	+2.86%
311	Plasma	No significant change
103	Plasma	+10%
312	Plasma	+5.2%
	B-propriolactone	+0.3%

is used. The use of Liposol to decrease lipemia was shown, by Lacher and Elsea,[83] to affect serum albumin. Mean serum albumin of 26 randomly selected sera increased from 34.7 g/L to 39.3 g/L after shaking with Liposol, when analyzed using the Beckman Ideal analyzer.

ANTICOAGULANTS

Although one report claimed that heparin did not interfere with estimation of albumin using a dye-binding method,[781] several groups found that there is a significant effect.

Lum and Gambino, using a HABA dye method on the Technicon SMA 12/60 analyzer,[391] obtained mean levels 1.2 g/L higher than on corresponding heparinized plasma specimens. Bonvicini et al.[792] and Perry and Doumas,[793] investigating BCP and BCG methods, found that an insoluble precipitate formed, using heparinized plasma. After centrifugation, manual methods gave a low result compared with serum, and the turbidity gave a high result in automatic methods. The turbidity was prevented by adding hexadimethine.

Hill and Wells considered that the turbidity was due to precipitation of fibrinogen[794] and showed that this could be prevented by incorporating 0.15 M sodium chloride into the buffered dye reagent.

VENOUS STASIS

An increase in serum albumin similar to that found with serum total protein would be expected following venous stasis. Statland et al.[38] found an increase of 3.3%, or a little over 1 g/L, due to hemoconcentration following application of a tourniquet for 3 min.

SAMPLE STABILITY

There is little change in serum albumin levels after periods of storage if the sample is tightly capped to avoid evaporation. Hanok and Kuo stored reconstituted lyophilized control serum at 15°C.[95] Analysis for albumin showed an apparent increase after 10 days of storage which was thought to be due to bacterial contamination.

Heating to 56°C

Several groups have investigated the effect of heating serum or plasma to 56°C to minimize the risk from HIV-positive samples (Table 115). Specimens of heparinized plasma become turbid due to a precipitate of fibrinogen. No explanation has been suggested for the apparent increase in serum albumin after heat treatment, which was found by two groups. The use of B-propriolactone has little effect.

PHYSIOLOGIC CHANGES

POSTURE

Serum albumin falls, in a way similar to total protein, when a subject moves from an upright

TABLE 116.
Change in Serum Albumin in a Group of Americans
Relocated from a Temperate Zone to the Arctic[a] (in g/L)

Month	Location		Mean
February	In Virginia		43.1
May	In Greenland soon after arrival		44.9
August	In Greenland after acclimatization		47.4
Summer	Eskimos in Greenland	Male	46.3
		Female	47.3
Winter		Male	48.7
		Female	45.9

[a] From Luzzio, A. L., *J. Appl. Physiol.*, 21, 685, 1966.

to a supine position. Statland et al. found that mean levels of serum albumin were 3% higher when subjects were standing than when they were sitting, and 6.7% higher when they were sitting than when they were lying down.[165] As noted under total protein, Whitehead et al. found that serum total protein and albumin changed by about the same amount,[739] suggesting no change in globulin, whereas Aull and McCord found that albumin and globulin changed similarly.[740] The results obtained by Statland et al. suggest a change in total protein of 8.6% in moving from lying down to standing,[38] and an alteration in serum albumin of 9.7%, suggesting that albumin and globulin vary similarly.

MEALS

There may be a small change in serum albumin after a meal, but reports are confusing. Statland et al. found no change,[38] but Annino and Relman[109] and Werner[795] reported a decrease of 1 to 2%. Steinmetz et al. found a similar fall if the meal was not strictly standardized,[796] but noted a rise of 1.7% after a standard meal. Two hundred office workers had a mean serum albumin of 44.70 ± 3.40 g/L at 12 noon, and a mean of 45.50 ± 3.50 at 2 p.m., after a 700-cal meal.

STRESS

Severe stress has been shown to increase serum albumin; this is linked to hemoconcentration and may be related to muscular tension. Dugue et al. found little change in mild stress,[745] but in a group of young healthy subjects, mean serum albumin in blood taken immediately before a first parachute jump was almost 10% higher than the mean of samples taken some days previously.

SEASONAL VARIATION

Lellouch and Claude found a tendency for serum albumin to increase in summer.[746] Others, however, have reported lower levels in spring and summer than in winter, although changes found by Gidlow et al. did not reach statistical significance.[691] Lyngbye and Krøll, estimating by immunoelectrophoresis,[797] found mean levels of 44.6 g/L in winter and 42.6 g/L in summer, in 149 males and 111 females from a group of ear and eye outpatients taking no medication. Similar results were reported by Ljundhall et al.,[128] who found serum albumin 2 to 3% higher in winter than in summer. The reason for any change is not known.

ENVIRONMENTAL CHANGE

Luzzio reported a change in serum albumin when a group of Americans were relocated from a temperate zone to the Arctic.[753] When 14 males and 14 females moved from Virginia to Greenland, the levels increased by about 10% and, after acclimatization, were similar to those found in Eskimo subjects (Table 116).

RANGE IN HEALTHY SUBJECTS

WITHIN- AND BETWEEN-PERSON VARIATION

One of the earliest reports on serum albumin levels was in 1903 by Lewinski,[798] who reported a range of 33.0 to 44.7 g/L in three cases. Higher levels in men than in women were probably first noted by Salveson in 1926,[747] who reported a range of 39.5 to 52.4 g/L in 16 "normal" men and 37.7 to 48.0 g/L in 16 "normal" women. Tables 117 and 118 show ranges found in several large studies. The differences may reflect the methods used or the use of plasma instead of serum.

It is agreed that there is a small fall with age in both men and women. Several workers have said that the distribution is approximately gaussian.

Although most textbooks generally agree on the range (Table 119), an overall range is usually given without any differentiation for age, sex, posture, or method. A detailed review of ranges found by a number of groups using different methods, with a comment on age differences, is given in the textbook edited by Henry, Cannon, and Winkleman.[803] The ranges appear to be generally lower than those of ambulatory subjects in Tables 117 and 118, suggesting that posture has not been standardized.

Between-Day Variation

Serum albumin remains reasonably constant over a period in an individual, with a coefficient of variation similar to that found in total protein (Table 120).

RACIAL DIFFERENCES

Several groups have reported different serum albumin levels in various racial groups. Rawnsley refers to studies in Africa, Jamaica, and the United States reporting lower albumin and higher globulins in blacks compared with whites.[749] Milam, using oxalated plasma,[751] found a mean serum albumin of 46.0 g/L (range of 38.4 to 53.1) in white subjects compared with 44.0 (range of 37.7 to 50.3) in black subjects. Bronte-Stewart et al.,[752] in Cape Town, found serum albumin (estimated by electrophoresis, staining with azo carmine) and elution a little lower in Bantu subjects than in European or Cape colored subjects.

Racial group	Serum albumin (g/L)	N
European	5.31 ± 0.46	46
Cape colored	5.32 ± 0.43	68
Bantu	5.15 ± 0.61	117

Those with an ESR of more than 8 mm/h were excluded. This included 30% of the Bantu subjects.

CHILDREN

Early reports suggest that serum albumin increases after birth and reaches adult levels after 6 to 12 months of life. Haas, in a large study, found that there is an increase throughout childhood in both girls and boys (Table 121).[804]

NEONATES

Serum albumin at birth is a function of gestational age[805,806] (Table 122). The newborn baby experiences a transfer of intravascular liquid to the interstitial space. This leads to hemoconcentration and an increase in serum albumin during the first hours of life. By the fourth day the level falls by about 40% and then remains constant for several months.[857]

TABLE 117.
Serum and Plasma Albumin Levels in Healthy Men (in g/L)

Reference		<20	Age (years) 21-25	26-30	31-35	36-40	41-45	46-50	51-55	56-60	61-65	66-70	71-75	76-80
140[a]	Range		32.86-43.48	32.86-43.48	32.40-43.03	32.40-43.03	31.95-42.57	31.95-42.57	31.50-42.12	31.50-42.12	31.40-41.67	31.40-41.67	30.59-41.21	30.59-41.21
141[b]	Mean		44.1	44.1	43.5	43.5	42.9	42.9	42.4	42.4	41.9	41.9	41.3	41.3
	Range		40.1-48.1	40.1-48.1	39.3-47.7	39.3-47.7	38.7-47.1	38.7-47.1	48.0-46.8	48.0-46.8	37.5-46.3	37.5-46.3	35.3-47.3	35.3-47.3
142[c]	Mean	48.5	48.5	47.5	47.5	45.9	45.9	44.5	44.5	43.4	43.4			
	N	31	77	63	54	35	32	29	23	27	11			
Coventry[d]	Mean	46.71	45.99	45.81	45.74	44.46	43.63	44.17	44.00	43.01	43.64			
	SD	1.49	1.81	1.77	2.01	2.01	2.06	1.98	2.11	2.22	1.57			
	Range	44-49	42-50	42-50	41-49	38-48	40-47	41-50	40-57	38-48	41-46			

[a] 278 Caucasian employees and subjects without complaints undergoing routine checkups. Fasting and recumbent. Analysis by paper electrophoresis followed by staining with amidoschwartz.

[b] 3700 males attending a well-population screening center. Exclusively Caucasian. Estimation using bromcresol green.

[c] About 500 blood donors. Specimen taken into lithium heparin. Analysis using a continuous-flow analyzer and a bromcresol green method.

[d] Healthy hospital staff. Specimen collected seated. Analysis using bromcresol purple, using the American Monitor "Parallel" analyzer Range given 2.5-97.5 percentile

TABLE 118.
Serum and Plasma Albumin in Healthy Women (in g/L)

Reference		<20	21–25	26–30	31–35	36–40	41–45	46–50	51–55	56–60	61–65	66–70	71–75	76–80
140	Range		32.86–43.48	32.86–43.48	32.40–43.05	32.40–43.05	31.95–42.57	31.95–42.57	31.50–42.12	31.50–42.12	31.40–41.67	31.40–41.67	30.59–41.21	30.59–41.21
	Mean		43.0	43.0	42.4	42.4	42.0	42.0	41.8	41.8	41.5	41.5	41.3	41.3
141	Range		38.6–47.4	38.6–47.4	37.8–47.0	37.8–47.0	37.4–46.6	37.4–46.6	37.8–41.8	37.8–41.8	37.1–45.9	37.1–45.9	37.1–45.5	37.1–45.5
142[a]	Mean	46.7	46.7	45.3	45.3	44.8	44.8	44.1	44.1	44.7	44.1			
Coventry	N	650	575	311	309	255	252	172	112	83	17			
	Mean	44.78	44.52	44.14	43.95	43.69	43.25	42.59	43.35	42.62	42.75			
	SD	2.46	2.30	2.51	2.41	2.09	2.19	2.12	2.04	2.37	2.65			
	Range	39–49	40–49	39–49	39–49	39–48	39–47	38–46	39–47	39–48	39–49			

[a] Subjects taking oral contraceptives excluded.

TABLE 119.
Range for Serum Albumin (in g/L) in Some Well-Known Textbooks,
Showing that Most Give a Lower Limit Less than that Found
in Ambulatory Subjects

Reference	Range	Comment
149	34–67	
152	36–58	
799	38–46	42 normal persons. Analysis biuret after globulin ppt with 20.8% sulfate, 7% sulfite
800	35–55	Analysis by paper electrophoresis
801	42–55	Distribution normal
802	38–46	
159	37–53	
162	32–50	
788	35–50	

TABLE 120.
Intraindividual Variation of Serum Albumin

Reference	Subjects	Method	N	Individual variation (mean cv)	Comment
163	Male and female white and black subjects 20–59 years old	Fasting specimen taken at 9 a.m. weekly for 10–12 weeks.	68	3.9%	After allowing for analytic variation of 3.3%
164	White doctors	One fasting specimen taken weekly for 10 weeks. Stored frozen and all analyzed on same day	9	2.8%	After allowing for analytic variation
165	Male students 21–27 years old	Five fasting samples taken within 3 weeks. Analysis using the "Autochemist" analyzer.	18	2.8%	

RANGE DURING PREGNANCY

After the first trimester there is a fall in serum albumin throughout the pregnancy, with levels at term 5 to 10 g/L lower than nonpregnant levels (Table 123).

OTHER CHANGES

BODY WEIGHT

Wingerd and Sponzilli, found serum albumin to decrease approximately linearly with an increase in body weight, in a study of about 5000 women.[807] The mean in those with a body weight 80% of the mean for the population was 41.5 g/L and was 39.5 g/L in those with a body weight 130% of the mean for the population.

SMOKING

Serum albumin is lower in smokers than in nonsmokers (Table 124). This may be due to the antidiuretic effect of nicotine.

Mean serum albumin estimated by an immunodiffusion method was also found, by Das,[808] to be lower in smokers than in nonsmokers (Table 125). It is thought that this and other changes in serum protein may represent a compensatory mechanism to the inflammatory condition.

TABLE 121.
Serum Albumin in Children[a] (in g/L)

	Boys			Girls		
Age (years)	N	50 percentile	2.5–97.5 percentile	N	50 percentile	2.5–97.5 percentile
5	68	44	39–48	83	44	41–48
6	138	45	40–49	120	45	42–48
7	130	44	41–48	146	45	40–48
8	142	44	39–48	132	45	41–50
9	131	45	41–49	135	46	43–50
10	140	45	42–50	123	45	41–49
11	171	45	42–48	130	45	42–50
12	170	46	41–50	162	46	43–51
13	148	46	42–52	143	46	42–51
14	130	47	43–53	128	48	43–53
15	103	48	43–53	134	48	44–53
16	78	49	42–53	105	48	44–53
17	78	49	43–55	76	48	43–54

[a] From Haas, R. G., in *Paediatric Clinical Chemistry Reference (Normal Values),* 3rd ed., Washington, AACC Press, 1989, 38. With permission.

TABLE 122.
Serum Albumin (in g/L) in Neonates of
Different Gestational Age

Gestation (weeks)	At birth mean[a]	N	At 24 h range[b]
27	26	4	15.1–26.7
28		7	14.3–28.7
29		5	14.3–23.5
30	24	10	14.7–26.3
31			
32	30	6	18.8–25.2
33		5	19.0–27.8
34	32		18.4–30.4
35			
43	45		22 full-term babies at 6 days 24.9–33.5 BCP method

[a] From Karlsson, B., et al., *Acta Paediatr. Scand.,* 61, 133, 1972.
[b] From Fleetwood, J. A., et al., in *Paediatric Clinical Chemistry, Reference (Normal Values),* 3rd ed., AACC, 1989, 41.

TABLE 123.
Serum Albumin (in g/L) During Pregnancy

Weeks of pregnancy	Mean[a]	Mean[b]	Mean[c]	Mean[d]	SD	N	Mean[e]
4–8	43.1	43.28	42.0	36.90	5.66	2	
9–12	43.1	43.28	42.0	31.22	5.64	5	38
13–14	43.1	43.28	42.0	25.70	5.13	10	
15–16	43.3		42.0				
17–18	44.0	37.62	39.1	26.21	5.75	14	
19–20	41.3	37.62	39.1				
21–22	41.3	37.62	39.1	26.69	5.51	12	
23–24	39.5	37.62	39.1	27.49	5.05	12	
25–26	39.5	37.62	33.4	27.18	4.77	9	
27–28	40.9	28.82	33.4				
29–30	40.9	28.82	33.4	24.49	5.98	10	30
31–32	40.9	28.82	33.4				
33–34	38.1	28.82	33.4	23.96	5.80	7	
35–36	38.1	28.82	33.4				
37–38	38.1	28.82	33.4	22.10	1.92	11	
39–40	38.1	28.82	33.4				30
1–6 days postpartum							34
6–7 weeks postpartum				32.70	5.01	9	38
Nonpregnant		41.86					

a Method based on that of Howe using 22.2% sodium sulfate to precipitate globulin.[762]
b Normal healthy pregnancies. Estimation by paper electrophoresis and optical scanning of bromphenol blue-stained strip.[759]
c Estimation by optical scanning of azocarmine-stained strip after paper electrophoresis.[760]
d Estimation by paper electrophoresis followed by optical scanning of bromphenol blue-stained strip.[763]
e Nine subjects throughout pregnancy. Paper electrophoresis followed by densitometry of bromphenol-stained strip.[761]

DRUGS AFFECTING SERUM ALBUMIN

Hepatotoxic Drugs

A number of drugs affect serum albumin, as a consequence of hepatic toxicity.[56] In some, such as methyl dopa, pyrazinamide, niacin, and nitrofurantoin, the effect is reported in individual cases, and in others the hepatic damage is found in a significant number of those given the drug, as with asparagine, azothiaprine cyclophosphamide, and hydralazine.

Estrogen

A fall in serum albumin is found in subjects taking estrogens. Several groups have shown this in those taking oral contraceptives (Table 126). It has been demonstrated that the progesteronic component has little effect.

Ibuprofen

Treatment with ibuprofen has been noted to result in a fall in serum albumin.[811] Using a bromcresol green method before treatment with 600 to 1600 mg/day, mean serum albumin was 4 g/L (SD 6.35); after treatment for up to 12 weeks, the mean was 37.5 g/L (SD 5.10).

Gemfibrozil

Stringer et al. found a small but significant increase in serum albumin in 27 hyperlipidemic patients,[812] age 35 to 70 years, with occlusive peripheral arterial disease, who were given a placebo for 2 weeks followed by 600 mg of gemfibrozil twice daily for 12 weeks. Serum albumin changed from 44.1 ± 4.0 g/L to 46.0 ± 3.2 g/L.

TABLE 124.
The Effect of Cigarette Smoking on Mean Serum Albumin (in g/L)

References		Age (years)	Male		Female	
			Smokers	Nonsmokers	Smokers	Nonsmokers
47	Subjects taking a health examination. Analysis by a HABA dye method.	15–19	42.2	41.7	39.3	40.0
		20–29	42.8	42.9	38.8	38.9
		30–39	42.5	42.9	39.4	39.8
		40–49	41.3	42.8	39.4	39.8
		50–59	40.7	41.7	39.6	40.2
		60–69	39.3	40.6	39.5	40.0
		70–79	38.4	39.2	39.1	38.8
808	Women smoking more than 1 1/2 packs a day		Mean level 0.6 g/L lower in smokers than in nonsmokers			

TABLE 125.
Effect of Smoking on Serum Albumin[a] (in g/L)

Subjects	Age (years)		N	Mean	Range
Smokers 90% smoking more	20–40 Median 32	Male	32	31.1	25.5–37.8
than 20 cigarettes per day		Female	32	30.5	25.0–46.0
Nonsmokers	20–40 Median 29	Male	20	39.0	31.7–61.0
		Female	12	34.5	26.0–42.6

[a] From Das, I., *Clin. Chim. Acta,* 153, 9, 1985. Estimation using an immunodiffusion method.

TABLE 126.
Serum Albumin (in g/L) in Subjects Taking Oral Contraceptives (O.C.)

Reference	Method	Dosage		N	Mean	SD
			Before		32.9	3.0
809	Analysis bycellulose acetate	Placebo	After		33.4	3.9
	electrophoresis staining with	0.1 mg mestranol	Before		32.3	4.0
	Ponceau S and densitometry	+ 1 mg norethindrone	After		31.1	3.4
	Oral contraceptives taken 20 days	0.1 mg mestranol	Before		32.1	3.6
	each cycle for 3 months		After		27.0	4.1
		10 mg medroxy	Before		36.4	3.0
		Progesterone acetate	After		33.3	5.5
810		Control group		12	41	3
		Ethinyl estradiol				
		10 μg daily		12	38	3
		20 μg daily		10	35	3
		50 μg daily		11	33	2
		75 μg daily		10	32	3
		Ethinyl estradiol +				
		norethisterone acetate				
		50 μg + 1 mg daily		12	34	3
		50 μg + 3 mg daily		12	33	2
767		150 mg depoprovera		133	41	4.2
		injected every 3 months				
		Oral contraceptive		117	35	3.5
		(Ovulen 21)				
		Nonoral contraception		147	39	3.4
		(IUCD)				
142	Blood donors	Taking oral contraceptives				
		Age 18–25			43.7	
		26–35			44.4	
		36–45			41.8	
		Not taking oral contraceptives				
		Age 18–25			46.7	
		26–35			45.3	
		36–45			44.8	

Chapter 10

TOTAL BILIRUBIN

Bilirubin occurs in blood, either free or as water-soluble conjugates, and is transported bound to serum albumin. The earliest attempts to estimate bilirubin in serum used the Gmelin reaction with nitric acid.[813] Van den Bergh, in 1913,[814] applied the Ehrlich diazo reaction to the analysis, and this became the basis of most methods. However, accurate methods were not developed until means of avoiding the precipitation of protein became available in the 1930s.

Total bilirubin is the sum of free bilirubin and conjugated bilirubin. Conjugated bilirubin reacts promptly with diazo reagents at an alkaline pH and has been termed "direct-reacting" bilirubin. Free or unconjugated bilirubin, which has been termed "indirect-reacting" bilirubin, reacts slowly with diazo reagents, and the reaction only goes to completion in the presence of an accelerator.

ANALYTIC CONSIDERATIONS

Methods of estimation of total bilirubin are based either on the conversion to azobilirubin followed by spectrophotometry, or by measurement of the absorption of bilirubin itself at 450 to 470 nm.

Early diazo methods included a protein precipitation stage using ethyl alcohol, which also accelerated the conversion to azobilirubin. Adsorption of azobilirubin onto the precipitate gave low results. Methods were developed to avoid protein precipitation, using compounds such as methanol, urea and benzoate, caffeine and benzoate, diphyllin acetate, or dimethyl sulfoxide as accelerators. A good account of the methods available is given by Winkelman et al.,[815] and a critical review is given by Billing et al.[816]

Most laboratories using the diazo method use diazotized sulfanilic acid to react with bilirubin, although diazotized dichloraniline has been used. Modern discrete analyzers frequently use diazotized 2.4 or 2.5 dichloraniline, as the reagents are more stable.

Some methods measure absorption of red azobilirubin at an acid pH, but measurement of the blue dye obtained under alkaline conditions has the advantages that the color is more intense and the absorption curve is not affected by the protein matrix.

The preferred manual method is based on the procedure of Jendrassik and Gröf.[817] A procedure similar to that of Michäelson et al.[818,819] was recommended by Billing et al.[816] Diazotized sulfanilic acid at a pH near 6.5 is used with caffeine and sodium benzoate as accelerator. Occasional problems due to turbidity are minimized by diphyllin, and the pH is adjusted to near 13 with alkaline tartrate before spectrophotometry.

The instability of bilirubin, and the varying purity of available preparations, makes the satisfactory calibration of methods for serum bilirubin difficult. Problems associated with the preparation of the calibrant are reviewed in detail by Turnell.[820]

Direct spectrophotometric estimation is based on use of the maximum absorbance at about 460 nm.[821] Corrections can be applied for hemoglobin derivatives, carotenoids, and turbidity. The procedure is most used for serum bilirubin estimation in neonates with hemoglobin derivatives, the main substances requiring correction. It has been suggested that bilirubin and conjugates of bilirubin have absorption maxima at different wavelengths. In the first edition of his book, in 1974, Henry quoted work in support of this.[822] However, in the second edition, in 1974,[815] Winklelman et al. stated that they believed that the available evidence suggested that the different bilirubin compounds found in serum have the same absorption peak.

ACCURACY AND PRECISION

The average between-batch cv for serum bilirubin estimation is approximately 6% for manual methods and about 4% for automatic methods, at 50 μmol/L.[823] This is in line with the median imprecision in United Kingdom laboratories, quoted by Fraser as 2.6 μmol/L,[824] without giving the bilirubin level.

Blijenberg et al. found the between-laboratory precision for the estimation in neonates in Holland[825] to be about 8% at approximately 300 μmol/L. It is important to be aware of the precision of estimations in the neonate, as serial estimations are frequently performed, and important clinical decisions are based on the results.

SI UNITS

To convert serum total bilirubin from mass to molar units,

$$\text{mg/100 mL} \times 17.1 = \text{μmol/L}$$

INTERFERENCE WITH ANALYSIS

HEMOLYSIS

Engel showed that the presence of hemoglobin in serum gives a low apparent bilirubin content when assayed using the diazo reaction.[826] Table 127 shows the effect on five methods found by Watson,[827] who concluded that the method of Lathe and Ruthven[830] was probably the method of choice for the estimation of serum bilirubin in neonates by a diazo method.

Later, Michäelson, in a modification of the Jendrassik and Gröf method,[818] used diphyllin as an activator and eliminated the effect of hemoglobin by adding ascorbic acid after the diazo reaction. Billing et al. adapted this method,[816] giving a satisfactory procedure. Schull-Lees et al. explained the mechanism by showing that the conversion of oxyhemoglobin to acid hematin under the assay conditions is associated with rapid destruction of bilirubin,[832] possibly by an oxidative reaction involving hydrogen peroxide. The effect could be prevented by adding a reducing agent.

SERUM FROM UREMIC PATIENTS

Andrews, in 1924,[833] reported a peculiar diazo reaction in sera from uremic patients. Most laboratory workers familiar with the manual method of analysis will have observed the brownish color obtained when diazo reagent is added to certain sera. Harrison and Bromfield believed that the color was due to a reaction with an indoxyl compound that they presumed to be indican or a conjugate of indican.[834] Many years later, in 1979, Stone et al. reinvestigated and could find no abnormality when testing serum with added indican,[835] using a modification of the Jendrassik and Gröf method. The cause of this reaction remains uncertain.

OTHER INTERFERING SUBSTANCES

In vitro experiments using the Technicon SMA 12/60 analyzer, by Singh et al.,[82] showed that methyl dopa at concentrations thought to occur in serum gave a small increase of about 1 μmol/L in apparent serum bilirubin levels, which was considered to be due to a colored product obtained by reaction of the drug with sulfanilic acid. The change is insufficient to affect interpretation of the result.

Stone et al. found that 16 of 132 chronic dialysis patients had an apparent increase in serum bilirubin,[835] using a method based on the Jendrassik and Gröf method. Interference was also demonstrated using the Malloy and Evelyn procedure. A spectrophotometric peak at 540 nm was found, distinct from that given by diazotized bilirubin at 600 nm. Propranolol was the only drug given in common to all 16 patients, and the peak was not found in serum from uremic

TABLE 127.
The Effect of Various Amounts of Hemoglobin (g/L) in Serum
on Some Methods of Estimation of Serum Bilirubin[a]

Reference	Method		Serum hemoglobin			
			<0.3	2	10	40
828	Diazo and benzoate-urea	Apparent bilirubin[b]	8.55	0	—	—
			171	73.5	49.6	0
			342	305	265	154
829	Based on Powell using a blank correction	Apparent bilirubin	8.55	5.13	0	—
			85.5	66.7	47.9	—
			171	125	111	—
830	Diazo and methanol	Apparent bilirubin	8.55	8.55	10.3	—
			85.5	75.2	73.5	82.1
			171	164	168	154
			342	342	359	300
831	Diazo and methanol with blank correction	Apparent bilirubin	8.55	8.55	6.84	—
			85.5	66.7	80.4	66.7
			171	161	145	117
			342	339	306	311
817	Diazo and methanol. Color measured at alkaline pH.	Apparent bilirubin	8.55	5.13	13.7	1.71
			85.5	71.8	56.4	46.2
			171	159	137	101

[a] From Watson, D., *Clin. Chim. Acta,* 5, 613, 1960.
[b] Apparent bilirubin in μmol/L.

patients not on propranolol. The effect was considered to be a phenolic metabolite of propranolol. Serial determinations gave varied results and potentially misleading information.

Serum from patients given dextran may give a turbidity when methods using methanol, ethanol, or isopropanol are used.[836] No turbidity is given using the Jendrassik and Gröf method, as alcohols are not used.

Analytic interference with drugs such as phenazopyridine, rifampicin, theophylline, and caffeine and with substances such as histidine, tyrosine, vitamin A, and xanthophylline is mentioned by Notler.[837]

PREANALYTIC ERROR

COLLECTION OF THE SPECIMEN
The specimen for serum total bilirubin estimation is usually collected without any special preparation of the patient, although factors such as the time of day and posture have a small effect on the level. Serum or plasma from anticoagulated blood can be used.

VENOUS STASIS
As bilirubin is transported bound to protein, excessive venous stasis may be expected to alter the serum level. Notler found that application of a tourniquet for 3 min,[837] instead of 1 min, increased serum bilirubin by over 8%.

Contamination
Soft glass pipettes used to transfer sera were investigated by McCormick et al.,[395] who found surface contamination with a hydroxide equivalent of 0.1 to 0.2 μmol per pipette. Bilirubin dissolved in chloroform decreased by 5% for each pipetting, due to the reaction with alkali. No experiments were performed on sera where the effect would be expected to be less

TABLE 128.
Serum Total Bilirubin (in μmol/L) After a Low-Calorie Diet

Reference	Subjects	Diet	N	Increase after mean	Maximum range
842	Normal subjects	300-cal diet	8	6.84	
	Mild unconjugated hyperbilirubinemia		7	51.28	56.43–123.12
843	Healthy subjects	400-cal per	12	5.2	
	Gilbert's syndrome	day for 48 h	12	29.0	
	Liver disease		12	2.5	
	Hemolysis		12	3.4	

due to buffering. Differences can be important if standards in chloroform are used for comparison.

SAMPLE STABILITY

Both direct- and indirect-reacting pigments are dehydrogenated on exposure to light, particularly wavelengths between 400 and 600 nm, leading to low results. Cremar et al. found that the indirect-reacting pigment is two to three times more sensitive to light than is the direct reacting pigment;[838] they reported that serum bilirubin may fall by 50% after exposure to sunlight for 1 h. After collection, bilirubin in serum is preserved if cells are not removed by centrifugation. After separation, samples must be kept from exposure to light.

For optimal stability, darkness and a low temperature are necessary. Samples stored in the dark are stable for at least 3 months if frozen and for 4 to 7 days at 4°C.

Heating to 56°C

Investigations of the effect of heating samples to 56°C for 30 min to minimize the risk from HIV-positive samples have shown different results that are difficult to explain. Ball found a fall of 19.4% in serum total bilirubin,[312] whereas Gouldie et al. reported a small rise of 2.3%.[101] Collinson et al.[103] noted a small negative bias of 3 μmol/L on samples containing 3 to 376 μmol/L of bilirubin.

PHYSIOLOGIC CHANGES

FASTING

An increase in serum total bilirubin due to fasting was noted as long ago as 1906 by Gilbert and Hersher,[839] who said that the level was maximal in normal adults after an overnight fast. A study of ten healthy individuals, by Broun et al in 1925,[840] found that seven had a higher serum bilirubin when fasting than after a high-fat breakfast. This was confirmed 2 years later by Perkin,[841] who observed a fall of about 8 mmol/L during the glucose tolerance test. A much greater rise is reported in patients with Gilbert's syndrome, and a test for the condition has been suggested based on the change when given a low-calorie diet (Table 128). Some workers have doubted the efficacy of a fasting diet as a diagnostic test for Gilbert's syndrome. This can be explained by the work of Dawson et al.,[844] who showed examined groups of patients with unexplained hyperbilirubinemia. One with electron microscopic abnormalities of liver biopsy showed a mean increase of about 100% when given a fasting diet, whereas others with no abnormality showed a mean increase of about 40%, similar to that found in normal subjects.

The increase has been linked to lipid withdrawal. Gollan et al. studied 29 patients with Gilbert's syndrome.[845] Following a normal diet, the patients received glucose intravenously for 2 days; plasma bilirubin increased by a mean 127%. Administration of intralipid and a return to a normal diet both caused a prompt return to previous levels. Then giving a "standard fasting diet" containing 1.6 mJ (400 cal) for 2 days, a mean increase of 135% was observed. On increasing the lipid content from 33 to 85%, the mean increase in serum bilirubin fell to 49%. It can be concluded that there is an increase of about 5 to 7 μmol/L on fasting in the healthy adult and a greater increase in some patients with Gilbert's syndrome, which is linked with lipid withdrawal. The uncertainty concerning the efficiency of using this response as a diagnostic test for Gilbert's syndrome could be linked to the presence of two groups of patients: some with, and others without, liver changes.

EXERCISE

A small increase in bilirubin has been found following severe exercise. Riley et al. estimated plasma bilirubin in five trained athletes running a marathon,[317] and reported an increase in the mean level from 9.6 to 15 μmol/L at the end of the run.

SUNBATHING

Broderson et al. suggested that exposure to sun reduced serum total bilirubin,[846] following a study of six healthy women that was designed to investigate the influence of steroid hormones as an explanation of why lower levels of bilirubin are found in women than in men. No variation during the menstrual cycle was found, but it was observed that the mean value on Monday was lower than that on Wednesday or Friday, in each of the 4 weeks studied. On enquiry it was found that each subject had spent several hours sunbathing on the Saturday and Sunday of each of the weeks. Either irradiation of the skin or increased ACTH during sunbathing were proposed as the cause. Irradiation of neonates, to reduce serum bilirubin, has been used therapeutically, and it may be that the same effect occurred in these adults.

POSTURE

Bilirubin in serum is protein bound, and changes with the posture of the subject can be expected. Dixon and Paterson, in a study of eight male and four female healthy students,[591] found mean serum total bilirubin was 10.10 μmol/L after the subjects stood for 30 min and 8.61 μmol/L after lying down for 60 min. This small change is unlikely to affect the interpretation, but indicates that reference intervals should be obtained using standard conditions.

RANGE IN HEALTHY SUBJECTS

WITHIN- AND BETWEEN-PERSON VARIATION

The level of bilirubin in the serum of healthy individuals has been studied for many years. In 1905 Gilbert and Hersher found a range of "0.25 to 3.57 centigrams per liter" (0.15 to 6.1 μmol/L).[839] Since methods avoiding protein precipitation were developed during the 1930s, there has been reasonable agreement on the range, and most reports state that the distribution is skewed.

Tables 129 and 130 show ranges found in several large series that considered levels at different ages in men and women. Mean values show higher levels in men than in women, with little change with age. The upper limit is difficult to define, reflecting the tail of a skewed distribution, the need to standardize collection procedures, the different composition of groups, and the sensitivity of the percentile method to outliers.

In a survey of samples from 50 male and 50 female staff, taken 1 h after breakfast, Vaughan and Haslewood, in 1938,[849] found a range up to 29.07 μmol/L, with 93% between 3.42 and 13.68 μmol/L. In a later study (by Bailey et al.[850]) of 18,454 men and 5471 women attending a screening center, the 98th percentile was found to be 25 μmol/L for men and 19 μmol/L for women. Levels given in commonly used textbooks have often suggested that the upper limit

TABLE 129.
Serum Total Bilirubin in Healthy Males (in µmol/L)

Reference		<20	21–25	26–30	31–35	36–40	41–45	46–50	51–55	56–60	61–65	66–70	71–75	76–80	81–85	86–90	91–95
847	Mean	11.80	12.31	12.31	11.11	11.11	10.60	10.60	10.43	10.43	9.41	9.41	11.46	11.46			
141[a]	Mean		10.94	10.94	11.11	11.11	10.77	10.77	10.43	10.43	10.26	10.26	11.63	11.63			
848[b]	N	68	351	513	522	473	520	696	696	786	907	907	794	662	304	124	20
	Mean	9.23	10.60	10.43	9.58	9.06	9.06	9.23	9.23	9.06	8.89	8.89	8.89	8.72	8.72	8.21	7.87
	2.5–97.5 percentile	2.05–20.50	2.91–27.87	1.54–29.07	2.56–23.94	2.22–19.67	3.08–19.67	2.05–19.84	2.39–20.35	2.39–20.35	2.22–18.64	2.22–18.64	2.39–19.84	2.91–18.64	2.22–1.17	1.37–15.22	0.34–14.54
Coventry[c]	N	122	296	280	152	125	113	106	82	67							
	Mean	11.2	11.4	10.3	10.6	9.2	9.9	10.7	9.45	9.15							
	2.5–97.5 percentile	5–22.5	6–30	5–30	6–31.5	2.5–30	5–31	4.5–30	3.5–22	5–29							

[a] Men from a well-person's clinic.
[b] From outpatients, excluding those with liver disease and hemolysis.
[c] Healthy hospital staff, as described in Chapter 7.

TABLE 130.
Serum Bilirubin in Healthy Females (in µmol/L)

Reference		<20	21–25	26–30	31–35	36–40	41–45	46–50	51–55	56–60	61–65	66–70	71–75	76–80	81–85	86–90	91–95
847	Mean	10.43	8.72	8.72	7.89	7.89	8.04	8.04	7.87	7.87	8.21	8.21					
141	Mean		9.41	9.41	8.72	8.72	9.23	9.23	8.89	8.89	8.38	8.38					
848	N	305	843	1023	996		986	946	987	1127	1088		1183	1052	469	171	39
	Mean	7.18	7.52	7.52	7.35		7.01	6.84	6.84	7.01	7.01		7.01	7.01	7.01	7.08	6.50
	2.5–97.5 percentile	2.57–17.61	1.88–16.20	2.74–18.30	2.74–16.59		2.91–14.88	1.88–13.51	2.74–14.88	2.74–14.88	3.08–13.68		2.74–14.54	2.05–13.51	2.74–15.05	2.74–15.05	0.34–12.14
Coventry	N	502	401	213	186	193	177	116	90	59							
	Mean	8.4	7.6	7.6	8.4	9.2	8.0	7.7	7.4	7.1							
	2.5–97.5 percentile	4–22	4–21	4–24	4–22	4–23	2.5–20	3–16	4–16.5	2–16.5							

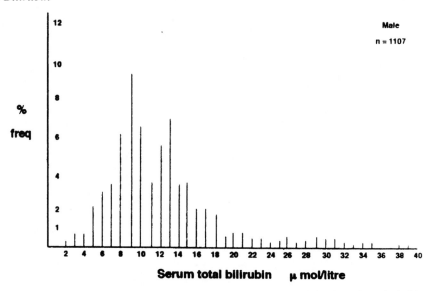

FIGURE 5. Distribution of serum bilirubin in 1107 healthy males 17–60 years old, from the author's laboratory.

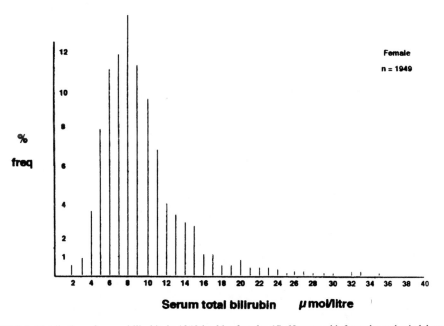

FIGURE 6. Distribution of serum bilirubin in 1949 healthy females 17–60 years old, from the author's laboratory.

is 17 μmol/L (1 mg/100 mL), although Henry, in 1974,[815] gave the range as "up to" 25.7 μmol/L (1.5 mg/100 mL), and Wells, in the 1988 edition of Varley's book,[823] said that there is a sex difference, with reported upper reference limits varying from 13.7 to 16.3 μmol/L in females and 20.5 to 24.0 μmol/L in males.

Skewed Distribution and Bimodality

The skewed distribution of serum total bilirubin in healthy subjects has been described as log normal by some workers, but a close study of large series suggests that the distribution departs from log normality at higher levels.

Bailey et al., in a large series,[850] claimed that there was no evidence of bimodality, and they believed that Gilbert's syndrome (constititional hyperbilirubinemia) may be merely reflecting the upper end of the normal range. Earlier, Owens and Evans,[851] in a series of 197 males and 102 females,[910] considered that the distribution in both sexes was bimodal. Figures 5 and 6 show the

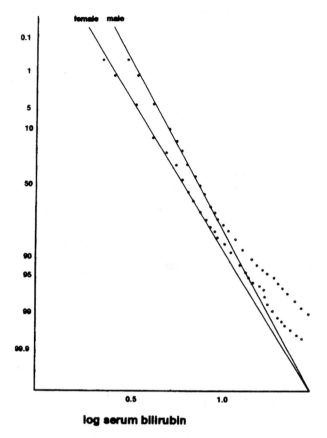

FIGURE 7. Plot of cumulative frequency against log serum bilirubin of distribution shown in Figures 5 and 6 on probability paper. Gaussian distribution is represented by the straight line.

TABLE 131.
Diurnal Variation in Serum Bilirubin (in μmol/L)

Reference	Subjects	N	Time	Mean
852	Healthy volunteers	20	8:30 a.m.	8.5
			12:30 p.m.	8.2
			4:30 p.m.	7.2
416	Men 40–49 years old from G.P.'s registers.		9 a.m.–3 p.m.	9.2
	Nonfasting samples		3 p.m.–6 p.m.	6.4

distribution in over 3000 healthy subjects from a study in the author's laboratory. Figure 7 shows a plot of the frequency against the log of serum bilirubin, showing that in 95% of males, total bilirubin is below 25 μmol/L, and in 95% of females, it is below 17 μmol/L. The distribution is near log gaussian up to these levels, with a deviation showing more than the expected number at higher levels. This appears to support the finding of Owens and Evans.

Diurnal Variation

Table 131 shows reports of a fall in serum bilirubin during the day. It is probable that food intake during the day leads to the changes found.

THE ELDERLY

Figures in Tables 129 and 130 suggest that there is little change in serum bilirubin with increasing age and that the lower level in females persists. This is confirmed by the study of 300 elderly patients living at home, by Leask et al.[166] (Table 132).

TABLE 132.
Serum Bilirubin in the Elderly[a] (in μmol/L)

Sex	Age	Mean	Range
Male	65–74	11.46	5.13–25.82
	Over 74	11.46	5.81–22.91
Female	65–74	9.58	4.45–20.18
	Over 74	9.58	4.79–17.10

[a] From Leask, R. G. S., et al., *Age Aging,* 2, 14, 1993. Three hundred subjects living at home, excluding any taking benzodiazepines or diuretics.

TABLE 133.
Serum Total Bilirubin (μmol/L) in Healthy Children[a]

	Male		Female	
		Range		Range
Age (years)	50 percentile	2.5–97.5 percentile	50 percentile	2.5–97.5 percentile
5	5	3–14	5	2–14
6	5	3–14	5	3–15
7	7	3–17	7	3–17
8	7	3–17	7	3–19
9	7	3–15	7	3–21
10	7	3–19	7	3–21
11	7	3–19	9	5–24
12	7	3–17	7	5–22
13	9	3–31	9	3–22
14	9	5–24	5	3–19
15	10	3–27	9	5–24
16	12	3–32	9	5–27
17	10	5–26	9	3–26

[a] From Haas, R. G., in *Paediatric Clinical Chemistry Reference (Normal Values),* 3rd Ed., Meites, S., Ed., Washington, AACC Press, 1989, 69. With permission. Fasting samples taken from mainly Caucasian children in Mansfield, WI. Range was 2.5–97.5 percentile.

CHILDREN

There are few detailed reports of serum bilirubin levels in children. Werner et al. found mean levels in children, up to 10 years of age, lower than in adults,[847] with little difference between girls and boys. Haas found that levels increased at puberty,[853] particularly in males (Table 133). Similar figures were reported by Werner,[847] who found mean levels in boys, age 0 to 12, of 6.67 μmol/L, and in girls, 7.35 μmol/L, compared with mean levels of 11.80 and 10.43 in boys and girls, age 13 to 18 years.

NEONATES

Serum total bilirubin is increased in the newborn[854] (Table 134). In full-term infants, mean levels fall to less than 34 μmol/L by the fifth to the seventh day of life. Higher levels, which take longer to fall, are found in preterm babies.[855] In clinical practice the level requiring action is probably more important than the reference range, which is affected by a number of factors such as maturity and anoxia at birth.

Anttolainen et al. reported a curious finding;[856] serum bilirubin was significantly lower in Scandinavian infants born during periods of continuous daylight than in those born during periods of little daylight.

TABLE 134.
Serum Total Bilirubin in
Neonates[a] (in μmol/L)

Age (hours)	Range
0–12	15–115
12–24	21–169
24–48	10–181
48–72	9–162
72–96	22–171

[a] From Clayton, B.E., et al., in *Paediatric Chemical Pathology*, Blackwell Scientific, Oxford, 1980, 38.

TABLE 135.
Serum Bilirubin (in μmol/L) in Subjects
with Impaired Vision[a]

	N	Mean	SD
Normal vision	50	9.4	3.5
Blind	220	12.3	3.5
Severly impaired (1/35 to 1/10 vision)	140	10.9	3.5

[a] From Hollwich, F. and Dieckhues, B., *German Med.*, 1, 122, 1971.

RANGE DURING PREGNANCY

There are few reports of serum bilirubin during pregnancy. The author's impression is that levels are lower than in nonpregnant subjects, but he has not been able to find any published detailed study. Notler stated that small increases in plasma bilirubin were found toward the end of pregnancy,[837] but did not give any figures. O'Kell and Elliott found little difference in the mean values in pregnant subjects at term (8.6 μmol/L) and in nonpregnant women of the same age (10.5 μmol/L).[144]

OTHER CHANGES

BLINDNESS

Hollwich and Dieckhuis reported serum total bilirubin levels in blind and partially sighted people higher than in those with normal vision[329] (shown in Table 135).

DRUGS AFFECTING SERUM BILIRUBIN

Malageau states "numerous medications increase the level of bilirubin in blood, chloroquine, isoniazide, methyl dopa sulfonamides," but gives no details or references.[857] No doubt, liver toxicity is the main cause, as with the drugs referred to by Young.[55,56]

Nicotinic acid given intravenously was shown to increase unconjugated bilirubin, due to increased catabolism of hemoglobin.[858] This was developed as a test for Gilbert's syndrome, by Davidson et al.,[859] who gave 50 mg by intravenous injection over 30 s and took blood samples over the next 5 h. The peak in normal subjects was found after 90 to 180 min, with an increase in the range of 2 to 19 μmol/L, whereas in patients with Gilbert's syndrome, the peak was at 180 min, with an increase in the range of 5 to 42 μmol/L.

There is a yellow pigmentation of the skin and sclera after administration of novobiocin. Sutherland and Keller showed that the pigment in infants with severe neonatal jaundice and treated with novobiocin was indistinguishable from bilirubin.[860] This was supported by Hargreaves and Holton,[861] who studied the rate of bilirubin glucuronide formation, using rat liver slices. Finland and Nichols attributed the pigmentation to an unidentified metabolic product.[862] Fekety considered it to be due to a pigmented lipochrome degradation product that is extractable with ethyl acetate and chloroform,[863] but said that true hyperbilirubinemia with a clinical picture resembling Gilbert's syndrome had also been observed and that in some other cases, hepatocellular damage, with or without cholestasis, had also resulted from the use of novobiocin.

* Blondes and brunettes — In 1927 Perkin reported that mean serum total bilirubin was 50% higher in brunettes than in blondes,[841] in a study of 50 healthy subjects. No definition was given of blonde and brunette, and the levels in those with other hair coloring (red, brown, silver, none!) was not stated. Further references to this curious finding are absent from the literature. As a protein precipitation method was used, with levels much lower than by other methods, the finding was probably linked to the use of an unsatisfactory method.

Chapter 11

UREA

In humans, urea is formed in the liver from ammonia obtained by deamination of amino acids. It has a rapidly diffusible molecule that permeates all tissue fluids. Because urea is the chief end point of nitrogen metabolism, its plasma concentration depends on the dietary intake of protein and the caloric balance; on the endogenous catabolism of protein as a result of stress, trauma, infection, or adenocortical activity; on the absorption of products of intestinal bleeding; on the ability of the liver to synthesize urea; and on the effect of drugs such as tetracycline, steroids, and thyroxine, as well as the glomerular filtration rate and any excretion through the skin.[864]

ANALYTIC CONSIDERATIONS

Urea has been estimated in body fluids for many years, with reports of the estimation in blood given by Strauss in 1902[865] and by Widal and Javal in 1904.[866] Reviews of the methods available are given by DiGordio[867] and by Taylor and Jadgama.[868]

HYDROLYTIC METHODS

Enzymic action using urease found in soya and jack beans, followed by quantitation of the ammonia formed, has been widely used for urea estimation. This procedure was first described in 1913 by Marshall.[869]

A suitable urease reagent, stable for long periods if refrigerated, can be prepared by extraction from the beans, with glycerol. Highly purified preparations are available commercially, but a fresh suspension must be prepared daily, as the enzymic activity quickly declines. A number of methods for quantitation of the ammonia produced have been used:

1. Titration with acid after separation by steam distillation, as in the original Marshall method, or by diffusion, as in the technique developed by Conway[870]
2. Use of the color reaction with phenol and hypochlorite, first described by Bertholet in 1859[871]
3. Production of a color, with Nessler reagent[872]
4. Reaction with oxoglutarate under the influence of glutamate dehydrogenase, and measurement of the change in absorbance at 340 nm, due to the conversion of NADH to NAD[873]
5. Use of a sequence of reactions with glutamate synthetase, pyruvate kinase, and pyruvate oxidase, followed by measurement of hydrogen peroxide formed using the Trinder reaction[874]
6. Conductimetric estimation using an ammonia electrode.

The procedure using Nessler reagent was used by many hospital laboratories until the introduction of continuous-flow analyzers, which utilize direct-reacting methods, despite problems with instability, nonlinearity of the color, and the formation of turbidity. Nessler reagent was simple and convenient to use. It is interesting that in a recent review of urea methods, Nessler reagent is not mentioned.[868]

DIRECT-REACTING METHODS

The reaction of urea with diacetyl monoxime in hot acid solution, described by Fearon in

1939,[875] has been adapted for use in continuous-flow analyzers. When used manually, the method has the disadvantage of nonlinearity and nonspecificity, but conditions in continuous-flow analyzers can be standardized to enable precise assays to be made. Variation of acid concentration and the use of semicarbazide or ferric ions are used to improve specificity and increase color intensity. Haslam added urea to the reagents to give a more linear standard curve at lower urea concentrations.[876]

Other direct-reacting methods have been used. Morin and Prox used the reaction with *p*-dimethyl amino benzaldehyde.[877] Condensation with *o*-phthaldehyde, followed by the reaction with a substituted quinoline derivative to give a colored product, has been used in manual, continuous-flow, and kinetic methods[868] and is used in the American Monitor Parallel and Perspective discrete analyzers.[878]

GASOMETRIC METHODS

Some early workers used the measurement of nitrogen produced by the reaction of urea with hypobromite,[879] but this method has now been abandoned.

"DRY" CHEMISTRY METHODS

Methods designed for ward or emergency work use ammonia, obtained by urease impregnated on sticks, to change the color of an indicator. Measurement of that length of the stick that was altered in color gives a measure of the urea concentration. "Urostat" (Warner) uses serum and bromcresol green as the indicator, and "Azostix" (Ames) uses whole blood and bromthymol blue. A similar principle is used in "dry" chemistry analyzers such as the Boehringer "Reflectron" and the Kodak "Ectochem." The Ames "Seralyzer" uses the reaction with *o*-phthaldehyde.

REFERENCE METHOD

A candidate reference method for urea, based on the urease reaction after removal of protein with $Ba(OH)_2$ and $ZnSO_4$ and estimation of ammonia, using the reaction with oxoglutarate under the influence of glutamate dehydrogenase, was proposed by an AACC Study Group.[880] The method gave accurate results, with little effect from interfering substances.

ACCURACY AND PRECISION

Direct-reacting methods have been reported to give slightly higher results than methods using the more specific urease procedures, although not all workers agree on this.

Marsh et al. found serum urea results 2 to 3% higher, using a diacetyl monoxime method than with techniques using hypobromite or urease.[881] Zilva and London, comparing diacetyl and urease methods,[882] found a good comparison up to urea levels of 16.6 mmol/L, but at higher levels diacteyl monoxime methods gave higher results (on one occasion a discrepancy of 25% was noted). They suggested that in some uremic patients, the blood contained a substance that either gave the diacetyl reaction or inhibited the urease reaction. In contrast, Searcy et al. could not demonstrate significant differences between the diacetyl method and a manual urease/Bertholet reaction method,[883] either with normal sera or with specimens from azotemic patients.

Quality control surveys suggest that mean levels obtained by either end-point or kinetic urease methods and by diacetyl monoxime methods using continuous-flow analyzers are similar,[868] although, in general, samples with very high urea levels will not be used. *O*-phthaldehyde methods using the direct reaction with serum give a positive bias when compared with indirect methods,[868] whereas results by the Kodak Ectochem procedure give results up to 1 mmol/L lower than other methods.

In some cases the "stick" tests may give different results from those obtained by other methods. Hall and Preston, using "Azostix,"[884] found levels lower than by a diacetyl monoxime method, in cases of acidosis, and lower levels in cases of alkalosis. The difference related to changes in blood pH.

The precision of blood urea assay is said to be about 8.5% for manual estimation and about 5% for estimation using continuous-flow analyzers, at 12 mmol/L.[159]

SI UNITS

The earliest workers were primarily interested in nitrogen balance and often reported nitrogen content as blood urea nitrogen. Urea (molecular weight 60) contains 46.67% nitrogen; so levels given as urea nitrogen in mg/100 mL must be multiplied by 2.143 to give urea content. Conversion to molar units is by the equation

$$\text{urea mmol/L} = 0.166 \times \text{urea mg/100 mL}$$

INTERFERENCE WITH ANALYSIS

HEMOLYSIS

Hemoglobin does not introduce error in procedures for the estimation of blood or serum urea, involving protein precipitation or dialysis.[292] Methods that do not include protein removal may be affected. Fales found apparent urea concentration 1.8 mmol/L higher, using serum and diacetyl monoxime than when using a protein-free filtrate with sufficient hemoglobin present to give serum a deep-red color.[885] Bertholet reaction methods are affected if the color is measured at wavelengths less than the peak at 630 nm,[886] whereas methods using dimethyl aminobenz–aldehyde give high results, with more than 1 g/L of hemoglobin present in serum.[877]

High levels of hemoglobin in serum have a small effect on the glutamate dehydrogenase method.[873] A level of 10 g/L decreases apparent serum urea by about 2%.[880]

BILIRUBIN

Serum bilirubin of 180 μmol/L increases apparent urea by about 1.1 mmol/L when estimated by a continuous-flow diacetyl monoxime method.[867] The effect is not observed using a manual procedure and may be due to the different reaction conditions used. Results up to 20% higher are obtained when serum bilirubin is more than 54 μmol/L, with dimethyl amino-benzaldehyde methods using nonprotein removal.[877]

Very high bilirubin levels give a small decrease in apparent serum urea, with the glutamate dehydrogenase method.[873] A 4% error is found with serum bilirubin of more than 1000 μmol/L.[880] The enzymic method using the Trinder reaction shows a slight interference with serum bilirubin of more than 300 μmol/L.[887] Results are about 0.4 mmol/L low;[874] the error may be reduced by including ferricyanide in the reaction mixture.

LIPEMIA

Methods reacting with serum directly are liable to be affected by lipemia. Sera with milk-like lipemia have apparent urea of up to 2.5 mmol/L lower using serum and diacetyl monoxime than using a protein-free filtrate.[885] Turbidity from lipemic sera persists throughout nonprotein removal methods based on urease followed by the Bertholet reaction.[888] The error can be eliminated by use of a blank with urease added after the phenol reagent or extraction of the final solution with ether. Some lipemic sera affect the *o*-phthaldehyde reaction, and bichromatic absorbance measurement has been suggested to overcome the problem.[887]

OTHER INTERFERING SUBSTANCES
Urease Methods

In some early work, variable results when using whole blood were found that were considered to be due to arginase producing ammonia from arginine in the urease prepara-tion.[889,890] Arginase can be destroyed by heat before urease is added, or avoided, as proposed by King and Allott,[891] by measuring the sample into isotonic sodium sulfate so that the cells remain intact. Modern urease preparations are purer, and as serum is usually used, the problem is unlikely to occur.

Oral administration of chloral hydrate was found to give an increase in apparent blood urea of 0.7 to 1.0 mmol/L, using a urease-Nessler method.[892]

Formaldehyde used as a preservative inhibits urea.[893] Problems may arise with estimation in urine, but this substance is rarely, if ever, used in blood.

Actetone used to dry pipettes and other glassware gives a turbidity with Nessler reagent, and care must be taken to avoid contamination.[894]

Diacetyl Monoxime Methods

A number of substances, such as guanidines, semicarbazide, allantoin, tryptophan, citrul-line, indoles, and indican, give a color with diacetyl reagent, but are not found in sufficiently high concentration in serum to give higher results than by a urease method.[882] Christian states that acetohexamide and the sulfonyl ureas give a color,[347] but does not give details of the quantitative effect. Sodium azide at a concentration of 1 mg/mL, which may be used as a preservative, reduces urea, estimated by diacetyl methods, by more than 50%.[888]

Methods Using the Bertholet Reaction

A color with Bertholet's reagent is given by *p*-amino phenol and substituted *p*-amino phenols.[888,895] Although not often used therapeutically, a blank correction can be made, if necessary, by adding urease after the phenol reagent.

O-Phthaldehyde Reaction

Sulfonamides interfere with the *o*-phthaldehyde reaction. A dose of 1 mmol/L of sulfon-amide added to serum gives a color equivalent to 15 mmol/L of urea.[878] The color forms quickly and then fades.

Sulfamethoxazole, a constituent of cotrimoxazole, was found to interfere in serum from patients treated with a high dose (1920 mg qid orally or 120 mg/kg/day intravenously), by Levitt et al.[896]

Dimethyl Aminobenzaldehyde Reaction

Dextran reacts as urea in the dimethyl aminobenzaldehyde reaction, and sulfonamides and *p*-amino salicylic acid also interfere.[877]

CONCLUSION

Surveys suggest that the kinetic urease and direct-reacting methods using diacetyl monoxime give similar results. It is possible that higher results are obtained, with some uremic samples, with the diacetyl method. For urease methods, a satisfactory enzyme preparation must be used. Direct-reacting methods are all subject to interference from hemoglobin, bilirubin, lipemia, and some drugs. Little interference has been reported with urease methods.

PREANALYTIC ERROR

COLLECTION OF THE SPECIMEN

Plasma urea was first reported to be a little higher than blood urea, by Wu in 1922.[897] Urea diffuses through the body fluids so that its concentration per unit of water is the same as in plasma and the cells. Due to the difference in water concentration, urea expressed per 100 mL will differ in plasma or serum from that in red cells. Ralls found that the ratio of urea in erythrocytes to urea in plasma[898] was 1.04:1 and said that it may decrease to 0.96:1 postprandially, due to an increase in plasma urea. As the water content of serum is higher than that of the erythrocytes by chance, there should be little difference between the concentration of urea in whole blood or plasma. However, Sacre and Walker found mean blood urea was 7% lower than the corresponding serum level,[899] in 51 specimens with urea up to 15 mmol/L.

Difficulties sampling whole blood, due to mixing problems, have been found using continuous-flow analyzers.[899-901] Due to this and other analytic problems on some instruments and possible differences with whole blood, most workers now prefer to use serum or plasma for the estimation of urea.

Collection of the sample into oxalate, heparin, or EDTA is acceptable, although anticoagulants using ammonia cannot be used with some methods. Fluoride and Thymol must be avoided if a urease method is used. Satzmann and Male[400] warned about errors due to evaporation when small amounts of blood (about 0.5 mL) was centrifuged in uncapped tubes. Three minutes of centrifugation increased plasma urea from 4.8 to 5.6 mmol/L.

SAMPLE STABILITY

Urea in serum is stable for at least 1 day at room temperature, several days at 4°C, and at least 6 months if frozen.[867] Fluoride (6 mg/mL) preserves the sample at room temperature for about 5 days, but interferes with urease methods.

Lyophilized serum is more stable. Hanok and Kuo stored reconstituted lyophilized serum (Hyland Laboratories) and found urea levels to be stable for 11 days at 10°C and for at least 22 days at −15°C.[95]

Heating to 56°C

Heating serum or plasma to 56°C to minimize the risk from HIV-positive samples has only a small effect on the urea concentration. Ball found that heating for 30 min gave a mean decrease of 1.4% in serum urea,[312] compared with a mean increase of 4.3% when B-proprio–lactone was added.

PHYSIOLOGIC CHANGES

MEALS AND DIET

Annino and Relman found no increase in serum urea after a standard breakfast.[109] Ralls only found an increase from a mean of 4.55 mmol/L in fasting males to a mean of 4.65 mmol/L 1 to 3 h after breakfast.[878]

It has been known for many years that the urea concentration in blood depends on the protein content of the diet. MacKay and MacKay noted in 1927 that in a population of healthy, mainly young subjects,[902] blood urea was in the range of 2.99 to 6.31 mmol/L, but if a diet of 1.1 g of protein per kilogram of body weight was taken, the range narrowed to 3.32 to 5.81 mmol/L. Table 136 shows the variation of blood urea, found by Addis et al.,[890] with different amounts of dietary protein: 0.5 g/kg body weight per day represents the amount required for nitrogen equilibrium, 1.5 g/kg/day represents the average protein consumption, and 2.5 g/kg/day represents a high-protein diet.

EXERCISE

Resting serum urea is higher in athletes in training than in young nonathletes. Figure 8 shows levels found in 114 athletes in training compared with 81 young nonathletes, by Haralambie.[903] The levels in athletes were up to 9 mmol/L, compared with the highest level of a little over 6 mmol/L in nonathletes.

DIURNAL VARIATION

Over 60 years ago MacKay and MacKay noted a tendency for blood urea to increase during the day and fall during periods of sleep. Changes were in the range of 0.1 to 0.5 mmol/L. This

TABLE 136.
Blood Urea (in mmol/L) at Different Dietary Protein Levels[a]

Subjects	Method	Diet Protein (g/Kg body wt. per day)	Mean	Range
Medical students	On appropriate diet for 5–6 days	0.5	3.20	2.16–4.15
	Samples taken before meals	1.5	6.41	4.15–8.80
	Analysis by urease-aeration method	2.5	7.55	5.15–9.96

[a] From Addis, T., et al., *J. Clin. Invest.,* 26, 869, 1947.

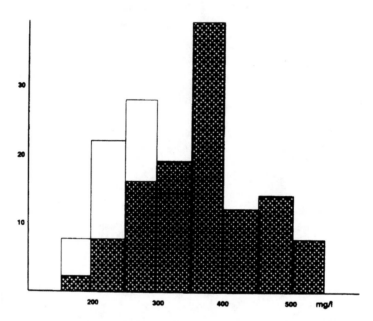

FIGURE 8. Frequency distribution of resting serum urea level in male control subjects (white bars, n = 81) and in athletes in training (black bars, n = 114) (Reproduced from Maralambie, G., in *Reference Values in Human Chemistry,* Siest, G., Ed., Karger, Basel, 1973, 249. With permission.)

was confirmed many years later by Pocock et al.,[409] who compared serum urea in 7735 men, 40 to 59 years old, with the time of collection. Mean levels in the morning were 5.10 mmol/ L, and at 6 p.m. they were 5.63 mmol/L. The increase may not be consistent throughout the day, as Statland et al., studying 11 healthy male nonsmokers age 21 to 27,[904] found mean levels of 4.62 mmol/L at 8:00 a.m., of 4.24 at 11:00 a.m., and of 4.34 at 2:00 p.m.

SEASONAL CHANGES

A slight increase in blood urea was claimed by Lellough and Claude, in a study of French civil servants,[905] but quantitative details were not given. It has been suggested that possible seasonal variation could be due to a change in eating habits.[906]

RANGE IN HEALTHY SUBJECTS

WITHIN- AND BETWEEN-PERSON VARIATIONS

Attempts have been made to establish the range of blood urea in healthy subjects from the earliest work. MacKay and MacKay[902] found large differences in a number of reports from 1913 to 1926 and proceeded to estimate the range in a large group of mainly young adults.

They obtained a range of 4.28 to 7.67 mmol/L in 58 men, which was higher than the range of 1.83 to 6.47 mmol/L obtained in 58 women. They also suggested that levels increased with age, although the number of older subjects was not great.

Later, large series using various methods all showed higher levels in males and an increase with age (Table 137 and 138). A distribution skewed toward the lower value was consistently reported. Differences obtained by the different groups might be due to method differences and dietary variation in the population studied. Figures quoted in textbooks reflect the varying ranges found by different workers (Table 139). Some of the earliest books use the range 15 to 40 mg/100 mL (2.49 to 6.64 mmol/L), although Peters and Van Slyke give blood urea nitrogen of 13 to 23 mg/100 mL (4.62 to 8.18 mmol/L).[150] Ranges given in later books rarely agree. Some state that the range is higher in men than in women, but the change with age is less frequently indicated.

DAY-TO-DAY VARIATION

The blood urea level in individuals varies considerably over a period of time. Several groups have found that the average intraindividual variation has a cv of more than 10% (Table 140). It is possible that the variation reflects changes in the protein content of the diet and in the degree of hydration. The mean intraindividual variation is higher in diseased individuals than in healthy individuals.[911]

CHILDREN

Definition of the range in children is difficult to determine, because of variation in dietary nitrogen and because information about levels in young children is scarce. Table 141 shows a number of published ranges. There appears to be little variation in the mean level in boys from the age of a few months to adulthood, but in girls, the mean level falls about 0.4 mmol/L at the age of about 11 years.

NEONATES

Serum urea falls during the first days of life and has been found to be lower in black babies than in white babies (Table 142). Higher levels are found in premature babies (Table 143). Blood urea varies with the nitrogen content of the diet in premature babies[917] (Table 144).

CORD BLOOD

Slemons and Morris, as long ago as 1916,[918] reported that the mean cord blood urea was similar to the mean urea of the maternal blood at birth. This was confirmed by Josephson et al.,[912] who found that the mean urea in the cord blood from 25 healthy babies was 3.58 mmol/L (range of 2.66 to 4.77), similar to that of their mothers' blood at term, but a little lower than the level in nonpregnant adults.

RANGE DURING PREGNANCY

It has been known from the earliest work on the subject that the concentration of urea in the blood during pregnancy is lower than that in nonpregnant women. Table 145 shows some reported levels. The decrease is due to reduced protein catabolism and increased clearance of urea by the kidney.

OTHER CHANGES

BLOOD PRESSURE

There appears to be a negative correlation between blood urea concentration and blood

TABLE 137.
Blood or Serum Urea in Healthy Men (in mmol/L)

Reference		Age (years)										
		15–20	21–25	26–30	31–35	36–40	41–45	46–50	51–55	56–60	61–65	66–70
907[a]	Mean						4.60	4.45	5.24	4.91	4.84	
	Range						3.73–5.69	2.49–5.87	4.16–6.44	3.63–6.12	2.45–6.51	
908[b]	Mean	4.54	4.71	4.87	5.02	5.18	5.34	5.50	5.66	5.81	5.97	
	Range	2.15–7.93	2.32–8.10	2.48–8.36	2.63–8.51	2.79–8.67	2.95–8.83	3.11–8.99	3.27–9.15	3.42–9.30	3.58–9.46	
140[c]	Range		2.64–7.85	2.64–7.85	2.86–8.07	2.86–8.07	3.07–8.28	3.07–8.28	3.29–8.50	3.29–8.50	3.50–8.72	3.50–8.72
145[d]	Range		3.56–7.42	3.56–7.42	3.20–9.26	3.20–9.26	3.20–9.61	3.20–9.61	3.56–9.61	3.56–9.61	3.56–13.53	3.56–13.53
141[e]	Range		3.38–7.42	3.38–7.42	3.57–7.49	3.57–7.49	3.66–7.38	3.66–7.38	3.65–7.69	3.65–7.69	3.78–8.18	3.78–8.18
Coventry[f]	N	93	194	170	151	146	126	111	93	89	46	
	Range	3.2–6.9	3.1–7.5	3.0–7.3	3.2–7.2	3.4–7.3	3.3–7.4	3.6–7.6	3.6–7.4	3.5–7.9	3.5–7.9	

[a] Blood urea.
[b] Blood urea derived from hospital population and calculated from regression equation.
[c] Serum urea from 298 Caucasian men in good health.
[d] Serum urea from 603 men subsequently found not to have any clinical abnormality.
[e] Serum urea from 3600 men from a well-persons' clinic.
[f] Coventry hospital staff, healthy, as described in Chapter 2.

TABLE 138.
Blood and Serum Urea in Healthy Women (in mmol/L)

Reference		Age (years)												
		15–20	21–25	26–30	31–35	36–40	41–45	46–50	51–55	56–60	61–65	66–70	71–75	76–80
908[a]	Mean	4.69	4.75	4.81	4.87	4.92	4.98	5.04	5.10	5.16	5.21			
	Range	3.00–6.38	3.06–6.34	3.12–6.40	3.18–6.46	3.23–6.51	3.29–6.57	3.35–6.63	3.41–6.69	3.47–6.95	3.52–6.80			
140[b]	Range		2.03–6.37	2.03–6.37	2.31–6.66	2.31–6.66	2.59–6.94	2.59–6.94	2.87–7.22	2.87–7.22	3.15–7.50	3.15–7.50	3.42–7.79	3.42–7.79
145[c]	Range		2.49–7.48	2.49–7.48	2.84–7.48	2.84–7.48	3.24–8.90	3.24–8.90	3.56–10.68	3.56–10.68	3.56–10.68	3.56–10.68		
141[d]	Range		2.71–7.23	2.71–7.23	3.23–6.67	3.23–6.67	3.15–7.11	3.15–7.11	3.40–7.60	3.40–7.60	3.69–7.97	3.69–7.97	3.57–7.53	3.57–7.53
Coventry[e]	N	682	573	314	313	258	233	169	117	84	27			
	Range	2.6–6.4	2.6–6.2	2.6–6.6	2.8–6.6	3.0–6.6	2.8–7.2	3.2–7.0	3.2–7.6	3.8–9.0	3.4–8.2			

a 908 blood urea derived from hospital population and calculated from regression equation

b 140 serum urea from 278 Caucasian women in good health

c 145 serum urea from 603 women subsequently found not have any clinical abnormality

d 141 serum urea from 1100 women from a well women's clinic

e Serum urea from healthy Coventry hospital staff described in Chapter 2.

TABLE 139.
Range for Blood and Serum Urea Given in Various Textbooks

Reference	Range in mmol/L	Range and information given in text
149	2.49–6.64	Blood urea 15–40 mg/100 mL
150	4.62–8.18	Blood urea nitrogen 13–23 mg/100 mL
152	2.49–6.64	Blood urea 15–40 mg/100 mL; a little higher in older people
909	2.49–6.39	Blood urea 15–38.5 mg/100 mL
867	2.85–9.30	Higher in men than in women
193	2.3–8.3	Persons on a full ordinary diet
910	1.78–6.08	Men higher than women. Slow rise with age

pressure, in the general population. Lellough et al., in a study[905] of 4422 French civil servants 46 to 52 years old, found

Systolic blood pressure (mm Hg)	Mean serum urea (mmol/L)
110	6.14
150	5.81
210	5.15

SMOKING

Nonsmokers have higher mean blood urea levels than smokers[924] (Table 146). The effect is related to the number of cigarettes smoked and is greater in inhalers than in noninhalers, suggesting a relationship with nicotine or with carbon monoxide and other products of combustion.

DRUGS AFFECTING BLOOD UREA CONCENTRATION

Many drugs have been reported as nephrotoxic and thus are liable to give an increase in blood urea. Young gives references to a large number of reports;[56] this publication should be consulted for details of individual drugs. A number of reports are of individual cases, and others are of the proportion of treated patients showing nephrotoxicity. The action on the kidney may be

- Direct: as with heavy metals, carbon tetrachloride, or cellusolve
- Ischemic: as with hypertensive drugs that reduce circulatory perfusion
- Hypersensitive: as with sulfonamides
- Predisposing: aggravate preexisting renal disease

Some drugs, such as corticosteroids and anabolic steroids, stimulate protein metabolism, leading to an increase in blood urea. Particularly large increases are found when very-low-birth-weight babies are given dexamethazone therapy. Henderson and Dear reported that they had observed a highly significant increase of nearly 5 mmol/L in the mean.[65]

TABLE 140.
Intraindividual Variation of Serum Urea

Reference	Subjects	Method	N	Individual variation mean	cv
163	Male and female white and black subjects, 20–59 years old	Fasting specimen taken at 9 a.m. once a week for 10–12 weeks. Analysis by diacetyl method on continuous-flow analyzer	68	11.9%	After allowing for analytic variation of 7.4%
164	White doctors	One fasting specimen taken once a week for 10 weeks. Stored, frozen, and analyzed on same day.	9	13.6%	After allowing for analytic variation
165	Male students 21–27 years old	Five fasting samples taken within 3 weeks. Analysis using the "Autochemist" analyzer	18	12.3%	

TABLE 141.
Serum Urea in Children (in mmol/L)

Reference		Sex	Age	N	Mean	Range
			(Days)			
912	Children less than 1 year old from Stockholm orphanages	M + F	30–150	18	3.70	3.34–4.26
			150–335	24	4.50	3.63–5.59
			(Years)			
913	Australian children analysis using Technicon SMAC analyzer		Less than 1	136		1.0–7.5
			1–5			2.0–8.0
			6–10			2.0–7.0
		Male	10–19			2.5–8.0
		Female	10–19			2.0–7.0
914	3600 children from a screening program in Marshfield, U.S.	Male	(Years)		50 percentile	
			5		4.6	2.9–7.9
			6		4.6	2.9–6.4
			7		4.3	2.5–6.1
			8		4.6	2.9–7.1
			9		4.6	2.9–6.8
			10		4.6	3.2–6.8
			11		4.6	2.9–6.8
			12		4.6	2.9–6.8
			13		4.3	3.2–6.4
			14		4.3	2.9–7.5
			15		4.3	2.9–7.1
			16		4.6	3.2–8.2
			17		4.6	3.2–7.5
		Female				
			5		4.6	2.9–6.8
			6		4.3	2.5–6.1
			7		4.3	2.9–6.4
			8		4.3	2.9–6.1
			9		4.3	2.9–6.4
			10		4.3	2.9–6.4
			11		3.9	2.1–6.4
			12		3.9	2.9–6.1
			13		3.9	2.5–5.7
			14		3.9	2.5–6.8
			15		4.3	2.9–6.1
			16		4.3	2.9–5.7
			17		3.9	2.5–6.8
		Adult				2.5–8.2

TABLE 142.
Serum Urea in the First Days of Life (in mmol/L)

References	Subjects	Sex	Race	Age (days)	N	Mean	SD	Range
915	Healthy full-term babies	M + F		3–3.5	12	4.83		3.07–6.57
				6–6.5	12	3.27		1.68–4.55
				8	12	2.71		1.73–4.15
181	Healthy babies	F	White	0.5	15	4.52	0.47	
		F	Black	0.5	7	3.39	0.46	
		M	White	0.5	11	4.55	0.53	
		M	Black	0.5	6	2.69	0.58	
		F	White	1.5	14	3.06	0.49	
		F	Black	1.5	8	2.74	0.46	
		M	White	1.5	11	3.33	0.49	
		M	Black	1.5	6	2.82	0.56	
		F	White	2.5	12	2.54	0.55	
		F	Black	2.5	8	2.60	0.48	
		M	White	2.5	13	2.82	0.56	
		M	Black	2.5	5	2.19	0.49	
		F	White	3.5	10	2.08	0.56	
		F	Black	3.5	4	1.74	0.66	
		M	White	3.5	17	2.60	0.49	
		M	Black	3.5	9	3.30	0.50	

TABLE 143.
Blood Urea (in mmol/L) of Babies of Different Birth Weights[a]

Birth weight (g)	N	Mean	Range
690–1350	17	3.65	1.49–5.98
1440–1905	25	3.15	1.33–5.98
1920–2395	31	2.66	1.39–5.31
2415–4020	12	2.49	1.16–4.98

[a] From Pincus, J. B., et al., *Paediatrics*, 18, 39, 1956. Babies less than 1 day old before any fluid or food. Analysis of heel puncture specimens by a diacetyl method.

TABLE 144.
Blood Urea (in mmol/L) in 60 Premature Babies, Mainly Black, with Birth Weight 1500–1750 g, showing Variation with Change in Nitrogen Content of Diet[a]

Age (weeks)	Nitrogen intake (g/kg/day)	Mean
1–3	6.60	8.00
	4.43	4.55
	3.21	1.21
3–5	6.72	6.54
	5.08	5.08
	3.60	3.60
5–7	6.89	7.04
	5.32	5.37
	3.96	2.21

[a] From Thomas, J. L. and Reichelderfer, T. E., *Clin. Chem.*, 22, 272, 1968.

TABLE 145.
Blood Urea During Pregnancy (in mmol/L)

Reference	2 Mean	2 SD	3½ Mean	3½ SD	6 Mean	6 SD	8 Mean	8 SD	Term Mean	Term SD	Nonpregnant Mean	Nonpregnant SD	Comment
919	4.62						3.56						During latter months of pregnancy, nonprotein nitrogen of blood falls slightly below the usual nonpregnant levels
920													Urea nitrogen fell in first 6 months of pregnancy
921					2.13								
152											4.98		"Commonly between 2.49 and 3.32, rarely higher than 4.15"
922					3.09	0.53			3.56	1.10	4.66	1.10	Nonpregnant 4–6 weeks postpartum
923											4.17	1.17	

TABLE 146.
Effect of Smoking on Blood Urea (in mmol/L) in a Study of over 6000 Male Frenchmen[a]

Age (years)	Taxi drivers Nonsmokers N	Mean	Smokers N	Mean	Sewer workers Nonsmokers N	Mean	Smokers N	Mean	Employees of a Paris firm Nonsmokers N	Mean	Smokers N	Mean
<30	24	5.71	46	5.83	18	5.53	53	5.26	159	6.56	282	5.99
30–39	53	5.78	134	5.56	53	5.25	261	5.05	142	6.52	346	6.62
40–49	391	5.88	108	5.74	56	5.84	213	5.06	125	6.61	605	6.14
50–59	91	6.03	210	5.76	36	5.83	80	5.28	282	6.37	822	6.37
>60	119	6.42	227	5.96	—	—	—	—	35	6.74	101	6.44

Cigarettes daily	Noninhalers N	Mean	Inhalers N	Mean
1–10	641	6.51	469	6.39
11–20	609	6.31	1079	5.91
21–30	62	6.51	161	5.73
>31+	38	6.13	60	5.69

[a] From Lellough, J., et al., *J. Chr. Dis.*, 22, 9, 1969.

Chapter 12

CREATININE

Creatine phosphate in muscle acts as a reservoir of high energy and is readily converted to creatinine. The formation of creatinine is directly related to total muscle mass and roughly related to body weight. Creatinine is solely the waste product of creatine and is not utilized in the body. It is excreted in urine and feces. Serum creatinine levels depend on the rate of production of creatinine and on the renal clearance of creatinine and thus are linked to total muscle mass and to kidney function.[925]

ANALYTIC CONSIDERATIONS

Colorimetric, kinetic, enzymic, and chromatographic methods are used to estimate creatinine in serum. A number of good reviews of these methods are available.[925-928]

METHODS USING THE JAFFÉ REACTION

Estimation based on the formation of a red complex with alkaline picrate, first described by Jaffe in 1886,[929] has been used for many years. A procedure for the estimation in blood was described by Folin in 1914,[930] and many modifications have since been published that attempt to improve linearity and specificity.

As the maximum absorbance of the colored complex at 493 nm is close to that of alkaline picrate, a narrow-band instrument to measure absorbance is required, to avoid error caused by the decrease in color as picrate is consumed by the reaction. Linearity is improved if a wavelength greater than 500 nm is used. Owen et al. found linearity of up to about 400 μmol/L.[931]

Temperature must be controlled, as changes during analysis can introduce errors due to the absorbance of the reagent and colored complex changing to a different degree.

The Jaffé reaction is not specific for creatinine. Any compound with an active methylene group can potentially react with picrate under the assay conditions. About 20% of the reaction in serum is not due to creatinine, and the amount is higher in whole blood.

Various procedures have been used to attempt to improve specificity:

1. Creatinine has been adsorbed onto hydrated aluminum silicate (Lloyd's reagent) or onto cation exchange resins, with creatinine estimated after subsequent elution.
2. Dialysis, as used in continuous-flow analyzers, removes some interference, but glucose, pyruvate, and other keto acids that react are still present.
3. The pH has been varied to obtain conditions giving the maximum specificity.
4. Using methods measuring reaction rate, a time interval has been selected during which the reaction is mainly from creatinine, as some interfering substances, such as aceto acetate, react more quickly than creatinine, and some, such as glucose, react more slowly.

ENZYMIC METHODS

A number of enzymic methods of estimation have been described that are claimed to be specific for creatinine and show no interference from other substances, although hemolysis and lipemia have been shown to affect some methods.

1. Masson et al.[932] used a method based on earlier work published in 1937 by Miller and

Dubos,[933] which measured creatinine as the difference between Jaffé chromogens before and after the enzymic conversion of creatinine to creatine.

2. Janes et al.[934] measured the change in absorption at 340 nm following the reaction sequence:

$$\text{creatinine} + H_2O \xrightarrow{\text{creatinase}} \text{creatine}$$

$$\text{creatine} + ATP \xrightarrow{\text{creatine kinase}} \text{creatine phosphate} + ADP$$

$$\text{phosphoenol phosphate} + ADP \xrightarrow{\text{pyruvate kinase}} \text{pyruvate} + ATP$$

$$\text{pyruvate} + NADH \xrightarrow{\text{LDH}} \text{lactate} + NAD$$

3. Fossati et al.[935] used the peroxidase reaction after the sequence

$$\text{creatinine} + H_2O \xrightarrow{\text{creatinase}} \text{creatine}$$

$$\text{creatine} + H_2O = \text{sarcosine} + \text{urea}$$

$$\text{sarcosine} + O_2 + H_2O \xrightarrow{\text{sarcosinase}} \text{glycine} + \text{formaldehyde} + H_2O$$

$$H_2O_2 = H_2O + O$$

4. Tanganelli et al.[936] estimated ammonia formed by the action of creatinine deaminase, using the change in absorption at 340 nm in the reaction

$$NH_4^+ + NADH + 2 \text{ oxoglutarate} = \text{glutamate} + NADP + H_2O$$

5. Sugita et al.[937] used the sequence of reactions used by Fossati et al., but measured using the formaldehyde obtained by the reaction

$$HCHO + NAD^+ + H_2O \xrightarrow{\text{formaldehyde dehydrogenase}} HCOOH + NADH + H^+$$

HPLC

Estimation of serum creatinine by an isocratic high-performance liquid chromatography (HPLC) method has been proposed, by Rosano et al., as a candidate reference method.[938]

METHOD DIFFERENCES

The lowest results are obtained using enzymic and HPLC methods, and these are considered to be measuring true creatinine. Jaffé reaction methods give results in the order

on protein-free filtrate > after using Lloyd's reagent > after dialysis > kinetic reaction

By carefully choosing conditions, using the Jaffé reaction, results can be obtained reasonably close to those using enzymic methods[939] (Table 147).

Consideration of creatinine levels in the literature should take into account differences in method, because much early work used nonspecific methods.

TABLE 147.

Serum Creatinine (in μmol/L) in Healthy Subjects, Using Various Methods[a]

	Men		Women	
Method	50 percentile	2.5–97.5 percentile	50 percentile	2.5–97.5 percentile
Enzymic	71.61	48.62–97.24	58.35	41.55–80.45
Kinetic Jaffé	78.68	50.59–99.89	63.95	53.93–90.17
SMA 6/60 Jaffé	88.40	70.72–106.08	70.72	53.54–97.24

[a] From Börner, V., et al., *J. Clin. Chem. Clin. Biochem.*, 17, 679, 1979.

ACCURACY AND PRECISION

Serum creatinine is overestimated by about 20% for levels less than 90 μmol/L, and by about 10% for higher levels, when using the Jaffé reaction on continuous-flow analyzers.[940] Enzymic methods give results close to the true level. The precision of creatinine estimation using the Jaffé reaction is approximately ±5% for levels within the normal range.[941] The precision of enzymic methods is similar.

Between-assay cv reported by the Wellcome Quality Control Scheme is approximately 6% for continuous-flow methods, approximately 5% for kinetic methods using discrete analyzers, approximately 11% for manual kinetic methods, and approximately 8% for other manual methods.[925]

SI UNITS

Serum creatinine in mass units as milligrams per 100 mL are converted to molar units as micromoles per liter by multiplying by 88.4.

INTERFERENCE WITH ANALYSIS

HEMOLYSIS

Tausskey found no interference by hemoglobin,[942] using a protein precipitation and Jaffé reaction method. Bryden and Roberts found no interference using a continuous-flow analyzer with dialysis followed by the Jaffé reaction.[292] Munz et al.[943] found that hemoglobin of more than 0.5 g/L interferes with an enzymic method, although Weber and Zanten[944] considered the effect negligible on an enzymic method based on the peroxidase reaction.

BILIRUBIN

Interference with the estimation of creatinine by bilirubin has been found using both the Jaffé reaction and enzymic methods that use the peroxidase reaction. Accounts of the interference with the kinetic Jaffé method are confusing. Lustgarten and Wenk[945] and Knight and Trainer[946] found negligible interference when adding bilirubin obtained from the American Monitor Co. to serum, whereas Daugherty et al. found a depression of about 20% when adding 17 μmol/L from another source.[947] Dorwart, using pooled sera,[948] found a reduction of 88 μmol/L in apparent serum creatinine at bilirubin levels of 60 μmol/L. It was noted that interference was found with samples brown or green in color, but not with those yellow in color, suggesting that different pigments acted differently.

A depression of about 30% with mainly conjugated bilirubin, and little change with conjugated bilirubin, was reported by Soldin et al.[949] However, Knapp and Hadid found different results and obtained interference with both conjugated and unconjugated bilirubin.[950] Osberg and Hammond suggested that results were affected by different reagents,[951] as apparent serum creatinine was depressed by bilirubin, using reagents from Electro Nucleonics Inc., but not when reagents from the Beckman Co. were used. Bilirubin interference was eliminated by the inclusion of borate, phosphate, and a surfactant, in the reagent. This was supported by Knapp and Halid,[950] who found that reagents used on the Beckman creatinine analyzer, which include borate/phosphate in the alkaline reagent, inhibit the formation of biliverdin and appear to give the best results among the methods tested.

It can be concluded that kinetic Jaffé methods of estimation give variable results for serum creatinine, depending on the bile and hema pigments present and the reagents used. Inclusion of borate and phosphate in the alkaline reagent reduces the interference.

Scott investigated the colorimetric method using serum from the neonate and compared results with different picrate concentrations,[952] with a HPLC reference method. He concluded that acceptable results could be obtained provided the picrate concentration was above 12 mmol/L, although they were somewhat high compared with the reference method.

Four commercial enzymic methods based on using the peroxidase reaction were studied by Weber and Zanten.[944] Bilirubin was found to cause a reduction in apparent serum creatinine, which varied between the methods used and increased with creatinine concentration.

Little interference is found using other enzymic methods, although Sugita et al. noted positive interference with over 171 μmol/L.[937]

LIPEMIA

Munz et al. found that lipemia of more than 20 g/L total lipid interfered with an enzymic method,[923] although Weber and Zanten[924] reported negligible interference by Intralipid of enzymic methods based on the peroxidase reaction.

PROTEIN INTERFERENCE

Aberhalden and Kanen stated that some proteins give the Jaffé reaction.[953] de Haan found considerable reaction of albumin at higher picrate concentrations.[954] Human albumin does not react at a final concentration of 5 to 20 mmol/L of picrate, which covers the range used in reaction-rate methods.[955]

Some paraproteins depress the Jaffé reaction. Jaynes et al. found low results in sera containing paraprotein,[956] when estimating using the Beckman Astra 8 analyzer, compared with a dialysis method. Datta et al. found a 50% depression in serum creatinine of some myeloma patients,[957] when using the Astra 8 and the Multistat III analyzers, compared with results obtained using the ACA Dupont and Ectochem 400 analyzers.

OTHER INTERFERENCE WITH THE JAFFÉ REACTION

Any compound possessing an active methylene group has the potential to react with picrate under the assay conditions. Some substances, such as acetoacetate and pyruvate, react more quickly than creatinine, whereas others, such as glucose, react more slowly. Reaction conditions must be chosen to minimize the interference.

An interval can be selected during which the reaction is mainly from creatinine. This has been applied to reaction-rate methods to measure the change in absorption during the most appropriate period.

Glucose

Glucose is a Jaffé chromogen. After an induction period, the color develops more slowly than with creatinine. Glucose has also been shown to inhibit the formation of alkaline creatinine picrate. Using reaction-rate methods, glucose has little effect on creatinine estimation. Fabini and Ertinghausen found that glucose at a concentration of 30 mmol/L did not interfere if the change between 20 and 80 s was measured.[958]

Keto Acids

Normal levels of acetoacetate do not affect analysis, but some methods are affected by abnormal keto acid concentrations. It is the concentration of alkaline picrate and the time of measurement of the color that mainly determine any errors produced. The effect on various methods has been reviewed by Blass and Ng.[959] Larsen compared results obtained using a reaction-rate method, with those obtained using a Lloyd's reagent method.[960] The error was greatest when readings were made at 10 to 60 s, but disappeared when made at 60 to 120 s. Although high keto acid concentrations are infrequently found in serum, it is desirable that methods chosen for serum creatinine estimation show minimum interference.

Acetohexamide

The sulfonylurea acetohexamide given to treat maturity onset of nonketotic diabetes mellitus was found to affect serum creatinine estimated by a method based on the Jaffé reaction, by Baba et al.[961] In five subjects given the drug, the mean apparent serum creatinine increased from 73 to 104 μmol/L at 2 h and fell at 5 h to 80 μmol/L. The effect was considered to be caused by reaction of the methylene group in the drug with alkaline picrate. Roach et al. confirmed the interference in a study of five methods[962] and showed that there was no interference with the other sulfonylureas, tolbutamide and tolazamide.

Ascorbic Acid

Interference of ascorbic acid, using the Technicon SMAC analyzer, was reported by Vinet and Letellier,[570] who stated that there was no increase at normal ascorbate levels. A small increase in apparent serum creatinine, compared with a control period, in ten subjects given 3 g of ascorbic acid per day for 18 days was found by Van Steirteghem et al.[963] Using the Technicon AA2 analyzer, the mean increase was 24 μmol/L, and using the Technicon SMAC analyzer, it was 20 μmol/L. The change was attributed to analytic interference.

Bromsulphthalein and Phenol Red

Dyes such as Bromsulphthalein, used to measure liver function, and phenol red, used to measure renal function, are red in alkaline solution and so will interfere with the Jaffé reaction. If it is not possible to wait until the dye has been removed from the circulation, Tillson and Schuchardt suggest that the interference can be eliminated by heating the dye with zinc dust in a boiling water bath, to convert the dye to a colorless base.[964]

Cephalosporins

Some cephalosporins react with the Jaffé reagent, and the error produced has been shown to vary with the method used and the cephalosporin given[965] (Table 148). The error is not great at usual therapeutic levels, but misleading results are possible with peak drug levels. Cefoxitin interference with different methods is shown in Table 149. The therapeutic level of cephalosporin is about 0.1 g/L,[965] and the peak level of cefoxitin reached after a rapid infusion is about 0.25 g/L.[966]

Lactulose

A discrepancy in serum creatinine between analyses using the Beckman Astra analyzer and the Technicon SMAC analyzer, of up to approximately 100 μmol/L in serum from a patient treated orally with lactulose for hepatic encephalopathy, was reported by Bruns et al.[967] They showed that addition of pure lactulose to serum affected the assay and concluded that in the patient, some had been absorbed through the gastrointestinal tract.

Methyl Dopa

Apparent serum creatinine estimated using a dialysis method was increased by about 60 μmol/L with 25 mg/L of serum methyl dopa and by about 140 μmol/L with 50 mg/L.[968] Using

TABLE 148.
Interference of Various Cephalosporins with the Direct Jaffé.
Reaction Read at 8 Minutes[a]

Reaction with Jaffé reagent	Cephalosporin	mmol/L	g/L	Error induced color equivalent to μmol/L creatinine
React quicker with Jaffé reagent than creatinine	Cephalothin	10	(4.2)	698
	Cephaloridine	10	(4.2)	283
	Cephacetrile	10	(3.2)	583
React similarly to creatinine with Jaffé reagent	Cephaloglycin	10	(3.9)	336
	Cefoxitin	10	(3.9)	796
No reaction with Jaffé reagent	Cefazolin cefamandole			
	Cephalexin cephaprin			
	Cephradine penicillin G			

[a]   From Swain, R.R. and Briggs, S.L., *Clin. Chem.*, 23, 1340, 1977.

TABLE 149.
Interference of Cefoxitin with Various Methods of
Estimating Serum Creatinine, Based on the Jaffé Reaction[a]

Method	Increase with 250 mg/L of cefoxitin
Protein ppt + Jaffé reaction	300%
Beckman creatinine analyzer	75%
Centrifugal analyzer	150%
Technicon SMAC analyzer	25%
Du Pont ACA analyzer	170%

[a]   From Saah, A. J., Koch, T. R., and Drusano, G. L., *JAMA*, 247, 205, 1982.

a Fuller's Earth method, no interference was found with up to 1000 mg/L of methyl dopa. As methyl dopa in serum in patients taking the drug is usually about 2 mg/L and levels as high as 25 mg/L are rarely obtained, the interference should not cause a problem.

Nitromethane
De Leacy-Brown et al. described a case of a patient (who had ingested a fuel containing methanol and nitromethane)[969] with apparent serum creatinine, estimated using a Technicon SMAC analyzer, of 8000 μmol/L compared with 90 μmol/L, using a specific enzymic method. They showed that a Jaffé chromogen was produced with nitromethane.

Phenacemide
The anticonvulsant phenacemide causes positive interference with most methods using the Jaffé reaction, but negative interference with the method used on the Du Pont ACA analyzer.[970] There is an increase in color for 21 s and then a fall, which explains this finding.

INTERFERENCE WITH ENZYMIC METHODS
Creatine, dopamine, and ascorbic acid interfere with methods for serum creatinine that use the peroxidase reaction.[970] Doses of 0.1 mmol/L of dopamine and 0.5 mmol/L of ascorbic acid reduce apparent serum creatinine significantly.

Sundberg et al. found that the antifungal drug 5-fluorocytosine reacted with 80% of the same molarity of creatinine,[971] using the Ectochem thin-film two-slide method. Cytosine also reacts, but is not usually present in serum. The later single-slide method using sarcosine oxidase and the peroxidase reaction is not affected.

Using the single-slide method on the Ectochem 700 analyzer, a 15 to 37% increase in apparent serum creatinine was found in patients treated with lignocaine for ventricular arrhythmias, compared with results using the Astra analyzer.[972] No interference was found when lignocaine was added to serum, suggesting that a metabolite affects the analysis. Roberts et al. later showed that *N*-ethyl glycine is the metabolite interfering with the method.[973]

CONCLUSION

A number of substances in serum interfere with methods based on the Jaffé reaction and on enzymic methods. Kenny has recently suggested that acetoacetate and bilirubin interfere significantly with methods used in many laboratories.[974] In a study of 51 laboratories in Ireland, errors of from −28 to +221% were found when serum spiked with 10 mmol/L of acetoacetate was analyzed; in a sample with serum bilirubin of about 350 μmol/L, serum creatinine was reported from 0 to 280 μmol/L.

Procedures should be developed to minimize the interference, and laboratory staff should be aware of the situations giving interference in the method used and advise clinicians accordingly.

PREANALYTIC ERROR

COLLECTION OF THE SPECIMEN

Plasma from anticoagulated blood or serum can be used for the estimation of creatinine by most methods. Plasma or serum should be separated soon after collection and stored refrigerated. Oxalate/fluoride and EDTA specimens gave significant increases in apparent plasma creatinine when analyzed using a two-slide coated-film method on the Ectochem analyzer.[971] No error was found using a later single-slide method based on sarcosine oxidase and the peroxidase reaction.

Use of the commercially available product Liposol, which decreases lipemia when shaken with serum, was found to decrease mean creatinine levels from 200 to 185 μmol/L, by Lacher and Elsea.[83] Salzmenn and Male warned about errors introduced when small amounts of blood from pediatric patients (about 0.5 mL) were centrifuged in uncapped tubes.[400] Three minutes of centrifugation increased plasma creatinine by about 10% due to evaporation.

SAMPLE STABILITY

Creatinine is stable in separated serum for at least 1 day at room temperature[961] and for 2 days at 4°C. It is stable for long periods if frozen.[25] A significant decrease is reported in plasma creatinine after 24 h,[942] although Pearce and Bosomworth found that the mean decrease was only about 3% if plasma is stored at 4°C.[975] There is an apparent increase in serum creatinine on storage at room temperature, which is not found on storage at 4°C or when enzymic methods of estimation are used. The change varies with the method used. Laessig et al., using a dialysis method and the Jaffé reaction on a Technicon SMA analyzer,[976] found an apparent increase of 5% on storing at room temperature for 48 h, whereas Rahak and Chiang, using a Technicon SMAC analyzer,[977] found the apparent increase to be about 25% after 24 h. Simpson, using a Du Pont Dimension analyzer and a kinetic Jaffé reaction method,[978] found an apparent doubling after 48 h and an increase of about 40%, using a Technicon Dax 72 analyzer. Harrison considered that the effect was probably due to the formation of pyruvate in stored blood.[979]

Reconstituted lyophilized serum appears to be more stable, and the level of creatinine does not change after 8 days at 10°C or at least 22 days at −15°C.[95]

Heating to 56°C

Heat treatment of serum or plasma to minimize the risk from HIV-positive samples has only a small effect on the creatinine, which is probably not significant (Table 150).

TABLE 150.
Effect of Heating Serum or Plasma for 30 min to 56°C,
on Creatinine Level (in μmol/L)

Reference	Method	Serum or plasma	Change mean
102	Kinetic method on Astra 8	Plasma	−15.6%
		Serum	−1.9%
104	IL 508 analyzer	Plasma	−33%
312		Plasma	−1.3%
	B-propriolactone added	Plasma	No change

TABLE 151.
Changes in Serum Creatinine (in μmol/L) after Eating Meat

Reference	Method	N	Meat content	Before mean	1 h after mean	3 h after mean
982	Protein precipitation followed by Jaffé reaction	1	400 g of beef	90	130	
			450 mg of creatinine	92	122	
983		6	300 g of raw beef		No change	
		6	300 g of fried beef	83.5		109.5
		6	300 g of boiled beef	80		180
		6	300 g of pork in stew		Similar increase	

PHYSIOLOGIC CHANGES

MEALS AND DIET

Although Annino and Relman found no change in serum creatinine following a standard breakfast,[109] others have found a change following meals. Rapoport and Husden found that mean serum creatinine was greater in specimens taken at 4 p.m. than in fasting specimens taken at 8 a.m.[980] Pasternak and Kuhlbäch found no change during the day in fasting subjects,[981] but when normal meals were taken, serum creatinine was about 30% higher at 7 p.m. than when fasting at 7 a.m.

The differences are probably explained by the changes found after ingesting cooked meat (Table 151). It is probable that the cause is related to the conversion of creatine in meat to creatinine by cooking. It is desirable when collecting samples for creatinine estimation that either meat is omitted from the previous meal or fasting samples should be used. This is particularly important during performance of the creatinine clearance test, as changes in serum creatinine can significantly affect the calculation.

EXERCISE

Houet gives references suggesting that serum creatinine can increase by up to 20% after periods of intense exercise.[984] This was thought to be due to increased creatinine production and reduced glomerular filtration.

RANGE IN HEALTHY SUBJECTS

WITHIN- AND BETWEEN-PERSON VARIATION

Early workers estimated creatinine in whole blood, by nonspecific methods. For example, Gettler and St. George, in 1918, reported a range of 9 to 70 μmol/L for blood creatinine in

TABLE 152.
Serum Creatinine in Healthy Subjects (in μmol/L)

Reference	Method	Subject	Sex	N	Age (years)	Mean	50 %ile	Range
413	Jaffé reaction	Morning specimen	M	102				74–124
	after dialysis	from blood donors	F	123				62–106
142	Jaffé reaction	Blood donors,	M		18–25	89.2		
	after dialysis	excluding women	M		26–35	94.9		
	on heparinized	taking oral	M	500	36–45	98.3		
	plasma	contraception	M		46–55	98.5		
			M		56–65	102.1		
			F		18–25	75.0		
			F		26–35	78.0		
			F	500	36–45	79.2		
			F		46–55	82.8		
			F		56–65	86.1		
984	Jaffé reaction	Fasting specimen	M	3100	18–55		89	65–115
	after dialysis	from healthy	M	273	55		91	63–122
		subjects	F	2600	18–55		69	48–95
			F	100	55		76	57–94
937	Enzymic method	Adult blood donors,	M		20–65	76.0		54.8–96.4
		donors, excluding	F		20–65	53.0		39.8–66.3
	Jaffé rate	for renal disease	M		20–65	91.9		73.4–109.6
	reaction method	drug and alcohol abuse	F		20–65	69.8		60.1–79.6

healthy subjects.[985] Plass, by 1917,[986] had recognized that the levels are different in men and women; most reports suggest that mean levels are about 20% higher in men than in women. The difference may be related to muscle mass. Table 152 shows the range of serum creatinine found in some large series.

Roberts[412] and Houet[984] found little change with age, whereas McPherson et al. noted a small increase.[142] Little change directly related to menopause was found by McPherson, and this was confirmed by Gardner and Scott, in a study of randomly selected adults in Scotland.[987] Both Roberts and McPherson et al. reported a log gaussian distribution.

Day-to-Day Variation

Serum creatinine remains fairly constant in a healthy individual over a long period, with a day-to-day cv of about 5% (Table 153). There may be some seasonal variation. Gidlow et al. found lower levels during the summer months in a study of 1500 workers over a 2-year period (Table 154).[691] The variation was more marked in those more than 45 years of age.

CHILDREN

There is a linear increase of serum creatinine with age in children until adult levels are reached at about 16 to 18 years. Tables 155 and 156 show reasonable agreement in the ranges found in several large series. Cherian and Hill found a deviation from the gaussian of the distribution,[326] but despite this, the ranges in the series of Schwartz[992] and of Savoury[989] are given as mean ± 2 SD. Haas used the percentile method to define the range,[990] and these may be the more reliable figures.

Donkerwolke et al. found that mean serum creatinine increased in relation to body surface area (Table 157).[991] Houet gave figures showing that in girls age 12 to 14, there was an increase in the mean of postpubescent subjects (Table 158).[984] The increase with age in children seems to be mainly related to the increase in body size, as creatinine formation is a function of muscle mass, however, there is a small contribution in girls attributable to puberty.

TABLE 152.
Serum Creatinine in Healthy Subjects (in µmol/L)

Reference	Method	Subject	Sex	N	Age (years)	Mean	50 percentile	Range
459	Jaffé reaction after dialysis	Morning specimen from blood donors	M	102				74–124
			F	123				62–106
142	Jaffé reaction after dialysis on heparinized plasma	Blood donors, excluding women taking oral contraception	M		18–25	89.2		
			M		26–35	94.9		
			M	500	36–45	98.3		
			M		46–55	98.5		
			M		56–65	102.1		
			F		18–25	75.0		
			F		26–35	78.0		
			F	500	36–45	79.2		
			F		46–55	82.8		
			F		56–65	86.1		
1042	Jaffé reaction after dialysis	Fasting specimen from healthy subjects	M	3100	18–55		89	65–115
			M	273	55		91	63–122
			F	2600	18–55		69	48–95
			F	100	55		76	57–94
995	Enzymic method	Adult blood donors, donors, excluding for renal disease	M		20–65	76.0		54.8–96.4
			F		20–65	53.0		39.8–66.3
	Jaffé rate reaction method	drug and alcohol abuse	M		20–65	91.9		73.4–109.6
			F		20–65	69.8		60.1–79.6

TABLE 153.
Intraindividual Variation of Serum Creatinine (in μmol/L)

				Individual variation	
Reference	Subjects	Method	N	Range	Mean cv
988	Single individual	22 samples taken over 12 months	1	115–141	
		Single sample taken 12 years later. Method estimating Jaffé reacting chromogen	1	115	
165	Male students 21–27 years old	Five fasting samples taken within 3 weeks. Analysis using the "Autochemist" analyzer	18		2.8%

TABLE 154.
Mean Seasonal Changes in Serum Creatinine (in μmol/L)
in 1500 Workers[a]

Jan	Feb	Mar	Apr	May	Jun
106	105	105	104	102	100
Jul	Aug	Sep	Oct	Nov	Dec
100	101	102	103	102	103

[a] From Gidlow, D. A., Church, J. F., and Clayton, B. E., *Ann. Clin. Biochem.*, 23, 310, 1986.

DRUGS AFFECTING SERUM CREATININE

The toxic effect of many drugs on the kidney results in increases in serum creatinine. References given by Young should be consulted for further information.[70]

Drugs such as gentamicin or methicillin may reduce the glomerular filtration rate by causing renal injury, or may induce volume depletion, as with diuretics. Changes may also be brought about in renal hemodynamics, as by indomethacin-induced inhibition of renal prostaglandin synthesis. These and other changes are discussed by Perrone et al.,[997] with a number of references given. Some drugs are discussed, such as phlorizin, cimetidine, probenecid, trimethoprin, and calcitrol, that interfere with renal tubular creatinine secretion and result in a functional and reversible increase in serum creatinine.

Administration of glucocorticoid results in an increase in the glomerular filtration rate and a reduction in serum creatinine. Chronic administration leads to a reduction in muscle mass, which is also responsible for lower levels of serum creatinine.

Anticonvulsant therapy may result in a fall in serum creatinine[998] (Table 160), which is also related to an increase in the glomerular filtration rate.

TABLE 155.
Serum Creatinine (in μmol/L) in Boys

Age (years)	991 N	991 Mean	991 Range	992 N	992 Mean	992 SD	989 N	989 Mean	989 ±2 SD	990 5 percentile	990 2.5–97.5 percentile
$1/12$–$1/4$							35	43	19–67		
$1/4$–$1/2$							23	45	28–62		
$1/2$–1							43	44	23–65		
1	10	32	20–41	89	36	9	58	58	22–74		
2	21	37	26–56	18	38	11	45	46	26–66		
3	27	38	29–53	30	41	10	40	44	32–66		
4	26	40	20–52	49	40	10	44	51	28–74		
5	24	43	29–57	50	44	10	49	53	34–72		26.5–79.6
6	21	43	28–55	62	46	11	40	55	34–76		
7	23	47	33–59	59	48	12	24	56	39–73		
8	33	50	37–69	60	50	14	34	57	38–76	44.2	
9	15	53	38–68	60	50	14	21	60	38–82	44.2	
10				58	54	20	27	64	40–88	44.2	
11				56	55	12	21	63	47–79	44.2	
12				67	57	14	38	66	46–86	53.0	
13				53	60	19	28	69	44–94	61.9	44.2–79.6
14				44	64	21	29	70	52–88	61.9	44.2–79.6
15				40	67	19	41	77	53–101	61.9	44.2–88.4
16				24	64	20	52	80	52–108	61.9	44.2–88.4
17				22	71	16	44	81	62–100	70.7	53.0–88.4
18							35	86	64–108	79.6	61.9–106.1
19				19	80	15	48	89	68–110	88.4	61.9–106.1
20							51	85	63–107	88.4	53.0–115

TABLE 156.
Serum Creatinine (in μmol/L) in Girls

Age (years)	991			992			989			990	
	N	Mean	Range	N	Mean	SD	N	Mean	±2 SD	50 percentile	2.5–97.5 percentile
¹/₁₂–¹/₄							24	44	29–59		
¹/₄–¹/₂							20	43	29–59		
¹/₂–1							29	43	20–66		
1				8	31	4	54	45	24–66		
2				13	40	6	40	46	21–71		
3				24	37	7	40	49	26–72		
4	16	34	26–43	28	42	10	40	51	35–67	44.2	35.4–70.7
5	22	35	25–50	44	41	11	30	50	32–68	44.2	35.4–70.7
6	22	38	26–50	44	42	10	19	51	36–66	44.2	35.4–70.7
7	34	39	24–60	50	47	11	31	54	36–72	53.0	35.4–61.9
8	22	42	30–53	61	47	10	31	58	43–73	53.0	44.2–70.7
9	20	44	30–61	61	49	10	23	57	45–69	53.0	44.2–79.6
10	25	44	28–59	46	49	11	31	60	47–73	61.9	44.2–79.6
11	32	50	32–74	57	53	11	44	63	44–82	61.9	44.2–79.6
12	15	52	45–71	54	52	11	28	60	51–69	61.9	53.0–79.6
13				41	55	12	32	66	53–79	70.7	53.0–79.6
14				30	57	11	41	69	48–90	70.7	61.9–88.4
15				22	59	20	54	69	54–84	70.7	61.9–88.4
16				16	57	13	67	72	51–93	79.6	61.9–88.4
17				12	62	18	57	76	59–93		
18							66	76	59–93		
19				15	64	17	74	77	59–95		
20							68	75	53–97		

TABLE 157.
Serum Creatinine (in μmol/L) in Boys and Girls 4–12 Years Old,
According to Body Surface Area[a]

Body surface area (cm²)	Boys				Girls			
	N	Mean	SD	Range	N	Mean	SD	Range
<6575	6	38	11	20–56	15	34	5	26–43
6579–7450	20	34	5	20–43	22	34	7	25–50
7450–8325	31	37	7	26–53	20	37	7	26–53
8325–9200	32	40	7	25–52	34	39	7	24–53
9200–10075	27	44	8	29–61	31	45	9	29–61
10075–10950	28	46	9	31–62	25	43	10	27–74
10950–11825	18	48	8	27–61	21	48	5	38–57
11825–12700	15	51	6	42–66	18	50	7	31–61
>12700	23	51	9	34–69	22	53	7	41–71

[a] From Donckerwolcke, R. A. M. G., et al., *Acta Paediatr. Scand.,* 59, 399, 1970.

TABLE 158.
Serum Creatinine (in μmol/L)
in Pre- and Postpubescent Girls 12–14 Years Old[a]

	N	50 percentile	2.5–97.5 percentile
Prepubescent	214	59.7	41–81
Postpubescent	313	62.1	42–85

[a] From Houet, O., in *Interpretation of Clinical Laboratory Tests,* Siest, G., et al., Eds., Biomedical Publishers, Foster City, CA, 1985, 231.

TABLE 159.
Serum Creatinine (in mmol/L) in the Neonatal Period

Reference	Subjects	Method	N	Age (days)	28 Mean	28 SD	29–32 Mean	29–32 SD	33–36 Mean	33–36 SD	37–42 Mean	37–42 SD	Comment
993	Low-birth-weight babies	Nonspecific manual manual Jaffé reaction		1–10			115						All below 88
				60–90			53						
994	Various exclusions	Kinetic Jaffé reaction method	56	1–5					Range 17–188				All below 62 at 5 days
			56	6–30					Mean 35	Range 12–62			
995	All babies		238	2	116	40	104	38	93	39	75	38	
	Breathed spontaneously			2	108	20	100	32	94	39			
	Ventilated			2	121	45	115	43	87	46			
	All babies		238	7	84	32	83	41	68	44	50	36	
	All babies		238	14	72	32	69	32	55	36	38	20	
	All babies		238	21	60	33	59	32	50	37	35	18	
	All babies		238	28	58	24	52	33	35	24	30	18	
989			36	0–2			106	64–148					
			50	3–5			83	45–121					
			17	6–7			80	46–114					
			17	7–30			74	49–99					
			51	0–2							105	70–140	
			66	3–5							75	41–149	
			17	6–7							63	33–93	
			43	7–30							56	31–81	
			35	30–90							43	19–67	

Gestation weeks

TABLE 160.
Change in Mean Serum Creatinine
in Patients Taking Anticonvulsants

	N	Change compared with control group
Phenobarbitone	32	–5.1%
Phenytoin + phenobarbitone	18	–18%
Other anticonvulsants	150	–12%

[a] From Bagrel, A., et al., *Drug Effects on Laboratory Tests Results,* Siest, G., Ed., Nijho Ed, The Hague, 1980, 201.

Chapter 13

URATE

Sydenham, in 1776, showed that uric acid was a constituent of some renal stones. Wolleston, in 1787, demonstrated urate in the tophi of gouty subjects. In 1854 Garrod reported excess urate in the blood of sufferers from gout. When Fischer, in 1898, showed uric acid to be a purine, the potential relationship to the nucleic acid constituents adenine and guanine became apparent.[999] Blood levels of urate reflect the equilibrium between purine elimination (mainly through the kidneys, with some fecal excretion) and purine formation.

ANALYTIC CONSIDERATIONS

In the earliest work, urate was separated from body fluids by precipitation as silver urate and estimated by reduction of phosphotungstic acid in alkaline solution. Folin and Denis, in 1912, used sodium carbonate as the alkalizing agent.[1000] Later, Benedict and Hitchcock used cyanide to increase sensitivity.[1001] Benedict applied the phosphotungstate reaction directly to a protein-free filtrate in 1922;[1002] most colorimetric methods have since been based on this procedure.

Procedures for the estimation of serum urate are reviewed by Watts in detail.[1003]

A number of difficulties when using reduction methods have been found. Some that use protein precipitation give low results due to adsorption onto the precipitate. Natelson found that there was no loss if tungstate and acid were mixed before the addition of serum.[1004] The use of carbonate as an alkaline reagent, although less sensitive than cyanide, gives a more reproducible color, linear with urate concentration, and has the advantage of being less toxic.[1005]

Turbidity has been found to interfere with measurement of the color. To overcome the problem, various reagents have been proposed, such as the addition of lithium salts to the color reagent; the use of sodium silicate, with or without the addition of glycerol, as the alkaline reagent; and the inclusion of urea in the alkaline solution.

Methods using automatic analyzers may depend on the reduction of phospho- or arsenophosphotungstate, or of a metal complex such as the copper salt of neocuproine or bathocuproine. Dialysis avoids the loss of urate in protein precipitate, but other interference remains possible. More specific methods have been developed based on the conversion of urate to allantoin and hydrogen peroxide, under the influence of uricase. The procedure suggested by Praetorius[1006] uses the fall in absorption at 292.5 nm, the maximum for urate. Protein absorbs at this wavelength, giving a high sample blank; thus, trichloracetic acid has been used to remove protein, shifting the peak to 283 nm. This procedure is the basis for a suggested reference method in which recovery of radioactive urate of 99 to 101%, and a precision of about 2%, is claimed.[1007]

Other uricase methods measure either the amount of oxygen consumed or hydrogen peroxide formed. The methods have been adapted for use with automatic analyzers.

Both reduction and enzymic methods can be affected by interference from hemolysis, bilirubin, and a number of drugs.

ACCURACY AND PRECISION

Enzymic methods should be capable of giving results close to the true urate content of serum. Watts states that results using reduction methods agree with those using enzymic methods,[1003] but some authors disagree. Lous and Sylvest found mean results, using a phosphotungstate method,[1008] about 60 μmol/L lower than with a Praetorius method, and using a ferricyanide reduction method (used particularly in Scandinavia at one time), about 180 μmol/L higher. Several groups[1009,1010] have said that results using the procedure suggested by Archibald,[1011] in which phosphotungstate is used both to precipitate protein and for color development, agree well with the enzymic method. Using results from Quality Assurance Schemes to assess accuracy, mean results by uricase methods are about 2.5 to 5% lower than those obtained using reduction procedures. This is a little higher than was suggested by the experiments of Caraway and Marabie,[1012] who used uricase to remove urate and found that nonurate chromogen was about 2%.

Precision of urate estimation has been reported to be from 4 to 8%, depending on the method. DiGorgio states that precision of manual and continuous-flow methods is about 5% and that precision of uricase methods is about 8%.[1013] McLaughlan found precision of 4.6% at 400 μmol/L using a phosphotungstate method on a continuous-flow analyzer.[1005]

SI UNITS

To convert from mass to molar units,

$$\text{serum urate mg/100 mL} \times 59.5 = \text{μmol/L}$$

A number of laboratories express serum urate as millimoles per liter. This appears contrary to the convention that figures should be between 1 and 1000 to minimize use of the decimal point. It is done to avoid the occasional problems caused when the figure in micromoles per liter is above 1000. To avoid confusion, laboratories do not then convert to millimoles per liter.

INTERFERENCE WITH ANALYSIS

HEMOLYSIS

Hemoglobin of about 2 g/L in serum increases apparent serum urate by 2 to 3%, using the phosphotungstate/carbonate method. At a serum hemoglobin concentration of 4.24 g/L, the error is over 10%. The increase is probably due to reducing substances, such as glutathione and ergothioneine from red cells, and is a potential source of error in all reducing methods. Up to 10 g/L of serum hemoglobin does not interfere with methods using dialysis on a continuous-flow analyzer.[292]

Most enzymic methods are not affected by hemolysis, although Duncan et al.[1007] found that 2 g/L of hemoglobin in serum reduced apparent urate by about 5%, using a method measuring the change in absorption at 283 nm.

Small amounts of hemoglobin do not affect peroxidase-linked assays. James and Price found that there was no interference with up to 7.4 g/L in serum,[1014] and Fossati et al. found none with up to 13 g/L.[1015] In contrast, Majic-Singh et al. found interference with up to 3 g/L, by their method.[1016] Using a catalase-linked assay, Nagayama found no interference with up to 3 g/L of serum hemoglobin.[1017] James and Price found no interference with up to 7.4 g/L.[1014]

BILIRUBIN

Up to 110 μmol/L of serum bilirubin does not interfere with the manual phosphotungstate method of DiGorgio.[1013] There is an error of about 6% at 145 μmol/L of bilirubin. Serum bilirubin of up to 170 μmol/L has been shown to have little effect, using a phosphotungstate method on a continuous-flow analyzer. Enzymic methods may also be affected by bilirubin. A reduction of about 5% in apparent serum urate was found by Duncan et al.[1007] using a method measuring the change at 283 nm with serum bilirubin of 170 μmol/L. However, Hullin and McGrane, using the loss at the peak of 292 nm,[1018] found no change with up to 120 μmol/L of bilirubin.

A considerable reduction in apparent serum urate due to bilirubin may be found in some uricase-peroxidase methods.[1019] Fossati et al. claimed that inclusion of potassium ferricyanide in the reagent eliminated the error with up to 170 µmol/L of bilirubin in serum,[1015] but Hullin and McGrane found that the error was reduced,[1018] but not completely eliminated. At 120 µmol/L of bilirubin, they reported that apparent serum urate was about 92% of the true level. The catalase method of Kageyama is not affected by up to 170 µmol/L of bilirubin. This has been confirmed by James and Price[1014] using a catalase/aldehyde dehydrogenase-linked assay.

OTHER INTERFERING SUBSTANCES

A number of substances can potentially interfere with methods based on reduction by urate. Watts lists the following:[1003]

1. Free thiols (thioneine, cysteine, glutathione)
2. Methylated purines (caffeine, theobromine, theophylline)
3. Gentisic acid — metabolite of acetyl salicylic acid
4. Homogentisic acid
5. Glucose

Quantitative effects are not given, but will vary with the method. Patel says that cysteine and glucose, at normal physiologic concentrations,[1020] do not interfere in a method using sodium EDTA as alkali and hydrazine as color intensifier.

Although ascorbic acid affects reducing methods, the highest level found in serum, even after the largest daily dose, will not significantly affect the apparent urate level.[1020] Enzymic methods are not affected, except those based on uricase with the second stage using copper reduction, which are prone to a large error even with physiologic levels of ascorbate. It should be noted that high doses of ascorbic acid increase urate excretion, thus, there is also a potential biologic effect from ascorbic acid therapy.

Allopurinol is given to prevent urate nephropathy in patients prone to high urate levels treated with cyclophosphamide. This leads to xanthine production. Serum xanthine levels increase in cases with reduced renal function, and this interferes with the uricase method. An error of up to 36.5% at 520 mg/L of xanthine has been found.[1021]

L-Dopa may affect both phosphotungstate methods and peroxidase-linked enzymic methods. Using the phosphotungstate method, Cawein and Hewins found a mean increase, above the pretherapy level, of 20% in 18 of 20 patients receiving 3 to 7 g of L-dopa per day.[1022] Bierer and Quebbman found that L-dopa and its major metabolites interfered,[1023] but at therapeutic L-dopa levels (% mg/L), the spurious increase was only 12 µmol/L. Using the peroxidase-linked uricase method, Sanders et al. found that 50 mg/L of L-dopa decreased urate by 80%,[1024] whereas Cawein and Hewins[1022] and Fossati[1015] found that there was no effect on the enzymic methods they used.

The chemotherapeutic agent eptoposide (Vapasid) interferes with the phosphotungstate method.[1025] Using the American Monitor "Parallel" discrete analyzer in one serum, the apparent urate level of the serum was 892 µmol/L compared with a level of 224 µmol/L when analyzed by a uricase method. The effect could be demonstrated by adding the drug to the serum.

Formaldehyde, which has been used to preserve aqueous urate calibration standards for many years, has been found to interfere with both the phosphotungstate reaction[1026] and the uricase reaction.[1027] At the concentration used in aqueous standards, the apparent standard level is increased by about 5%. Using the phosphotungstate reduction method in continuous-flow analyzers Beetham and Sanders showed that at pH below 8.5,[1028] the rate of dialysis of urate is affected due to formation of a pH-dependent addition product of urate and formaldehyde. Using the uricase-catalase method, the NSAIDs indomethacin and diclophenac, at about

TABLE 161.
The Effect of Paracetamol on Reduction Methods for Serum Urate (μmol/L)

Reference	Method	Dose (g)	Time after (h)	Change	Comment
82	SMA 12/60	2	2	+65	
1029	SMA 12/60	1	1	+120	Patient 1
		2	1	+180	Patient 2
		2	1	+240	Patient 3
1030	AA 1	Blood level	<0.04g/L	Small	Greatest effect using hydroxylamine/ tungstate method. Effect lesser using urea/cyanide and carbonate/
		Blood level	0.04g/L	+120	tungstate

10 × therapeutic concentration, increase apparent urate by about 7%. It is unlikely that this will affect interpretation of urate levels in patients taking these drugs.

Several groups have found that apparent serum urate is higher than the true level, in patients taking paracetamol, using the phosphotungstate method (Table 161). The much greater effect noted by Wilding and Heath[1029] is difficult to explain, as all used similar methods.

CONCLUSION

Hemolysis, bilirubin, some drugs, and a number of other substances introduce errors in both reduction and enzymic methods of estimation, and it is necessary to be aware of any interference with the particular method used, when interpreting serum urate results.

PREANALYTIC ERROR

COLLECTION OF THE SPECIMEN

Most early workers estimated urate, using whole blood. Levels are lower than those using serum, as erythrocytes contain only half the urate concentration of serum.[898] As the concentration of interfering substances, particularly glutathione, is greater in red cells, serum is now preferred.

ANTICOAGULANTS

Potassium salts give a turbidity with phosphotungstate,[1031] which DiGorgio suggested was due to insoluble potassium phosphotungstate.[1013] Thus, potassium edate, oxalate, citrate, and heparinate should not be used as anticoagulants if reduction methods are being used. A statistically significant, but clinically unimportant, difference of about 10 μmol/L between urate in serum and heparinized plasma was found by Lum and Gambino.[391] However, Hubsch differed,[1032] finding excellent agreement with no statistical difference demonstrated.

CONTAMINATION

The earliest phosphotungstate reagents were found to be contaminated with molybdenum, which is more sensitive to other reducing agents in serum than tungstate is. Folin and Trimble described the preparation involving precipitation of molybdenum as a sulfide.[1033] Reagents now available contain very low molybdenum levels, and contamination should rarely be a problem.

SAMPLE STABILITY

Some reports from the mid-1920s suggest that in mammalian blood there is a heat-stable catalyst that rapidly destroys urate.[1034] However, in 1939 Blauch and Koch,[1035] using human

TABLE 162.
Effect of Fasting on Serum Urate (in µmol/L)

Reference	Subjects	Day	Level		
1037	Healthy person taking only water	0	227		
		2	326		
		3	553		
		7	881		
		14	704		
1038	Three epileptic children		**Child 1**	**Child 2**	**Child 3**
		0	220	340	355
		1		290	252
		2	360	440	378
		3	433	700	257
		4		714	392
		5		730	390
		6	476	550	392
		7			383
		8			
		9	432		

blood, demonstrated that urate in an oxalated specimen is stable for several days if refrigerated, and for up to 1 day at room temperature. Desaty and Green showed that samples could be stored at 4°C for 4 days and at 20°C for 1 week.[309] Urate fell if these limits were exceeded.

Changes observed using reduction methods may be due to nonurate chromogen. Buchanan et al. reported that nonurate chromogen fell after heating serum or freezing it for 3 weeks.[1036] When compared with a Praetorius method, apparent urate was a mean of about 100 µmol/L higher in 1-day-old serum, compared with a mean of about 30 µmol/L higher when stored frozen for 21 days. The fall was mainly in the first few days and was almost complete after 3 weeks.

Heating to 56°C

Heating serum or plasma to 56°C to minimize risk from HIV-positive samples has been shown to have little effect on urate levels. After heating serum or plasma for 30 min, Gouldie et al. found a mean increase of 0.8%,[101] and Collinson et al. a mean increase of 0.2%.[102]

PHYSIOLOGIC CHANGES

POSTURE

Seated subjects are reported to have serum levels about 3% higher than in supine subjects,[1032] a difference that should not cause any problem in interpretation.

FASTING AND MEALS

It was shown many years ago that serum urate increases after a long period of fasting (Table 162). Urine urate decreases until a certain level of blood urate is reached, where excretion increases and blood urate no longer increases. It seems likely that the changes are caused by inhibition, by ketones, of tubular secretion of urate. There is a small increase of serum urate, following a standard meal. Steinmetz et al.[1039] found that a mean of 360 µmol/L at noon increased to 370 µmol/L 2 to 3 h later, after a 700-cal standard meal.

Diet

Ingestion of purine results in an increase of serum urate, which can reach 15%.[1032] Overeating can cause a similar increase. After 7 days on a purine-free diet, mean serum urate falls by about 10% in both healthy and gouty subjects.[1040] The fall may be up to approximately 30% in individual cases.

EXERCISE

In studies published in 1921, Rakestraw found an increase in serum urate of 55 µmol/L in subjects after brief exercise[1041] and 90 µmol/L after prolonged exercise. This was confirmed by later researchers. Levine found increases of from 25 to 155 µmol/L in subjects after a marathon run;[1042] Nicholls et al. found a rise of about 30 µmol/L in subjects after 30 min of running.[1043] Zachau-Christianson found an increase of up to 60 µmol/L after light exercise,[1044] such as gymnastics for 30 min. Hubsch found that exercise before blood collection resulted in a 4% increase in serum urate levels,[1032] but gave no details of the amount of exercise involved.

It seems unlikely that the modest exercise involved in attending a clinic would affect interpretation of results, but excessive exercise should be avoided.

SEASONAL VARIATION

Reports differ about the variation of serum urate during the year. Although Hubsch says that no annual rhythm has been described, Becker and Goldstein found significantly higher levels in summer,[1045] with the mean for 12 healthy men increasing from 280 to 359 µmol/L. Gidlow et al., in a study of 1000 workers over a 2-year period, found the highest mean levels in February and March,[691] but said that the changes did not reach statistical significance. The mean throughout the year varied from 320 to 341 µmol/L.

MENSTRUAL CYCLE

Mira et al. found mean serum urate levels to be 255 µmol/L (SD 54) during the luteal phase of the menstrual cycle, and 286 µmol/L (SD 50) during the follicular phase, in a group of apparently healthy women 25 to 40 year old.[411] These small changes are unlikely to cause any difficulty in interpretation.

RANGE IN HEALTHY SUBJECTS

WITHIN- AND BETWEEN-PERSON VARIATIONS

It is difficult to define a range for serum urate in healthy persons, without taking into account a number of factors, such as sex, body bulk, socioeconomic factors, and ethnic origin. All of these influence the level. Indeed, Newcombe claimed that defining normal serum urate is a didactic exercise[1046] and may not be relevant at all times to a patient with disordered urate metabolism. Large differences in serum urate have been reported in studies of people from different parts of the world and different ethnic groups[1047] (Table 163). Higher levels are consistently reported in men than in women, and the highest mean is about twice the lowest.

There is little change in serum urate with age in men, but usually the level is found to be higher in older women than in the younger age groups (Table 164).

Interpretation of Serum Urate

As a guide to serum urate in healthy European subjects, one can use the ranges found by Hubsch[1032] in a study of 32,000 French people, excluding obese subjects, and those suffering from gout, tumors, blood diseases, and renal disease, and those with high alcohol consumption (Table 165).

More important than the range in healthy subjects, in interpreting levels, may be the definition of pathologic levels. Hubsch gives references defining hyperuricemia as more than 420 µmol/L in men and more than 360 µmol/L in women. The maximum plasma concentration in plasma before saturation is reached is said to be 416 µmol/L for both sexes; below this concentration, the risk of gout is minimal. Approximately 90% of gouty subjects and 10% of other men have serum urate exceeding this level.

TABLE 163.
Serum or Plasma Urate in Various Populations and Ethnic Groups[a]
(figures converted to μmol/L)

Population	Male N	Male Mean	Male SD	Female N	Female Mean	Female SD
Tecumseh, MI	2987	292	83	3013	250	71
Framington, MA[b]	2283	305	66	2844	238	56
U.S. army inductees	817	301	56			
U.S. prisoners — white	90	298	66			
Denmark150	303	71	150	238	56	
Finland737	298	65	1048	238	60	
Wensleydale, England	436	265		475	220	
West Germany	265	289	79	119	241	77
Australian — White[b]	100	331	57	100	269	42
France	23923	350	71			
Thai recruits 20 years old	710	295	54			
Thai prisoners 15–50 years old	399	282	58			
Ethnic group						
American black	154	308				
North American Indian						
Pima	949	291	71			
Blackfoot	1018	251	71			
Haida	237	262	59			
Filipinos						
In Seattle	118	374	77			
In Hawaii	60	363	77			
In Philippines	483	309	77			
Hawaiians (full blooded)	49	321	65			
Micronesians						
Chamorros						
California	164	381	83	151	292	77
Guam	273	422	89	355	321	83
Rota	122	428	83	149	321	71
Palauans						
Koror	109	405	83	145	309	77
Paleliu	41	369	77	57	327	71
Nger	69	357	77	89	292	83
Polynesians						
Maori (New Zealand)	366	420	92	381	343	92
Rarotongans	243	414	83	228	355	71
Pukapukans	188	419		191	368	65
Australian aborigines						
Aurukun	82	359	74	135	284	73
Taiwan Chinese	247	297	54	120	230	46
Malayan Chinese	298	363	77	106	269	54
Malays	169	376	74	9	250	40
Indians	141	214	42			

[a] From Wyngaarden, J. B. and Kelley, W. N., in *Metabolic Basis of Inherited Disease*, 5th ed., Stanbury, J. S., Ed., McGraw-Hill, New York, 1983, 936. With permission.

[b] Colorimetric methods. All other values by enzymatic spectrophotometric methods.

Day-to-Day Variation

The coefficient of variation (cv) from day to day in healthy individuals is from 7 to 10% (Table 166). This is surprisingly high, as posture, exercise, and meals have only a small effect on serum urate levels and must be taken into account if serial estimations are being considered.

TABLE 164.
Serum Urate (in μmol/L) at Different Ages[a]

Reference		Men Age (years)					Women Age (years)				
		20–29	30–39	40–49	50–59	60–69	20–29	30–39	40–49	50–59	60–69
1048				Little effect with age				Level at age 60–64 higher than at age 32–39			
145	Median	363	357	369	369	369	268	256	268	286	292
	Range	244–494	244–494	244–518	196–524	226–595	167–422	155–416	167–482	196–464	

[a] Phosphotungstate methods used.

TABLE 165.
Range of Serum Urate (in μmol/L)
in 32,000 Healthy French People[a]

Sex	Age (years)	50 percentile	2.5–97.5 percentile
Male	18–65	339	238–458
Female	18–45	256	173–348
	45–55	250	178–363
	>55	262	190–375

[a] From Hubsch, G., in *Interpretations of Clinical Laboratory Tests*, Siest, G., et al., Eds., Foster City, CA, Biomedical Publishers, 1985, 428.

Inheritance

Ryckewaert found hyperuricemia to be present in 20 to 25% of patients with gout.[1049] This has been attributed to an autosomal dominant gene or group of genes. A simple mendelian mechanism is unlikely, as hyperuricemia is a continuously distributed variable, and the essentially unimodal curve suggests a multiple and cumulative etiology. There appears to be a complex genetic background influenced by multiple environmental factors.

A strong genetic element was suggested in a study by Prior et al.,[1050] which compared serum urate in Maoris from New Zealand, Raratongans from the Cook Islands, and subjects from Pukapuka, also in the Cook Islands. Despite very different life styles, ranging from a Western life style for many years to life at subsistence level with limited cash income, serum urate levels were similar. In other work it has been difficult to separate genetic factors from socioeconomic factors, sexual maturity, and muscle mass, as when Harlan et al. found a 10% difference between white and black American adolescents.[1051]

A link with blood groups has been found. Griebsch and Zollner found that serum urate in females with blood group AB was 12% higher, on average, than in those with blood groups A.[1052]

Social Status

An impressive list of prominent people in history have suffered from gout, including Alexander the Great, Charlemagne, Bacon, Milton, Darwin, Harvey, and Hunter. An uncommon frequency of high social class among gouty patients has been noted,[1053] and a number of attempts have been made to correlate urate levels with occupation, intelligence, drive, achievement, and leadership, with motivated school students, and with various personality traits. These have been reviewed with references.[1054]

Hubsch gives further references[1032] suggesting that town dwellers, professional staff and intellectuals have higher urate levels than have manual workers or those living in a rural environment. It is difficult to separate differences between groups from differences due to inheritance, life style, body weight, etc., when attempting to establish the reason for variations.

THE ELDERLY

In the elderly, cardiovascular disease and antihypertensive drugs tend to increase serum urate; reduced body mass, reduced physical activity, and changes in eating habits may have the opposite effect. There are few studies of serum urate in the elderly. In a study of a rural population in north Finland, Takala et al.[1055] found little change in men or women, from 65 to 89 years old (Table 167). A small difference in the mean serum urate of pre- and postmenopausal women of the same age has been noted (Table 168), suggesting that the increase found in older women is related to menopause.

TABLE 166.
Intraindividual Variation of Serum Urate

Reference	Subjects	Method	Individual variation N	Mean cv	Comment
163	Male and female white and black subjects 20–59 years old	Fasting specimen taken at 9 am once a week for 10–12 weeks	68	10.1%	After allowing for analytic variation of cv 3.5%
164	White doctors	One fasting specimen taken once a week for 10 weeks. Stored frozen and analyzed on the same day	9	8.3%	After allowing for analytic variation
165	Male students 21–27 years old	Five fasting samples taken within 3 weeks. Analysis using the "Autochemist"analyzer	18	7.3%	

CHILDREN

The serum urate level is lower in children than in adults and is similar in boys and girls up to puberty. At puberty the level increases more in boys than in girls, giving rise to the sex-based difference found in adults (Table 169).

CORD BLOOD AND NEONATES

Serum urate in cord blood is higher than in the corresponding maternal serum (Table 170). The level in neonates peaks at the age of 1 day and falls to the maternal level or below by the 2nd or 3rd day of life in full-term babies. In low-birth-weight babies, the peak is on the 1st day, but levels take longer to fall to maternal levels (Table 171).

RANGE DURING PREGNANCY

Early workers believed that blood urate did not change during pregnancy and that it rose during labor.[1060] However, Bunker and Mundell[919] and Harding et al.[1061] reported during the early 1920s that there was a rise during the later months of pregnancy. Table 172 gives results of some later work, showing that there is a fall during the first and second trimesters and then an increase during the third trimester, although the mean level does not reach that in nonpregnant women. The changes are considered to be due to altered renal handling of urate.

OTHER CHANGES

BODY WEIGHT

In most populations studied, serum urate is positively correlated with body weight and surface area, although exceptions are reported. Table 173 shows the results of some studies. An interpretation of serum urate, without consideration of the body weight, is likely to be misleading.

A statistical correlation can be shown between gout and hypertension, arteriosclerosis, and hypertriglyceridemia. As these are associated with obesity, the correlation is explained.

SMOKING

Two large studies, shown in Table 174, have shown that smoking tobacco has an effect on serum urate. The change is small and is unlikely to affect the interpretation of a single result.

TABLE 167.
Serum Urate (in µmol/L) in an Elderly Finnish Population[a]

| Sex | Age (years) | | | | | | | | | | | | | | |
| | 65–69 | | 70–74 | | 75–79 | | 80–84 | | 85–89 | |
	N	Mean	SD	N	Mean	SD	N	Mean	SD	N	Mean	SD	N	Mean	SD
Male	142	294	68	86	289	65	46	297	70	18	251	67	6	268	51
Female	129	275	96	80	264	64	44	283	65	22	241	71	5	298	63

[a] 89.8% of a rural population, with those taking diuretics excluded. From Takala, J., et al., *Scand. J. Rheum.*, 17, 155, 1988.

TABLE 168.
Changes in Serum Urate (in μmol/L) at Menopause

Reference	Subject and method		Age (Years)			
			36–45 Mean	46–55 Mean	45–55 50 percentile	45–55 2.5–97.5 percentile
142	Blood donors					
	Phosphotungstate reduction	Premenopausal	263	276		
	method on continuous-flow	Postmenopausal	276	303		
	analyzer					
1032	French women from a	Premenopausal			244	173–363
	health screen	Postmenopausal			262	179–387

TABLE 169.
Serum Urate (in μmol/L) in Children

Reference	Age (years)	Boys N	Boys Mean	Boys Range	Girls N	Girls Mean	Girls Range
1056[a]	4	29	205	107–363	32	205	131–357
	5–9	336	216	71–571	287	221	113–494
	10–14	429	255	77–524	360	243	107–583
	10		218			233	
	11		235			229	
	12		250			249	
	13		274			254	
	14		299			265	
	15–19	254	319	89–530	258	250	101–464
	15		325			245	
	16		327			261	
	17		337			246	
	18		293			246	
	19		299			252	
				2.5–97.5			2.5–97.5
1057[b]			50 percentile	percentile		50 percentile	percentile
	5		250	180–350		250	160–330
	6		240	160–320		250	180–330
	7		250	160–330		250	180–330
	8		250	170–330		250	170–330
	9		250	170–330		260	170–350
	10		250	170–370		250	180–360
	11		260	180–360		260	180–380
	12		270	190–430		270	190–380
	13		300	190–440		270	190–380
	14		360	210–440		260	190–360
	15		330	230–490		270	180–360
	16		360	270–480		270	180–360
	17		360	250–480		270	180–380
	Adult			210–460			170–420

[a] Children in Tecumseh, MI. Uricase method.
[b] Children in Marshfield, WI. Phosphotungstate method on Technicon SMAC analyzer.

BLINDNESS

Serum urate in blind and partially sighted people has been found to be higher than in those with normal vision (Table 175).

TABLE 170.
Serum Urate in Cord Blood (in µmol/L)

Reference	Method	Term	Mother			Cord		
			N	Mean	SD	N	Mean	SD
1058	Phosphotungstate/ carbonate method	Full-term	40	232	60	30	262	54
		Low-birth weight	28	214	77	30	286	77
1059	Uricase method					279	64	

TABLE 171.
Serum Urate (in µmol/L) in Neonates

Reference	Method	Age (hours)	Full term			Lowbirth weight		
			N	Mean	SD	N	Mean	SD
1058	Phosphotungstate/ carbonate method	0–24	28	333	48	34	405	107
		25–48	29	226	60	25	405	137
		49–72				21	303	107
		73–96				5	167	48
		97–120				11	184	54
1059	Uricase method	12–24	15	359	82			
		25–48	15	258	66			
		49–84	15	188	44			

ALCOHOL

The association of consumption of alcohol with hyperuricemia and gout was discussed by Garrod as long ago as 1863.[1067] A number of workers have shown that ethanol consumption increases serum urate. In 12 acutely intoxicated subjects studied by Lieber et al.,[1068] serum urate was above the normal range in five and fell to normal within 2 to 11 days. In the seven cases with normal serum urate, the level fell in each case. Alcohol given intravenously to produce a blood level of more than 200 mg/dL almost doubled serum urate in each of three subjects. Baker et al. found that mean serum urate of 107 healthy nongouty alcohol drinkers was 400 µmol/L (range of 250 to 605),[1069] which compared with a mean in 37 nonalcohol drinkers of 350 µmol/L (range of 200 to 545). The increase of serum urate by alcohol is reported to be greater in women.

The relation between ethanol metabolism and uric acid was reviewed by Newcombe.[1070] He noted that the primary cause of hyperuricemia after alcohol consumption was from increased lactate formation, which alters renal transport, leading to a fall in urate excretion.

ALTITUDE

Acheson and Florey, in a study of military recruits from Columbia,[1065] found a positive correlation between the altitude of previous domicile and serum urate:

- Altitude of less than 1000 ft, serum urate mean was 284 mmol/L
- Altitude of 1000 to 1999 ft, serum urate mean was 301 mmol/L
- Altitude of more than 2000 ft, serum urate mean was 316 mmol/L

These results were consistent with earlier work showing a correlation with blood hemoglobin,[1064] which increases in subjects living at higher altitudes.

TABLE 172.
Serum Urate (in µmol/L) During Pregnancy

Reference	Method	1st trimester			2nd trimester			3rd trimester			Nonpregnant		
		N	Mean	SD	N	Mean	SD	N	Mean	SD	N	Mean	SD
919	Phosphotungstate using whole blood					137			226				
1062	Phosphotungstate, with serum on continuous-flow analyzer	44	162	37	48	125	32	14	215	45	64	230	43
1063	Enzymatic on serum with reaction-rate analyzer	24	168	26	24	178	30	24	202	35	24	219	36

TABLE 173.
Some Large Studies of the Relationship Between Serum Urate (in μmol/L) and Body Bulk

Reference	Subjects and method	N	Results	Comment
1064	Five social classes in New Haven, CT. Phosphotungstate method on continuous-flow analyzer	2250		Men — strongest correlation with ponderal index (height/weight). Women — strongest correlation with weight. Little difference with social class
1065	Male army recruits from different countries	5047	Body wt. / Mean: Argentinians and Americans 110 lb 256; 175 lb 298. Brazilians <135 lb 238; 165 lb 256. Colombians — No association with body weight	
1066	Women. Uricase metho		(see table below)	
905	Male Parisian civil servants. Fasting samples at 8:30–10 am. Phosphotungstate method on continuous-flow analyzer	4422	Age 46–52: <8 kg fat body wt. 309; >30 kg fat body wt.; >30 kg fat body wt. 410	8 kg fat body weight 1.5% 476. 30 kg fat body weight 17.7% 476
1032	French subjects for health screen. Phosphotungstate method on continuous-flow analyzer			Hyperuricemia in obese males 45%. Hyperuricemia in obese females 21%. (Obesity 50% greater than ideal body weight. Obesity associated with urate >600 in

Results for reference 1066 (Women, Uricase method):

Age (years)	Body weight (lb) 55.0–59.9			60.0–64.9			65.0–69.9		
	N	Mean	SD	N	Mean	SD	N	Mean	SD
38	81	207	54	76	208	65	59	220	60
46	96	220	65	114	214	60	62	226	54
50	66	232	77	90	238	71	77	244	60
54	25	220	77	39	256	65	29	268	77
60	13	226	30	15	250	95	16	286	89

TABLE 174.
Mean Serum Urate (in µmol/L) in Smokers (S) and Nonsmokers (NS)

Reference	Subjects and method	Age (years)	White men NS Mean	White men S Mean	White women NS Mean	White women S Mean	Black men NS Mean	Black men S Mean	Black women NS Mean	Black women S Mean	NS N	NS Mean	S Not inhaling N	S Not inhaling Mean	S Inhaling N	S Inhaling Mean
47	Americans Phosphotungstate method on continuous-flow analyzer	15–19	336	338	254	244	323	317	226	222						
		20–29	342	337	246	244	328	321	223	230						
		30–39	347	337	248	248	334	330	242	244						
		40–49	353	343	259	258	341	339	260	262						
		50–59	355	344	284	283	358	346	289	295						
		60–69	353	343	299	293	375	350	303	314						
		70–79	368	355	302	305										
905	French										1106	369	1636	369		351

TABLE 175.
Serum Urate (in μmol/L) in Partially Sighted and Blind Subjects[a]

Subjects	N	Mean	SD
Normal vision	50	265	80
Blind	220	348	72
Severely impaired (1/35 to 1/10 vision)	140	300	87

[a] From Hollwich, F. and Dieckhues, B., *German Med.*, 1, 122, 1971. Analysis using a continuous-flow analyzer. Specimens collected at 8 am. No details given of control group or ratio of males to females, in each group.

DRUGS AFFECTING SERUM URATE

DRUGS USED TO TREAT GOUT

The alkaloid colchicine obtained from the corm of the meadow saffron was used by the Ancient Greeks to treat gout. It was rediscovered in the late 18th century and was used enthusiastically by 19th-century physicians to treat gout. Nicolaier and Dohrn, in 1908, reported that colchicine increased urine urate and reduced blood urate.[1071] From the middle of this century, it has been replaced by less-toxic drugs.

Acute gouty attacks are usually treated with anti-inflammatory analgesics. Some, such as phenylbutazone and indomethacin, have little effect on urate levels. For the long-term control of gout, a number of drugs have been used. Drugs such as probenicid and sulfinpyrazone decrease serum urate by inhibition of renal tubular urate absorption, leading to increased urine urate. Other drugs, such as allopurinol, reduce serum urate by inhibiting xanthine oxidase and by reducing the conversion of xanthine to urate.[1072]

OTHER DRUGS THAT DECREASE SERUM URATE
Nonsteroidal Anti-Inflammatory Drugs
Salicylate

For many years high doses of salicylate have been known to increase urine urate and to decrease serum urate.[1073] The retention of uric acid in response to low doses of salicylate was reported by Salome[1074] in 1885. On some occasions, observation of this increase has led to a misdiagnosis of gout in treated rheumatic patients. Table 176 shows findings from several groups. More than 2.5 g of salicylate per day decreases serum urate.

It is possible that salicylate in low doses inhibits renal tubular secretion of urate and that in high doses, both renal tubular secretion and reabsorption of urate are inhibited. This theory is difficult to test experimentally.

Diflunisal

Serum urate is reduced by up to 30% by diflunisal.[1077,1078] The change is dose dependent, with a mean fall of about 15% at 250 mg/day and a mean fall of about 40% at 1000 mg/day.

Fenoprofen

A large fall in serum urate is found with fenoprofen. Huskisson et al.[1079] gave 60 patients from 1600 to 2400 mg of fenoprofen per day and found a mean fall of 60 μmol/L.

TABLE 176.
Effect of Salicylate on Serum Urate (in μmol/L)

Reference	Subjects and method	Dose	N	Change		
1075	Aspirin given daily for 4 days	1.2 g/day		Males	+60–107	
				Females	up to +60	
1076	Gouty subjects	1 g/day	4	+6%		
		2 g/day	7	+7%		
		3 g/day	9	–8%		
		5.2 g/day	15	–26%		
		5.2 g/day (+5.2 g NaHCO₃)	7	–40%		
256	Healthy staff Analysis with SMA 12/60	0.625 g (single dose)		No change		
		0.625 g every 4 h			**Mean**	**SD**
				Before	298	77
				Day 1	255	101
				Day 2	202	107
				Day 3	173	95
		0.625 g every 4 h for 5 days		Before	309	58
				Day 5	238	118
		Discontinued for 8 days		Day 13	309	56
		0.625 g every 4 h for further 5 days		Day 18	262	107
		0.625 g every 4 h for 14 days		Before	292	60
				Day 7	232	97
				Day 14	238	99
		Discontinued for 7 days		Day 21	315	64
		0.625 g every 4 h for 14 days		Day 28	256	114
				Day 35	268	92

Ibuprofen

A similar fall is seen with ibuprofen. Mean levels fall by about 20% compared with the mean of an untreated group under similar conditions.[811]

Indomethacin

Little change in serum urate is produced by indomethacin. Goldfarb et al.[1080] gave five healthy adults 1.2 g/day and found mean serum urate changed from 315 to 327 μmol/L.

Oxaprocin

Treatment with oxaprocin causes a fall in serum urate. Goldfarb et al. gave 386 patients with rheumatoid arthritis 1.2 g of oxaprocin day and found that mean serum urate fell from 286 to 256 μmol/L,[1080] whereas in seven healthy subjects given the same amount, the mean fell from 345 to 286 μmol/L by the seventh day.

Oxametacin

Eight healthy volunteers given a single oral dose of 200 mg of oxametacin, a NSAID suggested for use in treatment of acute gouty attacks, were found, by Broekhuysen et al.,[1081] to show a small change in mean serum urate from 315 to 332 μmol/L.

Piroxican

Murphy gave 26 patients with gout the long-acting anti-inflammatory drug piroxican.[1082] After 4 to 6 days of treatment, mean serum urate was 480 μmol/L; 7 to 12 days later it was 420 μmol/L.

Steroids
Cortisone

Serum urate is decreased by cortisone. Ingbar et al. found a decrease of about 40% in two subjects given cortisone intramuscularly for 2 to 8 days.[344] Gutman and Yü reported a mean fall of 17% in ten patients given 20 to 100 mg of adrenocorticotropic hormone (ACTH) per day.[1083]

Stilbestrol

Nichols et al. found a mean fall of 40 μmol/L in serum urate in 15 of 22 transsexual men given stilbestrol.[1084] A fall was also noted in one given ethinylestradiol.

Lipid-Lowering Drugs
Clofibrate

Albert and Stansell found a mean decrease of 27% in serum urate in ten hyperlipidemic patients given 2 g of clofibrate per day for 1 to 10 weeks.[1085] Lisch et al., giving a similar dose,[1086] found a mean fall of 12% after 2 weeks, with no further fall for 48 weeks.

Halofenate

Lisch et al.[1086] also found a mean fall of 24% after 2 weeks, and no further fall for 48 weeks, in nine patients given 1 g of halofenate per day.

Gemfibrozil

There is a small but significant fall in serum urate in patients treated with gemfibrozil. Stringer et al.[1087] gave 27 hyperlipidemic patients 1200 mg of gemfibrozil daily for 12 weeks and found that the mean level fell by 13%, from 390 ± 100 μmol/L to 340 μmol/L.

Other Drugs
Ascorbic Acid

Very high doses of ascorbic acid have a uricosuric action. Stein et al.[1088] found that 2 g of ascorbic acid per day had little effect, but three subjects given 8 g/day for 3 to 7 days had a fall in serum urate of from 25 to 32%. As some subjects take very large doses of ascorbic acid on occasions, the serum urate may be affected.

Acetohexamide

Uricosuric properties are shown by the hypoglycemic drug acetohexamide. In 18 patients with gout and diabetes given 1 g of acetohexamide per day for 2 weeks by Yü et al.,[1089] the mean serum urate fell from 607 to 434 μmol/L.

Angiotensin-Converting-Enzyme Inhibitors (ACE Inhibitors)

Patients with mild hypertension given captopril and enanopril show a reduction in serum urate. The drugs have been given to partially compensate for the hyperuricemic response to thiazides. Leary et al. found that the mean reduction in serum urate in patients given captopril is about 20%.[1090] Enanopril was given to hypertensive patients taking both low sodium diets and diets with unrestricted sodium; it was found that in both groups, mean serum urate fell by about 10%. The effect has been shown to be due to an increase in the renal clearance of urate.

TABLE 177.
Effect of Anticoagulants on Serum Urate

Reference	Subjects and method	N	Anticoagulant	Dose (g/day)	Change	Comment
1091	Gouty and nongouty subjects	9	Ethyl biscoumacetate	1.2–1.5	Fall 12–46%	Greatest fall at 5 h
1092	Healthy subjects	4	Ethyl biscoumacetate	2	Mean fall 120 μmol/L at 6 h	
			Phenylindandione	0.35	Mean fall 90 μmol/L at 6 h	
1093	Healthy subjects Uricase method	4	Dicoumarol	0.4–0.5	Mean fall 65 μmol/L at 32 h	Minimum at 32 h

Anticoagulants

Most workers have found a fall in serum urate, after giving oral anticoagulants (Table 177). However, Batt et al. found no change.[1094] Renal urate excretion has been found to increase.[1091]

Aziocillin

The penicillin derivative aziocillin causes an approximately 40% fall in mean serum urate. Faris and Potts found that in 18 of 21 courses given to 16 patients,[1095] the mean serum urate fell from 325 to 190 µmol/L. A rapid increase to pretreatment levels occurred after discontinuing treatment.

Azothiaprine

In six healthy subjects given 100 mg of azothiaprine per day by Maly et al.,[1096] the mean serum urate fell from 344.5 to 294.5 µmol/L.

Chlorprothixene

Healey et al. found that the tranquilizer chlorprothixene decreased mean serum urate by 65 to 120 µmol/L in three healthy volunteers given 50 to 100 mg per day.[1097]

Glucose and Mannitol

Skeith et al. observed a small fall in mean serum urate from 320 to 298 µmol/L in seven adult male volunteers given 10% glucose intravenously for 20 min.[1098] After giving mannitol in the same way, the mean change was from 298 to 286 µmol/L.

Glycine

Yu et al. showed that a single oral dose of 100 mg of glycine caused a mean fall of 18 µmol/L after 4 h in 10 healthy men and in 17 subjects with primary gout.[1099] The change was attributed to an increase in the renal clearance of urate.

Methotrexate

Uric acid synthesis is inhibited in patients treated with methotrexate, leading to lower serum urate levels.[1100]

Piparazine

Dohrn, as long ago as 1912,[1101] found that piparazine used to treat worm infestation increased urate excretion and reduced the level of urate in blood.

Sodium Chloride

Expansion of extracellular fluid volume by giving isotonic sodium chloride affects serum urate levels. Steele[1102] gave 15 healthy subjects isotonic sodium chloride for up to 55 min until the body weight had increased by 2%,[1102] and found a decrease in mean serum urate of 12%.

Triacetyl Azauridine

Calbresi and Turner found a fall of from 30 to 200 µmol/L in 12 of 13 cases given the antimetabolite triacetyl azauridine.[1103]

X-Ray Contrast Agents

Mudge found that the X-ray contrast agents iopanoic acid and calcium ipodate had a uricosuric effect,[1104] which leads to a reduction in serum urate, with a potency similar to that of probenecid.

TABLE 178.
Effect of Various Diuretics on Serum Urate (in µmol/L)
in an Elderly Population[a]

Diuretics taken	N	Mean	SD
Frusemide + spironolactone	9	413	113
Hydrochlorthiazide + amiloride	72	390	126
Frusemide	60	358	98
Frusemide + triampterine	37	356	64
Chlorthalidone	11	345	78
Hydrochlorthiazide	132	334	104
Trichlormethiazide + triampterine	84	331	83
Triampterine	5	280	87
No diuretics	578	281	75

[a] Rural population in north Finland, age over 65 years. From Takala, J., et al., *Scand. J. Rheum.*, 17, 155, 1988.

DRUGS THAT INCREASE SERUM URATE
Beta-Adrenocepter-Blocking Drugs

Small increases in serum urate following administration of beta blockers has been reported.

Propranolol

Mean serum urate increased from 292 to 327 µmol/L after 2 months and to a mean of 321 µmol/L after 12 months, in 53 hypertensive men given 80 or 160 mg of propranolol by Berglund et al.[1105] A smaller increase was found by a Veterans Administration Study Group[266] in 340 hypertensives given up to 640 mg of propranolol daily, according to requirement. In white subjects, mean serum urate increased by 2.3%; in black subjects, the mean increase was 3.5%.

Atenolol

Reports of the effect of atenolol differ. Fagard et al. found a mean increase in serum urate of 7% in 55 hypertensives given up to 600 mg of atenolol per day for 3 weeks.[1106] Kjeldsen et al., who gave 50 to 100 mg of atenolol per day for 18 weeks found little effect.[1107] Mean serum urate only increased from 341 to 348 µmol/L.

Antituberculous Drugs
Ethambutol

Serum urate increased by 140 µmol/L or greater in 15 of 24 patients treated with ethambutol by Postlethwaite et al.[1108] Other workers have reported similar findings. Narang et al. found an increase of up to 50% in 30 of 52 patients,[1109] and Khanan and Gupta found a mean increase of 74% in 71 patients.[1110]

Diuretics

A number of diuretics cause urate retention by the kidney, leading to increased serum levels. Table 178 shows some comparative levels.

Thiazides

At low plasma levels, thiazides increase serum urate. Table 179 shows the changes found by several groups after oral administration of thiazides. High plasma levels, as obtained by intravenous administration, cause increased urate excretion, leading to lower serum urate.

TABLE 179.
Effect of Thiazides on Serum Urate

Reference	Subjects and method		Change Mean	Change Range
1111	Hydrochlorthiazide given to 12 subjects	0 h	275	161–351
		24 h	296	196–357
	Phosphotungstate method on	48 h	321	220–393
	continuous-flow analyzer	72 h	327	250–405
1112	1.5–2 g daily chlorthiazide given to		Increase	18–309
	gouty and nongouty subjects		(Increase in 7 of 8)	
1113	200 mg daily hydrochlorthiazide	Before	323	
	for 6 weeks to hypertensives	After	423	
266	200 mg daily hydrochlorthiazide	White subjects		
	to 343 hypertensives	Before	391	
		After	472	
		Black subjects		
		Before		
		After	484	

TABLE 180.
Effect of Ethacrynic Acid on Serum Urate (in μmol/L)

Reference	Dose	N	Before mean	After mean
1116	100 mg daily for 6–8 weeks	4 men 7 women	315	416
1113	200 mg daily for 6 weeks		323	469

Acetazolamide

Serum urate is increased by giving acetolamide; the effect is potentiated by hydro-chlorthiazide. Avyazian and Ayvazian gave 1 g of acetazolamide daily to healthy subjects and found that in 3 days, mean serum urate increased from 294 (range of 202 to 333) to 316 μmol/L (range of 220 to 363).[1111] In a group given 50 mg of hydrochlorthiazide daily, the increase was from a mean of 275 (range of 161 to 351) to a mean of 333 μmol/L (range of 250 to 405). In another group given 0.5 g of acetazolamide and 50 mg of hydrochlorthiazide daily, the increase was from a mean of 284 (range of 202 to 321) to a mean of 398 μmol/L (range of 286 to 482).

Bumetamide and Piretamide

Roberts et al. found a mean increase of 70 μmol/L (range of 30 to 80) in the serum urate of patients given 1 mg of bumetamide per day and a mean increase of 40 μmol/L (range of 10 to 80) in patients given 6 mg of piretamide per day.[1114]

Chlorthalidone

The thiazide-related drug chlorthalidone also increases serum urate. Bengstsson found that mean serum urate increased from 226 to 298 μmol/L in 36 women 38 to 65 years old who were given 50 mg/day for 3 months.[1115]

Ethacrynic Acid

Mean increases in serum urate of about 30% are found in patients with mild hypertension treated with ethacrynic acid (Table 180).

TABLE 181.
Effect of Frusemide on Serum Urate (in μmol/L)

Reference	Subjects	Dose	N		Change	
					Mean	Range
1118		80 mg daily	13	Increase in five patients		
1117	Hypertensives	80 mg daily	20	3 weeks	No change	
				3 months	+3.4%	
1114	Healthy males	40 mg daily	9	1 week	+70%	40–100
1119	Patients treated with frusemide		595	Urate >430 in 54 patients; gouty symptoms in 2 patients		
					Mean	SD
	Controls		578		281	75
1055	Elderly subjects treated with frusemide		60		358	98

Frusemide

Most reports show an increase in serum urate following treatment with frusemide, although little change was found by Jackson and Nellan[1117] (Table 181).

Others
Cimetidine

A small increase in serum urate has been reported in patients following treatment with cimetidine. Larsson et al. studied 33 treatment periods in 22 patients with renal failure who were given 400 to 1000 mg/day.[1120] Mean serum urate before treatment was 425 μmol/L and on day 7, it was 447 μmol/L. Three days after stopping the drug, the patients' mean level returned to 425 μmol/L.

Cytotoxic Drugs

Administration of any drug that leads to the breakdown of cells may increase serum urate, as there is a rapid release of purine nucleotides and nucleic acid, resulting in increased urate formation. This occurs when cytotoxic agents are used to treat malignant diseases.

L-Dopa

It has been noted earlier that L-dopa interferes with the estimation of serum urate, giving falsely high results. Some groups have reported increases in serum urate following L-dopa treatment, which they consider to be a true increase.[1121,1122] Honda reported three cases who developed gout, thus supporting this suggestion.[1123]

Fructose

Hyperuricemia induced by fructose has been reported by a number of groups,[1124,1125] whereas others found no effect.[1126,1127] This difference was explained by Heukenkamp and Zöllner,[1128] who showed, by giving fructose intravenously to healthy volunteers, that at least 1 g/kg/h was needed to induce an increase in serum urate (Table 182). The workers who found no effect had given less than this amount of fructose to their subjects. The increase is considered to be due to the action of urate formed by the kidney.

Halothane and Methoxyflurane

There is an increase in serum urate following anesthesia with halothane and methoxyflurane, which lasts for several days (Table 183). Robertson and Hamilton[1132] found that the response was dose-related; this may explain the different findings shown. The effect is probably caused by a transient change in distal tubular function.

TABLE 182.
Serum Urate (in μmol/L)
after Intravenous Infusion of Fructose[a]

Fructose given (g/kg/h)	Before Mean	Before SD	After 90-min infusion[b] Mean	After 90-min infusion[b] SD
0.25–0.5	310	30	310	35
1.0	275	10	330	40
1.5	300	40	380	30

[a] From Heukenkamp, P.-U. and Zöllner, N., *Lancet*, i, 808, 1971.
[b] The increase peaked at 90 min and then tailed off.

TABLE 183.
Serum Urate (in μmol/L) Following Anesthesia with
Halothane and Methoxyflurane

Reference	Subjects	Halothane N	Halothane Mean	Halothane SD	Methoxyflurane N	Methoxyflurane Mean	Methoxyflurane SD
1129	Preop.	10	310		12	310	
	Postop.	10	315		12	465	
1130	Children						
	Preop.		250	48		262	42
	Postop. 24 h		370	100		512	125
	Postop. 48 h		292	77		464	125
1131	Preop.		252			258	
	Postop. 24 h		217			315	
	Postop. 48 h		226			353	
	Postop. 72 h		239			357	

Nicotinic Acid

Hyperuricemia is found in about 50% of patients given 3 to 6 g of nicotinic acid daily to treat hypercholesterolemia.[1133] Solomon and Thomas[1134] gave subjects 4.5 g daily and found that serum urate increased for 3 weeks; the increase peaked at 75% of the pretreatment level, returning within 1 week after discontinuation of treatment. The mechanism is not clear. Becker et al. found that nicotinic acid increased the rate of purine synthesis,[1135] whereas Gershon and Fox found that there was a decrease in urine urate.[1136]

Pancreatic Extracts

High serum urate levels are found in children given pancreatic extracts to treat cystic fibrosis. Stapleton et al. found increased levels in 14 of 15 children taking pancreatic extract containing purine equivalent to 120 to 300 mg daily.[1137] In a study of 82 children who had taken 50 to 170 pancreolipase capsules or pancreatin tablets daily for up to 6 years (purine equivalent to 150 to 585 mg/day), Davidson et al.[1138] found that mean serum urate was 370 ± 105 μmol/L compared with a mean of 290 ± 96 μmol/L in 15 patients with cystic fibrosis, and a mean of 268 ± 77 μmol/L in children without pancreatic or renal disease. High levels of urate were found to correlate with age and the number of years since diagnosis.

Theophylline

A mean serum urate of 375 μmol/L in patients taking theophylline, compared with a mean of 255 μmol/L in controls, was found by Morita et al.[1139] Serum urate correlated with serum theophylline levels. The reason for the increase is not certain.

Chapter 14

TRIGLYCERIDES

Triglycerides are triesters of glycerin (glycerol), with saturated or unsaturated fatty acids. Mixed triglycerides contain more than one type of fatty acid per molecule. Serum triglycerides are "mixed" with mainly long-chain fatty acids, whose composition is influenced by that of the dietary fat. Each day about 100 g of triglyceride are ingested compared with about 1 g of cholesterol.[1140]

Triglycerides in serum are either held in solution as complexes with protein or circulate postprandially as chylomicrons. Chylomicrons contain about 85% triglyceride, are synthesized from dietary fat, and are transported via the lacteals and thoracic duct. Usually only small amounts are present in serum 12 to 14 h after ingestion of a fat-containing meal.

Increase in serum lipid is considered to be a risk factor for the development of atherosclerosis. Carlson and Böttinger, in a 9-year follow-up of 3168 men,[1141] concluded that serum triglyceride and serum cholesterol were risk factors independent of each other.

ANALYTIC CONSIDERATIONS

In the earliest work, serum triglyceride was estimated by the difference between total lipid estimated gravimetrically or as total fatty acid, with the contribution from other lipids estimated separately and subtracted. The need to use results from a number of assays resulted in poor accuracy and precision.

Most methods now estimate glycerol liberated either by saponification or by lipase, using a colorimetric or an enzymic method. One procedure, considered a reference procedure,[1142] after extraction with a nonane–isopropanol mixture, saponifies and glycerol is converted to formaldehyde, with the Hantsch reaction. Lutidine formed by condensing formaldehyde with acetyl acetone and ammonia is measured fluorimetrically. Another procedure uses the reaction of formaldehyde with chromotrophic acid.[1143] A widely used enzymic method estimates glycerol obtained by saponification or the action of lipase,[1144] using the following sequence of reactions:

$$\text{Glycerol + ATP} \quad \overset{\text{glycerol kinase}}{=} \quad \text{glycerol-1-phosphate + ATP}$$

$$\text{Phosphoenol phosphate + ADP} \quad \overset{\text{pyruvate kinase}}{=} \quad \text{pyruvate + ADP}$$
$$\text{Pyruvate + NADH} \quad = \quad \text{lactate + NAD}$$

The decrease in absorption at 340 nm is proportional to the glycerol content, as this is the rate-limiting substance. Another enzymic method, by Fossati and Principi,[1145] uses glycerol phosphate oxidase to give hydrogen peroxide, which is estimated by the peroxidase reaction.

A problem common to all these methods is that free glycerol present in the specimen is included as a triglyceride. In the healthy subject the level is low, and a common practice is to subtract 0.11 mmol/L to allow for this.[1145] A number of groups have suggested that this may introduce significant error. Carlstrom and Christenssen found that mean free glycerol exceeded 0.11 mmol/L in cardiac patients.[1146] Elin et al. showed that in healthy subjects, free glycerol would add 0 to 0.41 mmol/L (mean 6.1%).[1147] In unselected patients, it added 0 to 1.22 mmol/L (mean 8.9%), and in selected patients with liver disease or high lactate levels, 0.18

to 11.63 mmol/L (mean 35.7%) would be added. Ter Welle et al. found that free glycerol added 0 to 2.7 mmol/L to the triglyceride result in 810 sera from fasting cardiac patients.[1148]

For an accurate serum triglyceride assay, it is desirable either to include a blank correction or to use a method such as that of Neri and Frings,[1149] which removes free glycerol before saponification.

ACCURACY AND PRECISION

Accuracy depends on the use of a correction for free glycerol. If a blank correction is applied, results by the Soloni and enzymic methods are similar.[1150] Gowland found that the between-batch precision of a triglyceride assay is 0.06 mmol/L, using an automated enzymic method, and 0.11 mmol/L, using a similar manual system.[1145] Steinmetz found that the between-batch coefficient of variation did not exceed 4% at average levels,[1150] using an enzyme method on a discrete analyzer. Assay imprecision is greater if a blank is determined, as two assays are required.

SI UNITS

Triglyceride is usually related to a standard prepared from triolein, to convert from mass to molar units.

$$\text{mg/100 mL (as triolein)} \times 0.0113 = \text{mmol/L}$$

The molar concentrations of triglyceride (whether triolein or others) and of glycerol liberated from it are numerically equal.

INTERFERENCE WITH ANALYSIS

There are few reports of interference with analysis for serum triglycerides. Enzymic methods based on the estimation of hydrogen peroxide produced using the peroxide reaction are affected by bilirubin. To avoid interference, ferricyanide can be incorporated into the reaction mixture.[1145]

PREANALYTIC ERROR

COLLECTION OF THE SPECIMEN

For serum triglyceride estimation, most laboratories use serum from clotted blood. Those using plasma from anticoagulated blood often use a correction factor for the slightly lower results obtained. Subjects should have fasted for at least 12 h before collection of the specimen, to ensure that there is no effect from postprandial changes.[1151,1152]

VENOUS STASIS

As triglycerides are present in serum as part of lipoprotein complexes, excessive venous stasis can be expected to have an effect similar to that on protein. However, Tan et al., using relatively mild conditions,[1153] noted no change in serum triglyceride after venous occlusion for ½ to 1 min.

ANTICOAGULANT

Many years ago, plasma turbidity in random samples was found to be greater than in serum taken at the same time. This was attributed to "enmeshment during clot formation."[1154] Anticoagulants such as oxalate and citrate exert osmotic effects that cause water to shift from cells to plasma, giving lower values.[1152] Triglyceride is similar in serum and heparinized plasma. Henny et al. found that there is no difference,[1155] and Lum and Gambino[391] found a mean of 1.80 mmol/L in serum compared with 1.75 mmol/L in heparinized plasma: a difference considered to be statistically unimportant.

A Laboratory Methods Group of the Lipid Research Clinics found that serum triglyceride levels were higher than those in plasma from samples anticoagulated with EDTA salt,[1156] according to the formula

$$\text{Serum triglyceride} = 1.031(\text{plasma triglyceride}) - 0.0052$$

CONTAMINATION
Glycerol

Glycerol contamination of vacutainer tubes and stoppers has been noted.[1157] Soaps and detergents may contain glycerol and triglyceride, so all glassware used must be clean.[1142] Use of "Hemosol" followed by chromic acid and several washes with deionized water is recommended. Ryder et al. reported contamination by glycerol from hand lotion used by a laboratory worker.[1158]

Lipase

Lipase used in some methods may be contaminated with phosphatase.[1144] This introduces a competing reaction, leading to falsely high values for serum triglyceride. Lipase used in methods of estimation of triglyceride should be checked for purity.

SAMPLE STABILITY

Triglyceride in plasma decreases significantly after storage at room temperature for 3 days. Von Mühlfellner et al. found a fall of 6.7% in the mean level of 30 samples.[1159] No change was noted in specimens stored at 4°C or frozen.

Endogenous lipase causes an increase in free glycerol during storage, and a fall in triglyceride. There may be an apparent increase in triglyceride, using methods that do not remove or estimate free glycerol, but which subtract a fixed amount.

Schwertner and Friedman found that 3% of serum samples received by mail contained phospholipase-C-producing bacilli,[1160] experiments showed that doubling of the original triglyceride concentration was possible. EDTA was found to inhibit the bacterial activity.

PHYSIOLOGIC CHANGES

MEALS

Serum triglyceride increases after food is taken. In healthy subjects, chylomicrons reach a peak about 2 h after a meal, with a second increase in triglyceride after 4 to 7 h, which is related to an increase in VLDL.[1161]

The course of hypertriglyceridemia is variable, being influenced by the composition of the meal, the absorptive processes, and the metabolism of the chylomicra. For this reason it is desirable for subjects to have fasted for at least 12 h before collection of samples.

DIET

The level of triglyceride in serum is affected by the form in which carbohydrate is administered, with an increase if it is supplied as sucrose and a decrease if given as starch.[1162,1163] DenBesten et al. gave eight healthy volunteers from a penitentiary a fat-free diet with 80% of calories from glucose[1164] and found an increase in fasting serum triglyceride from a mean of 1.98 mmol/L to 3.19 mmol/L. There was no increase, given an intravenous diet.

Addition of bran to the diet decreases fasting serum triglyceride. Heaton and Pomere fed 14 healthy subjects a diet including a median intake of 38 g (range of 18 to 100 g) of unprocessed wheat bran, for 4 to 9 weeks and found that mean fasting serum triglyceride fell from 1.33 to 1.13 mmol/L.[114]

EXERCISE

The postprandial rise in serum triglyceride is affected by exercise. Cohen and Ginsberg noted that physical activity reduces plasma turbidity after a fatty meal,[1165] but did not include quantitative lipid analysis. Later, Nikkilä and Konttinen, in a study of 40 healthy army recruits,[1166] showed that vigorous exercise modified the postprandial rise in serum triglyceride. After fasting for 11 h, all ate a meal containing 55 g of fat. After moving freely indoors for 2 h, one group marched 16 km in 2 h and the other group rested in bed for the same amount of time.

Bed-rest group	
Fasting serum triglyceride	1.11 ± 0.07 mmol/L
4 h later after 2 h in bed	1.97 ± 0.18 mmol/L
6 h later after 2 h in bed	1.25 ± 0.10 mmol/L
Marching group	
Fasting serum triglyceride	1.13 ± 0.14 mmol/L
4 h later after 2-h march	1.42 ± 0.18 mmol/L
6 h later after 2-h march	1.11 ± 0.19 mmol/L

It was concluded that vigorous exercise probably reduced the postprandial rise in serum triglyceride, by accelerating the removal of chylomicrons from circulation.

Exercise has little effect on the level of serum triglyceride while the subject is fasting,[1167] but when individuals leading sedentary lives are given a program of exercise to follow over several months, fasting serum triglyceride is reduced (Table 184). These findings are supported by the lower levels found in athletes compared with healthy, less-active subjects (Table 185).

The studies on subjects given a program of exercise did not consider whether changes are linked to a change in body weight, as serum triglyceride is known to increase with an increase in fat body weight.

POSTURE

The change in serum triglyceride, with posture, is parallel to the change in serum protein. Tan et al.[1153] studied seven nonobese males 18 to 50 years old and found a mean maximum fall of 12.4% (range of 8 to 20%) in subjects lying down for 30 min after being upright for 10 min. The change was up to 5% after lying down for 5 min. These variations should be considered when interpreting results, and conditions must be standardized when determining reference intervals.

SEASONAL VARIATION

Some groups have reported changes in serum triglyceride during the year, but findings have been inconsistent. Fuller et al. found mean levels about 50% higher in summer than in winter,[1174] whereas Carlson and Lindstedt found levels in the period July to September to be about 25% lower than those in December.[1175]

SHIFT WORK

A study of shift workers in France found that they had higher fasting serum triglyceride levels than day workers did.[1176] Subjects were matched according to age, educational level, birthplace, and occupational physical activity, and shift workers had been employed for more than a year. Although serum cholesterol levels were similar, mean fasting serum triglyceride levels of shift workers was 1.26 mmol/L, compared with a mean of 1.03 mmol/L in day workers. There was no difference in the energy or nutrient intake of the two groups.

TABLE 184.
Relationship of Exercise and Fasting Serum Triglyceride (in mmol/L)

Reference	Subjects	Exercise	Change			Level	Comment
			N	Mean	Range	Mean	
1168	Professional men leading sedentary lives	Progressively more strenuous program for 6 months	15	Fall 0.74	Fall up to 3.8		Fall in 14 of 15
1169	Male Air Force officers classified according to estimated exercise taken	Moderate to high	229			1.13	
		Low to none	126			1.28	

TABLE 185.
Fasting Serum Triglyceride (in mmol/L) in Active and Less-Active Subjects

Reference	Subjects and age (years)	Exercise	N	Mean
1170	Male 52–56	Regular activity (skiing and cross-country running)	15	0.90
		Sedentary controls	45	1.23
1171		Long-distance runners	14	0.63
		Nonathletes	14	0.96
1172	Male 30–59	Long-distance runners	41	0.79
	Female 30–59	Long-distance runners	45	0.63
	Male 30–59	Nonathletes	747	1.65
	Female 30–59	Nonathletes	932	1.39
1173	Finnish lumberjacks	It was presumed that electricians are less active	12	0.60
	Finnish electricians	than lumberjacks	15	0.92

RANGE IN HEALTHY SUBJECTS

Serum triglyceride in healthy adults shows geographic differences that tend to vary parallel to serum cholesterol. Levels are often lower in communities with low-fat intake, high-carbohydrate intake, and infrequent ischemic heart disease. Lewis gives references to the differences between the populations of London, Nigeria, Japan, and India.[1177]

In general, levels are higher in men than women, and increase up to the sixth decade and then decrease. Tables 186 and 187 give reported findings for triglyceride in fasting subjects in some large series. The distribution is usually reported to be skewed toward the lower levels. Populations are not necessarily made up of patients with ideal or healthy values; in total-population studies, a substantial number of subjects with, or liable to have, cardiovascular disease may be included.

WITHIN-PERSON VARIATION

Large variations in fasting serum triglyceride have been reported on repeat sampling. Elveback et al.[1183] took three specimens in a week from six boys and four girls and found a mean cv of 25.9% (range 7.9–38.2). Haas[1184] also found a large variation when taking samples 3–7 months later in a subset of a Heartwatch study. 30% of subjects showed differences of more than 50%.

RACIAL DIFFERENCES

A number of groups have reported that serum triglyceride is higher in white than in black subjects in the same community in the United States. Tyroler et al.[1185] studied the residents of Evans County in the southern United States and found mean fasting serum triglyceride to be about 1.50 mmol/L in white males and 1.15 mmol/L in black males. Fredericks et al. reported that in a study of children in Bogalusa, LA, white boys had a mean of 0.78 mmol/L compared with 0.72 in black boys, and white girls had a mean of 0.87 compared with 0.69 in black girls.[1186] Similar results were obtained by Christenson et al.,[1187] who found mean levels of 0.76 mmol/L in white males 0 to 19 years old compared with 0.64 in black males, and a mean of 0.79 in white females compared with 0.69 in black females.

CHILDREN

Levels of fasting serum triglyceride change little with increasing age until puberty, with mean levels being a little higher in girls. Mean levels increase in both sexes from the age of about 11 or 12 years (Table 188).

TABLE 186.
Fasting Serum Triglyceride (in mmol/L) in Healthy Males

Reference		21-25	26-30	31-35	36-40	41-45	46-50	51-55	56-60	61-65	66-70	>70
1178[a]	N	17	35	35	27		31		29		12	
	Mean	1.05	1.15	1.15	1.37		1.48		1.41		1.31	
1179[b]	N	10		14		22		25				
	Mean	0.99		1.18		1.32		1.16				
	Range	0.49-1.99		0.55-2.55		0.74-2.38		0.25-2.56				
1180[c]	N	441	768	801	428	453	4072	1007				
	Mean	0.85	0.90	1.03	1.20	1.22	1.47	1.41				
1157[d]	N	29		115		171		133		19		
	Mean	1.07		1.40		1.72		1.62		2.01		
	Range	0.80-2.32		0.73-2.09		0.75-2.69		0.75-2.46		0.85-2.49		
1181[e]	Mean	1.16	1.34	1.49	1.68	1.75	1.76	1.76	1.64	1.65	1.59	1.51
	Range	0.51-2.34	0.53-2.89	0.58-3.09	0.62-3.74	0.63-3.73	0.67-3.81	0.67-3.73	0.67-3.32	0.67-3.39	0.65-3.11	0.67-3.00
1182	50 percentile	0.75					0.84					
	2.5-97.5 percentile	0.29-1.78					0.25-1.88					

Age (years)

[a] 237 Swedish men.

[b] 126 Danish men. Enzymic method of analysis.

[c] 1973 healthy French civil servants. Analysis using Technicon analyzer.

[d] Analysis by enzymic method on centrifugal analyzer.

[e] Study by 10 collaborating Lipid Research Clinics in U.S. Serum values calculated from plasma levels.

[f] 582 French men. Excess weight, tobacco, and alcohol consumption excluded. Enzymic method.

TABLE 187.
Fasting Serum Triglyceride (in mmol/L) in Healthy Females

Reference		21–25	26–30	31–35	36–40	41–45	46–50	51–55	56–60	61–65	66–70	>70
1179[a]	N	9		16		18		13				
	Mean	0.74		0.88		0.98		0.98				
	Range	0.51–1.06		0.45–1.72		0.47–2.05		0.60–1.58				
1157[b]	N	25		17		22		18				
	Mean	1.07		1.08		1.06		1.59				
	Range	0.81–1.33		0.69–1.44		0.57–1.56		0.76–2.43				
1181[c]	Mean	0.84	0.87	0.91	0.99	1.14	1.22	1.33	1.46	1.51	1.52	1.52
	Range	0.42–1.52	0.43–1.68	0.45–1.75	0.46–2.16	0.52–2.22	0.53–2.48	0.60–2.71	0.63–3.05	0.64–2.78	0.69–2.82	0.69–2.76
1182[d]	50 percentile	0.60		0.75								
	2.5–97.5 percentile	0.25–1.44		0.25–1.88								

a   102 Danish women.

b   Analysis by enzymic method on centrifugal analyzer.

c   Hormone users excluded. Other details as males.

d   2239 French women. Excess weight, tobacco, and alcohol consumption and hormone users excluded.

TABLE 188.
Fasting Serum Triglycerides (in mmol/L) in Children

Age (years)	Reference 1181				Reference 1184			
	Male		Female		Male		Female	
	Mean	Range	Mean	Range	50 percentile	2.5–97.5 percentile	50 percentile	2.5–97.5 percentile
0–1	0.79	0.35–0.93	0.88	0.35–1.11				
2–3	0.62	0.34–0.95	0.75	0.36–1.16				
4	0.62	0.32–1.03	0.67	0.36–1.10				
5					0.51	0.23–1.36	0.57	0.28–1.41
6	0.63	0.35–1.19	0.68	0.37–1.21	0.51	0.23–1.36	0.57	0.23–1.41
7					0.51	0.28–1.30	0.62	0.28–1.47
8	0.65	0.35–1.23	0.72	0.38–1.24	0.51	0.28–1.24	0.57	0.23–1.36
9					0.57	0.28–1.41	0.68	0.34–1.52
10	0.67	0.34–1.23	0.81	0.42–1.40	0.57	0.28–1.36	0.68	0.28–1.47
11					0.62	0.28–1.58	0.73	0.34–1.75
12	0.81	0.41–1.56	0.91	0.47–1.56	0.62	0.34–1.41	0.73	0.34–1.86
13					0.62	0.34–1.52	0.73	0.40–1.86
14					0.68	0.34–1.64	0.73	0.34–1.58
15	0.86	0.41–1.56	0.89	0.45–1.55	0.73	0.34–1.81	0.73	0.40–1.41
16					0.73	0.40–1.64	0.73	0.34–1.52
17	0.90	0.43–1.77	0.82	0.45–1.36	0.79	0.34–1.86	0.73	0.40–1.30
18–19	0.96	0.49–1.91	0.89	0.46–1.52				

TABLE 189.
Serum Triglyceride (in mmol/L) During Pregnancy

Reference	Subjects	Stage of pregnancy	N	Mean	SD
1191	After 12-h fast	Late	28	3.41	1.53
1192	Fasting	34–36 weeks	18	3.13	
		Non pregnant		0.41	
1193	Nonfasting	7 weeks		0.74	
	taken between	40 weeks		3.27	
	8 and 10 am				

CORD BLOOD

Serum triglyceride in cord blood is lower than in healthy adults. Brody and Carlson found a mean of 0.38 ± 0.19 mmol/L in cord blood from 52 infants.[1188] Tsang et al. obtained a mean of 0.41 mmol/L (range of 0.09 to 1.07) in cord blood from 60 infants in Cincinnati with parents having "normal serum lipids."[1189] Carlson and Hardell[1190] found a mean of 0.46 ± 0.05 mmol/L in the cord blood of boys and 0.46 ± 0.06 in the cord blood of girls.

RANGE DURING PREGNANCY

Serum triglyceride increases during pregnancy, with levels at term four or five times those found in nonpregnant subjects (Table 189). Darmady and Postle found that the level did not return to the pre-conception level until about 6 months after delivery and that the return was quicker in lactating mothers.[1194]

OTHER CHANGES

BODY WEIGHT

Fasting serum triglyceride increases with an increase in fat body weight. In a study of French civil servants 46 to 52 years old, Claude and Lellough found that the mean level in those with less than 8 kg of fat body weight was 0.87 mmol/L,[1180] with only 0.5% with levels more than 2.83 mmol/L. However, in those with more than 30 kg of fat body weight, mean fasting serum triglyceride was 1.94 mmol/L, with 15% having levels of more than 2.83.

BLOOD PRESSURE

There is also a relationship between systolic blood pressure and fasting serum triglyceride. Claude and Lellough[1180] found the following:

* Systolic BP less than 110 mm Hg, mean 1.04 mmol/L
* Systolic BP less than 150 mm Hg, mean 1.62 mmol/L
* Systolic BP more than 210 mm Hg, mean 1.92 mmol/L

It is possible that this finding is linked with obesity related to high blood pressure.

ALCOHOL

A number of groups have shown that ingestion of alcohol increases serum triglyceride[1188,1195] (Table 190). Ginsberg et al. studied the effect of adding ethanol to the diet.[1195] Four men and two women with normal serum triglyceride and six men and three women with hypertriglyceridemia were given the same liquid-formula diet (none of the carbohydrates were sucrose) for 7 days. Alcohol equivalent to 7.5 oz of whiskey per day was added to the diet for the next 7 days.

TABLE 190.
Effect of Alcohol on Serum Triglyceride Level

Reference	Group	N	Fasting serum triglyceride (mmol/L)	
			Mean	SD
1198	Nondrinkers	167	1.45	0.96
	1–15 drinks per month	99	1.45	0.87
	16–45 drinks per month	116	1.38	0.80
	46–135 drinks per month		1.58	0.89
	More than 135 drinks per month		2.24	1.77
1195	Days 5, 6, and 7 of control period			
	Normal-triglyceride group	6	0.79	
	High-triglyceride group	9	3.82	
	Days 12, 13, and 14 alcohol period			
	Normal-triglyceride group	6	0.93	
	High-triglyceride group	9	5.63	

The postprandial increase in serum triglyceride was found to be greater during the alcohol period in both groups (Table 190).

The effect of completely withdrawing alcohol from 13 alcoholic patients was considered by Chait et al.,[1196] who observed a fall in fasting serum triglyceride, of at least 25%. The level before withdrawal was 4.66 to 47.14 mmol/L and after withdrawal, 3.39 to 7.38.

Others have investigated levels in the general population, according to the amount of alcohol taken. Whitfield et al. found that the mean fasting triglyceride level increased from 2 mmol/L in men who stated that they had consumed 0 to 50 drinks per month, to almost 4 mmol/L in those admitting to more than 200 drinks per month.[1197]

Allen and Adena[1198] also noted an increase with increased alcohol intake (Table 190).

Although it has been demonstrated that an increase in serum triglyceride occurs after a subject drinks alcohol, none of the studies of the general population considered the possible contribution from obesity or smoking, both of which correlate with alcohol intake.

DRUGS AFFECTING SERUM TRIGLYCERIDE

Lipid-Lowering Drugs

Serum triglyceride is frequently affected, as well as serum cholesterol, during therapy with lipid-lowering drugs. Clofibrate,[1199] benzafibrate,[1200] gemfibrosil,[1201] and nicotinic acid[1202] reduce triglyceride and cholesterol. Halofenate reduces triglyceride, with little effect on serum cholesterol.[1203] L-Thyroxine, when given to hypothyroid patients, is reported to give an increase of about 20% in serum triglyceride.[1204] However, the synthetic compound D-thyroxine causes a fall of about 50%.[1205]

Ion exchange resins such as cholestyramine and colestipol do not decrease serum triglyceride. Howard et al. found no effect in three hypertriglyceridemic patients.[1206] Fallon and Woods found no decrease in seven hypertriglyceridemic subjects.[1207] Others have reported small increases. Berkowitz noted an increase in 7 of 15 hyperlipidemic patients,[1208] and Weitzel et al. noted a small but significant rise in five normolipidemic patients.[1209]

Oral Contraceptives

The effect of estrogens and progesterins on serum triglyceride are reviewed by Henkin et al.[1210] Synthetic, but not natural, estrogens increase the level by up to 90%, whereas progesterins either decrease serum triglyceride or have little effect. Older oral contraceptive preparations are usually reported to increase serum triglyceride. The effect is less with preparations with

TABLE 191.
Change in Fasting Serum Triglyceride (in mmol/L)
in Patients Taking Beta-Blocking Drugs

Reference		N	Baseline	6 months	24 months
1214	Atenolol 100 mg/day	25	1.30 ± 0.47	1.71 ± 0.54	1.62 ± 0.52
	Bisoprolol 10 mg/day	20	1.26 ± 0.48	1.64 ± 0.56	1.52 ± 0.51
	Mepindolol 10 mg/day	18	1.27 ± 0.49	1.60 ± 0.53	1.45 ± 0.51
	Propanolol 160 mg/day	17	1.28 ± 0.50	1.81 ± 0.52	1.74 ± 0.49
	Celiprolol 400 mg/day	19	1.30 ± 0.46	1.03 ± 0.41	1.12 ± 0.44
1215	Pindolol				**12 months**
	Mean dose 7.7 mg/day	82	1.83 ± 0.91	2.10 ± 1.24	2.02 ± 1.01

decreased doses or a modified proportion of estrogen and progesterin. Progestational oral contraceptives do not increase serum triglyceride.

Ascorbic Acid

Sokoloff et al. found that 50 of 60 patients with hypercholesterolemia improved when given 1.5 to 3 g of ascorbic acid daily.[1211] Serum triglyceride fell by 50 to 70%. Later, Cērnë and Ginter[1212] found a negative linear correlation between leukocyte ascorbic acid and serum triglyceride. Subjects with low leukocyte ascorbic acid had mean serum triglyceride of 1.51 mmol/L compared with 1.42 in those with medium levels and 1.16 in those with maximum levels.

Amioderone

A study of three patients with abnormal carbohydrate and lipid metabolism when treated with amioderone was reported by Politi et al.[1213] During oral treatment with 300 mg daily, serum triglyceride was 3.8, 7.8, and 14.7 mmol/L, respectively. Thyroid function was not found to be abnormal.

Beta Blockers

Most beta-blocking drugs cause an increase in fasting serum triglyceride, but little change in serum cholesterol. Fogari et al. compared five different beta blockers and found a mean increase of about 30% in patients taking atenolol, bisoprolol, mepindolol, and propranolol,[1214] but a decrease in those taking celiprolol (Table 191). Terent et al. found increases of over 10% in a group taking pindolol.[1215]

Chendeoxycholic Acid

Bell et al. gave 18 women and 4 men 0.75 to 1.5 g of chendodeoxycholic acid daily to dissolve gall stones.[1216] Fasting serum triglyceride was estimated before treatment and at monthly intervals during treatment, and an unexpected, unexplained fall from a mean of 1.36 ± 0.14 to 1.10 ± 0.08 mmol/L was found.

Corticosteroids

Several groups have reported an increase in serum triglyceride in patients on long-term steroid therapy. Doar and Wynn found the mean fasting serum triglyceride in 19 women taking 5 to 25 mg of prednisolone daily[1217] to be 0.98 ± 0.30 mmol/L compared with 0.84 ± 0.29 in 53 control subjects. Jefferys et al. found a mean of 1.84 ± 0.55 in 16 premenopausal women and 1.21 ± 0.42 in 15 men 24 to 38 years old, on long-term corticosteroid therapy,[1218] compared with 0.98 ± 0.28 and 0.87 ± 0.56 in healthy controls.

Danazol

There are different reports on the effect of danazol, given to treat endometriosis, on serum triglyceride. Luciano et al. found a fall in the mean level, from 1.07 to 0.72 mmol/L, in fasting serum triglyceride in 7 healthy women taking 800 mg daily for 2 months,[1219] whereas Fähraeus et al. found an increase from 0.92 mmol/L to 1.10 after 2 weeks, 1.02 after 8 weeks, and 1.08 after 24 weeks.[1220]

Diuretics

Several groups have noted an increase in fasting triglyceride after treatment with diuretics. Ames and Hill found a rise of about 25% in the mean fasting triglyceride level in 32 patients given chlorthalidone in various doses according to need.[1221] Schnaper et al. reported a rise of 13.8% in the mean level of 311 patients given 50 or 100 mg of chlorthalidone daily, and a rise of 4.3% in 325 patients given a placebo.[1222] A Veterans Administration Study Group found an increase of about 20% in the mean level of fasting serum triglyceride in 170 patients given hydrochlorthiazide for 12 months.[1223]

Enalapril

A decrease in fasting serum triglyceride is found in patients treated with the angiotensin-converting-enzyme inhibitor enalapril. Chandler et al. found a mean fall in six men and six women, 24 to 80 years old and with mild hypertension, from 1.48 ± 0.18 to 1.10 ± 0.11 mmol/L after 24 weeks' treatment.[1224]

Glucagon

Serum triglyceride is depressed in subjects given glucagon. Caren and Corbo gave 20 healthy subjects glucagon after they had fasted overnight.[1225] After receiving 1 mg of glucagon intravenously, the subjects' serum triglyceride fell by about 10% after 1 h and about 15% after 2 h. It was back to the baseline level after 3 h. After giving 1 mg of glucagon subcutaneously, the level was depressed by about 25% after 1 h, 35% after 2 h, and 44% after 3 h.

Phenothiazine

An increase in fasting serum triglyceride in a group of patients taking phenothiazines, compared with a control group, was reported by Sasaki et al.[1226] In 17 schizophrenic patients taking the drug, the mean was 1.84 ± 0.73 mmol/L compared with a mean of 1.43 ± 0.80 in 14 hospital employees.

Stanozol

The anabolic steroid stanozol has been shown to reduce fasting serum triglyceride, whereas testosterone has little effect. Thompson et al. found a fall from 1.50 ± 0.80 to 1.25 ± 0.59 mmol/L in subjects taking 6 mg of stanozol daily for 1 week, compared with an insignificant change from 1.48 ± 0.55 to 1.47 ± 0.90 in those given an injection of 200 mg of testosterone.[1227]

Chapter 15

CHOLESTEROL

Cholesterol is present in serum, combined with triglyceride and protein in lipoprotein complexes. In erythrocytes, cholesterol concentration is from 10 to 30% less than in serum and is located mainly in the cell membrane, largely in the free, nonesterified form.[1228] In serum, about 25% occurs as free cholesterol and about 75% as cholesterol ester with fatty acids.[1229] The serum level varies in different populations and seems to have a link with the frequency of coronary heart disease.[1230]

ANALYTIC CONSIDERATIONS

Early methods extracted cholesterol from serum or blood, with covalent solvents followed by estimation using a color reaction. Chloroform and ether extract only a small percentage when cold. The equipment devised by Soxhlet for the refluxing of organic material with heated solvents was used by some workers.

For extraction, dissociation of the link with protein is required; in 1914 Bloor introduced a reagent containing a mixture of ethanol and ether,[1231] which with the ratio of serum to reagent of from 1:25 to 1:50, splits the protein–lipid bond and also extracts cholesterol at room temperature. Others, such as Schoenheimer and Sperry,[1232] have used a mixture of ethanol and acetone similarly. Petroleum fractions extract free and ester cholesterol, giving an extract with few interfering substances and no change in volume;[1233] they have been used in some methods of estimation.[1234] Low boiling fractions (30 to 60°C) or hexane have been used.

Many techniques have been used to estimate serum cholesterol; gravimetric, nephelometric, turbidimetric, gas, thin-layer, and high-performance liquid chromatography and fluorimetric, colorimetric, and enzymic methods have all been described. Comprehensive reviews of the methods available have been published by Wybenga and Inkpen,[1229] Zak,[1235] and Richmond.[1236]

COLORIMETRIC METHODS

Several reagents giving a color with cholesterol have been used. The acetic acid/acetic anhydride/sulfuric acid reagent which gives a green color with cholesterol was introduced by Liebermann in 1885 and applied to the solution in chloroform by Burchard in 1890; it was used in a number of early methods after extraction and removal of solvent.

Schoenheimer and Sperry, in 1934,[1232] described a method in which hydrolysis of esters was followed by extraction and precipitation of cholesterol as digitonide, and quantitation using the Lieberman–Burchard reaction in acetic acid. A modification of this procedure, by Sperry and Webb,[1237] was used as a reference method for some years.

A simpler method giving similar results was introduced by Abell et al.[1234] and has replaced the Schoenheimer and Sperry procedure as a reference procedure. Cholesterol was extracted from serum, with a petroleum fraction, and after evaporating, the solvent color is produced with an acetic anhydride/sulfuric acid reagent. Acetic acid, instead of chloroform, is used in these methods, as ester cholesterol gives an equal color with free cholesterol, whereas in chloroform, ester cholesterol gives about 20% more color.

The purple color given by cholesterol with ferric chloride in sulfuric acid, described by Lipschitz in 1907, has been used in some methods.[1229] Equal amounts of color are given by ester and free cholesterol. Direct addition of serum to the color reagent has been used with both color methods.[1238,1239] The early direct methods were found to give results considerably higher than those obtained by reference methods, but later workers obtained better results. A modification, by Richardson et al.,[1240] of the procedure described by Watson[1241] that used dimethyl benzene sulfonic acid and sulfuric acid gave mean results only about 0.15 mmol/L higher than those obtained by the Abell method. Wybenga et al. found that a direct method using ferric perchlorate and sulfuric acid gave results comparable to those obtained by a reference method.[1242]

There are a number of limitations with the color methods; these limitations make color methods difficult to control. Temperature, water content, and the time of reaction are critical, and because the reactions are nonspecific, they are susceptible to interference. These factors, along with the hazardous nature of the reagents, have resulted in clinical laboratories looking for other methods.

ENZYMIC METHODS

The development of methods using cholesterol dehydrogenase[1243-1247] or cholesterol oxidase[1246-1248] has resulted in many laboratories changing from methods using strong acid. The procedures estimate either cholest-4-en-3one after extraction and measurement at 240 nm, or hydrogen peroxide, often by the reaction with 4-amino phenazone and peroxidase. Ester cholesterol must first be hydrolyzed using either ethanolic potassium hydroxide[1249] or cholesterol ester hydrolase.[1250]

OTHER METHODS

GLC

The use of gas liquid chromatography (GLC) for the estimation of serum cholesterol requires preliminary extraction for accurate and precise results and thus is unsuitable for routine use. It has, however, been proposed as a reference procedure.[1251] Several isotope dilution–gas chromatography–mass spectrometry procedures have been described,[1236] and it has been shown that a precision of better than the 0.5% advocated for a definitive method can be obtained.

HPLC

High-performance liquid chromatography (HPLC) has been used for the determination of free and ester cholesterol, using reverse-phase chromatography.[1236] The sample is first hydrolyzed with ethanolic potassium hydroxide and then extracted with hexane.

"Dry" Chemistry Analyzers

Analyzers that incorporate the application of blood samples to paper strips impregnated with reagents have been developed for use outside of laboratories. There has been controversy about their accuracy of estimation. A number of publications between 1986 and 1987 reported that cholesterol estimated by the "Reflotron" system (Boehringer, Mannheim, Germany) was low by about 10%.[1252,1253] A new set of serum calibrators were introduced, and when tested by Boerma et al.,[1254] a reasonable comparison with the NIH Consensus Development Conference (CDC) modification of the Abell method was found, with cholesterol values 2 to 4% higher.

The reliability of these methods when used by nonspecialist staff has been discussed. Nelson and Fraser studied the analytic imprecision using the "Reflotron" system.[1255] They found a cv of 3.0%, analyzing sera with cholesterol between 5.25 and 7.0 mmol/L, and a cv of 3.6%, with levels of more than 7.0%. However, when analysis was performed by medical staff in the coronary care unit, the cv was 12.6%. Strip analyzers appear to be capable of obtaining results with satisfactory accuracy and precision, but the use of trained staff and proper quality assurance is essential.

ACCURACY AND PRECISION

There have been a number of reports comparing results by different procedures. Cooper et al., using an enzymic method including enzymic hydrolysis,[1250] obtained results 5 to 7% lower than those obtained by the Abell procedure. The discrepancy was attributed to incomplete hydrolysis. However, Siedal et al. doubted this explanation,[1256] as the experiments had used different matrices, and it was shown that using "Monotest" reagents (Boehringer, Mannheim, Germany), 99.5% cleavage could be obtained.

Although Allain et al. claimed that absolute specificity was not obtained using enzymic methods,[1245] the procedure gave less error than the Abell method. Svensson et al. reported that using a carefully controlled procedure,[1257] enzymic methods were capable of giving results almost identical with those obtained using isotope dilution techniques. Whatever the methods are capable of, it seems that in practice, enzymic methods give significantly higher results than are obtained by the CDC method, which is based on the Abell procedure. This was shown by the 1986 American College of Pathologists survey and supported by Blank et al.,[1258] who found significantly higher results using enzymic methods on the Du Pont ACA and Technicon SMAC analyzers.

Kroll et al. obtained similar findings with 4 analyzers:[1259]

CDC reference method	Mean 2.19 (mmol/L)
Enzymic:	
Du Pont ACA	2.27
TDX	2.27
Technicon SMAC	2.24
Technicon RA 1000	2.18

In each case the calibrator supplied was used, and only one instrument gave results similar to the reference method. Blank et al. attributed 3% of the bias to the use of plasma for the reference method and serum for the enzymic methods.

Accuracy of estimation of serum cholesterol is important, as predictive values for possible heart disease are frequently based on studies by the American Centers for Disease Control (CDC) Lipid Research Clinics. These are based on analyses using a modified Abell procedure on plasma. The Laboratory Standardization Panel of the National (U.S.) Cholesterol Education Program points out that standardization of assays should enable results to be traceable to the CDC reference method.[1260]

Studies showing that blood cholesterol levels strongly influence the development of atherosclerosis have resulted in a national campaign in the United States to identify and treat subjects considered to be at risk.[1261] The NIH. Consensus Development Conference Panel recommended that action be taken if an adult was found to have a cholesterol level above the seventy-fifth percentile for the population.[1262] The limits of 2.00 and 2.40 mmol/L recommended by the National Cholesterol Education Program fall at about the fortieth and seventy-fifth percentiles.

A much larger fraction of the population in the middle of a distribution is affected by analytic error, compared to the population falling at the extremes of the distribution. From data given by Kroll et al.,[1263] the bias of a cholesterol assay must be kept below 1.6% in order to keep the misclassified percentage of the population below 3%. Although surveys of clinical laboratories suggest that this is rarely obtained, it is thought to be possible.[1264] The Lipid Research Clinics claim an overall bias of less than 1.7%, using the CDC reference method over an 11-year period,[1265] and the U.S. Air Force Heart Program claims to have achieved a mean bias of less than 1.3%, using the same method.[1266]

The need to attempt to achieve such stringent analytic standards was questioned by Boyd,[1264] as the intraindividual variation in serum cholesterol averages about 8%; in addition, the effects of postural changes and of anticoagulants on the sample can introduce further bias.

Consequently, more modest analytic aims have been suggested. The Laboratory Standardization Panel, in 1988,[1260] recommended that the bias of a cholesterol method currently in use should not exceed 5% and that developments should ensure that it does not exceed 3% by 1993. They also recommended that as a national (U.S.) goal, clinical laboratories should initially achieve an overall precision consistent with a cv of 5% or less; ultimately, a cv of 3% or less should be achieved. Reports from the mid-1980s[1260,1267] show that interlaboratory precision was about 6%, with mean intralaboratory precision of 3.5%. Broughton and Buckley suggested a target of 1% analytic imprecision to detect a clinically significant change of 5% in response to therapy.[1267]

SI UNITS
Conversion from mass to molar units is by the equation

$$\text{Cholesterol mg/100 ml} \times 0.0259 = \text{mmol/L}$$

INTERFERENCE WITH ANALYSIS

HEMOLYSIS
The effect of hemolysis on the estimation of serum cholesterol is minimal with most extraction and enzymic methods. Considerable interference has been reported with direct-reacting procedures, particularly those using iron reagents.[1268]

Richardson et al.[1240] found that a satisfactory correction, up to 2 g/L, could be applied with serum hemoglobin, with their dimethyl benzene sulfonic acid method. Haechel et al. found no interference with up to 7 g/L of hemoglobin for either enzymic methods or a Lieberman–Burchard method on the Technicon SMAC analyzer.[1269]

BILIRUBIN
Most methods for serum cholesterol estimation are liable to be affected by bilirubin. In both Lieberman–Burchard methods and those using iron salts in which serum is added directly to reagent, bilirubin reacts to give biliverdin, and the apparent serum cholesterol is increased.[1233]

Enzymic methods have been claimed to give a positive error,[1270] a negative error,[1245] and no error.[1271] Zak considered that bilirubin could give a positive error in the static mode and a negative error in the dynamic mode,[1235] but he found it difficult to rationalize no error at all for enzymic methods with colorimetric end points.

The extent and direction of interference is determined by the chemical interference and spectral interference. Bilirubin reacts chemically with an intermediary in the peroxidase reaction, reducing chromophore, and is also oxidized to biliverdin during the reaction, giving a fall in absorbance. Pesce and Bodourian[1272] studied five commercially available reagents, using enzymic methods based on the peroxidase reaction and incorporating a serum blank, and found that at serum bilirubin levels of 340 μmol/L, serum cholesterol was 12 to 73% lower than the true level.

Several procedures have been used to reduce interference. Preliminary alkaline action destroys the interference.[1273] Chemical interference can be reduced by including ferricyanide in the reagents,[1274] or bilirubin oxidase can be used to pretreat the serum.[1275] Spectral interference can be reduced by measuring at 520 nm, instead of at 500 nm, the absorbance maximum for the Trinder chromogen.[1235]

LIPEMIA
Direct-reacting methods are susceptible to interference from turbidity. Richardson et al. found in their *p*-toluene sulfonic acid method that turbidity was avoided by replacing acetic acid with phosphoric acid.[1240]

Enzymic methods may be affected if a surfactant is included in the reagent. Pesce and Bodourian found low results in these methods,[1272] due to the mixture partially clearing as the reaction proceeds, so that the blank is less at the end of the estimation than at the beginning. Small et al. reported false high levels of cholesterol obtained in patients with hyperglyceridemia,[1276] when estimated using Lipotrend (Boehringer, Mannheim, Germany; a desktop analyzer using principles similar to those of the Reflotron). Errors appeared to be proportional to the triglyceride concentration.

TRYPTOPHAN

There are early reports of interference by tryptophan in direct-reacting iron methods, due to a reaction with glyoxylic acid present as an impurity in acetic acid. The falsely high results can be corrected by refluxing acetic acid with potassium permanganate and distilling it before use.[1277]

NITRATES AND NITRITES

Absorbance of the Lieberman–Burchard color is depressed by nitrate and nitrite. Caraway and Kammeyer found that nitrite present in one lot of isopropanol was sufficient to depress the absorption by 25% at 6.48 mmol/L.[305] Rice showed that nitrate, which may be present in some lots of sulfuric acid, at 10 μg in the final reaction mixture, reduced apparent cholesterol by 30%.[1278]

THIOURACIL

Rice reported that apparent serum cholesterol was reduced by 0.75 to 1.0 mmol/L when thiouracil was used as a preservative.[1278]

SODIUM AZIDE

When developing a stable serum-based control for a cholesterol assay, Poon and Hinberg found that sodium azide added to serum interfered with the estimation using the "Reflectron" system.[1279]

	% decrease	
Sodium azide (g/L)	Serum A	Serum B
0	0	0
0.5	8	10
1	15	12
2	25	20

No interference was found when using a Liebermann–Burchard procedure or an enzymic method.

DRUG INTERFERENCE
Ascorbic Acid

Pesce and Bodourian, in a study of five commercially available reagents for estimating serum cholesterol, using enzymic methods,[1272] found that ascorbic acid added to serum, at a concentration of 100 mg/L, reduced the apparent level by about 20%. As the maximum concentration of ascorbic acid in serum is about a quarter of this, a significant effect will sometimes occur, and further investigation of the possible *in vivo* effect is desirable.

Bromide

Positive interference in methods involving the direct addition of serum to an iron reagent is given by bromide, which may occasionally be present in serum.[1280]

TABLE 192.
Cholesterol (in mmol/L) in Serum and Plasma from
Venous and Fingerstick Blood

Reference	Method		Venous		Fingerstick		Comment
			Mean	SD	Mean	SD	
1282	Enzymic	Serum	4.70	0.83	4.28	0.72	
1283	Enzymic	Heparinized plasma	4.66		4.87		
1284	Ectochem analyzer	Plasma					Plasma from venous blood 3.6% lower than from fingerstick blood

Salicylate

Tonks lists salicylate as possibly interfering with methods using an iron reagent,[1239] but Caraway and Kamneyer found that 1 g/L did not interfere when an isopropanol extract was used.[305] Jelić-Ivanović et al.[1281] added 8326 μmol/L of acetyl salicylic acid to reconstituted commercial lyophilized serum and found little effect on enzymic methods, but found a reduction from 3.31 to 3.08 mmol/L, using a Liebermann–Burchard method.

PREANALYTIC ERROR

Most laboratories estimate serum from clotted blood, although plasma may be used in some centers that also undertake lipoprotein analysis. A number of factors influence the result and should be taken into account. Also, the patients should be taking their normal diet and should not have, or be recovering from, an acute illness.

VENOUS BLOOD AND SKIN PUNCTURE

Although Kupke et al. found cholesterol in serum from skin-puncture blood lower than that from venous blood,[1282] later workers, using plasma, found higher levels (Table 192). The differences have not been satisfactorily explained.

VENOUS STASIS

Cholesterol in serum is bound to protein. Thus, excessive venous stasis will increase serum and plasma cholesterol. Koerselman et al. found an increase of from 0 to 22% (mean 14.8%) after venous occlusion for 5 min at 60 mm Hg.[1285] There was a parallel change in the packed cell volume. After occlusion for about 1½ min, an increase of up to 8% was found. Tan et al.[1153] observed no change when veins were restricted for ½ to 1 min.

ANTICOAGULANTS

Serum cholesterol has been known to be higher than cholesterol in plasma from anticoagulated specimens, at least since a report by Sperry and Schoenheimer in 1935.[1286]

Oxalate and Citrate

Sperry and Schoenheimer reported that cholesterol in oxalated specimens from three healthy adults was up to 15% lower than in the corresponding serum.[1286] In a single case of hypercholesterolemia, they found a 25% difference. Grande et al. found a 10%-lower level in oxalated plasma[1287] and noted a similar effect when citrate was used. Bachorik considered that the differences were due to osmotic effects that shifted water from cells to plasma, diluting plasma constituents.[1288]

Heparin

Sperry and Schoenheimer found no difference between serum and heparinized plasma,[1286] but Lum and Gambino reported that the mean level in heparinized plasma was 6% higher than in serum,[391] using a direct-reacting method. Little difference was noted using an extraction method of analysis. The higher level with a direct-reacting method was considered to be due to turbidity.

EDTA

A study by the Laboratory Methods Committee of the Lipid Research Clinics Program (United States) of 506 serum/plasma pairs analyzed by a modification of the Abell method[1156] found mean serum cholesterol to be 2.9% higher than mean plasma from EDTA specimens. The relationship was represented by the equation

$$\text{Serum cholesterol} = 1.036 \times (\text{plasma} - 0.138)$$

EDTA is the preferred anticoagulant if investigation is also to include lipoprotein analysis and the sample is to be stored.

Although Cloey et al. found plasma cholesterol to be 4.7% lower than serum,[1289] which they suggested was due to the higher concentration of disodium EDTA now used, Wickus and Dukerscheim,[1290] with Becton and Dickenson "Vacutainer" tubes (final concentration of disodium EDTA 4.46 mmol/L), found the difference with paired samples to be only 1.3%.

PRESERVATIVES

Briggs et al. reported that the antibacterial agent thimerosal,[1291] used to preserve isolated lipoprotein fractions, interfered with the cholesterol oxidase–aminophenazone method of estimating cholesterol. The catalase method was not affected. The problem can be overcome by replacing thimerosal with sodium azide.

SAMPLE STABILITY

Cholesterol is reasonably stable in serum. It is stable for up to 7 days at room temperature[1292] and for 2 weeks at 4°C.[1229] Crawford claimed stability for up to 6 months if there was only one freezing and thawing,[1293] although Henry stated that serum cholesterol has been reported to be stable for 5 years at –20°C.[1277] Wood et al. found that specimens frozen for 2 years were satisfactory when estimated by Liebermann–Burchard methods,[1294] but that apparent serum cholesterol increased by a mean of 2.5% per year when estimated by a method using iron salts.

PHYSIOLOGIC CHANGES

MEALS

Several studies have shown that although small changes in serum cholesterol have been noted after meals, they are probably not significant statistically (Table 193). It is not considered necessary to collect specimens from the fasting patient.

DIET

The effect of diet on serum lipids is complex, and detailed accounts are given in a number of publications.[1296] There is considerable public interest due to the acceptance that raised serum cholesterol is a primary risk factor contributing to the development of atherosclerosis.

Dietary Fiber

Cholesterol and other sterols are excreted into the intestinal tract in bile. Some are

TABLE 193.
Serum Cholesterol (in mmol/L) Following Meals

Reference	Subjects	N	Mean change
1295	Healthy men inactive for 2 h following a heavy breakfast		+0.13
	Healthy men with physical work after a heavy breakfast		−0.10
109	Healthy subjects 19–67 years old, after a breakfast containing 25 g of fat 15 g of protein and 50 g of carbohydrate	37	−0.11 45 min after −0.06 120 min after

TABLE 194.
Effect of Dietary Fiber on Serum Cholesterol (in mmol/L)

Reference	Subjects	N	Diet	Change Mean	SD
114	36–63 years old	14	18–100 g of bran per day	−0.23	0.13
1298	Healthy males	12	Similar diets with 36 g/day of wheat fiber	+0.17	0.18
			Similar diets with 36 g/day of guar gum	−0.76	0.25
			Similar diets with 36 g/day of pectin	−0.94	0.17
1299	Healthy males	3	Unprocessed wheat bran	No effect	
	Healthy females	3	Pectin	−15%	
1300	Psychiatric patients confined in a metabolic unit		Diet plus 15 g of fibre for 20 days	No effect	
			Diet plus 15 g of pectin for 20 days	−5%	

reabsorbed, the amount depending on the degree of binding to dietary fiber. Pectins and carrageenan, but not cellulose and lignin, bind and increase fecal excretion of bile acids and sterols.[1297] Serum cholesterol is consistently lowered by some water-soluble dietary fibers, such as pectin and guar gum, but water-insoluble wheat fiber and cellulose appear to have little effect.[1298] A number of accounts from the literature are shown in Table 194. Boyd suggested that the different effects are possibly due to hydroxy citrate found in pectin and guar gum, but not in bran.[1301] Later workers have shown that larger amounts, approaching 100 g of oat bran per day lower serum cholesterol. Kirby et al. found a mean reduction of 13% when the diet contained about 100 g of oat bran per day.[1302] Others have obtained similar results.[1303,1304]

Swain et al. gave a mean of 87 g/day of high-fiber oat bran,[1305] and a similar amount of low-fiber refined wheat products, for 6 months and found that both reduced serum cholesterol:

	Before	After 6 weeks
Oat bran (high fiber)	4.80 ± 0.80	4.44 ± 0.73 mmol/L
Refined wheat product (low fiber)	4.80 ± 0.80	4.46 ± 0.64 mmol/L

It was concluded that the fall in serum cholesterol was due to the diet containing less saturated fat and a higher proportion of unsaturated fat. However, some others in correspondence did not agree.[1306] It was claimed that the numbers were too small to make statistical conclusions, that the trial was not completely blind, and that fat intake was different in the two groups. In reply, Swain et al. answered the criticisms.[1306] They were supported by results, given by Birkeland et al.,[1307] of a similar experiment with a larger number of participants.

Dietary Fat

A link between low fat intake and low serum cholesterol came from early work studying vegetarian communities.[1308] Reducing fat intake to a maximum of 5 g/day and replacing

TABLE 195.
Cholesterol Levels in Subjects with Different Diets[1311]

| | Mean serum cholesterol (mmol/L) | |
	Male	Female
Vegan	5.00	4.84
Vegetarian	5.30	5.38
Fish eater	5.59	5.71
Meat eater	5.59	5.95

TABLE 196.
Saturated Fat and Polyunsaturated/Saturated Fat Ratio
in Different Diets[1311]

| | Saturated fat as % of energy intake | | Polyunsaturated/saturated fat ratio | |
	Male	Female	Male	Female
Vegan	33.5	36.2	1.85	1.77
Vegetarian	36.4	39.6	0.73	0.63
Fish eater	38.2	40.5	0.73	0.75
Meat eater	38.1	38.7	0.56	0.49

calories with carbohydrate produces a fall in serum cholesterol for about 1 week, and then no further fall occurs.[1309] Levels are affected by the nature of the dietary fats as well as their quantity. The ratio of unsaturated fatty acids to saturated fatty acids, stereoisomeric differences, and the chain length of fatty acids all alter the response of serum cholesterol to changes in dietary fat.

Saturated Fatty Acids

In a comparison of population groups in seven countries, Keys et al. found that there was a linear correlation between saturated fat intake and mean serum cholesterol.[1310]

A number of groups have noted that the ratio of polyunsaturated fatty acids to saturated fatty acids in the diet affects the serum cholesterol level. Thorogood et al., in a large study of 6000 non-meat-eating subjects (recruited through the Vegetarian Society) compared with 5000 meat-eating friends and relatives, confirmed this.[1311] Groups of 26 men and 26 women, classified as vegans, vegetarians, fish eaters, and meat eaters, were randomly selected and age matched (Table 195). The fat intake as a percentage of energy intake was not found to be significantly different in each group, but the ratio of polyunsaturated fatty acid to saturated fatty acid was much higher in vegans than in the other groups (Table 196).

Serum cholesterol can be reduced by an average of 20% by reducing fat intake and replacing half of the saturated fatty acid by polyunsaturated fatty acid. This is dietetically easier, as reducing fat intake alone is unpalatable and also causes an increase in serum triglycerides. Corn oil or cottonseed oil, or a blend of the two, can be used to replace animal fat. This also results in a relatively low cholesterol intake, as cholesterol is associated with animal fats. Ground-nut oil and olive oil contain mainly monounsaturated fatty acids and have less of an effect. Replacement of saturated fatty acids isocalorically by fat rich in polyunsaturates will produce a decrease in serum cholesterol of 15 to 20% in 2 to 3 weeks.

Chain Length

The cholesterol-raising effect of saturated fatty acids appears to be confined to those with 12, 14, and 16 carbon atoms.[1312] Palmitic (16 carbon) and myristic (14 carbon) acids increase serum cholesterol, whereas stearic acid (18 carbon) high in beef fat does not. Lauric acid (12 carbon) high in coconut oil increases serum cholesterol, which explains the effect of an apparent vegetable oil raising the level of serum cholesterol. Medium-chain saturated fatty acids with 8 or 10 carbon atoms do not increase serum cholesterol.[1313]

Stereoisomers

Different actions of stereoisomers have been reported. Elaidic acid, the transisomer of oleic acid (18 carbon), produced during the dehydrogenation of some oils, has been found to raise serum cholesterol in man, whereas oleic acid has little effect.[1314,1315]

Conclusion

The effect of dietary fat on serum cholesterol is complicated. Since not all saturated fatty acids increase the level of serum cholesterol, it may be desirable to follow the suggestion of Grundy[1313] that fatty acids should be grouped as cholesterol-raising fatty acids. This would include palmitic, myristic, lauric, and elaidic acid and noncholesterol-raising fatty acids.

Dietary Cholesterol

About 30% of the dietary requirement of cholesterol is obtained from the diet. However, if less cholesterol is eaten, more is synthesized by the liver.

Individual responses to a given change in dietary cholesterol appear to vary widely. It has been suggested that there may be a genetic element. Gotto[1316] refers to a study of 68 papers over 30 years in which it was calculated that there is a mean increase of 0.06 mmol/L in serum level for each 100-g increase in dietary cholesterol. Subjects varied widely. Kern had the opportunity to study an elderly man who ate 20 eggs per day[1317] and who maintained serum cholesterol between 3.88 and 5.18 mmol/L. Studies showed that only 18% of dietary cholesterol was absorbed and that bile acid synthesis was about twice the rate in normal volunteers. This suggested that there was a mechanism for adapting to high cholesterol intake, which involved decreased efficiency of cholesterol absorption and increased conversion to bile acids.

Atherosclerosis has been associated with high cholesterol intake. However, it is possible that this is fortuitous, as the high intake in Western society may be a consequence of a high meat intake and therefore a consequence of the intake of animal protein and saturated fatty acids.

In some populations, such as the Greenland Eskimo, the diet contains a high cholesterol content, mainly from fish and whale and seal meat, yet there is a low incidence of atherosclerosis. Nevertheless, in the population they considered, Shekelle et al.[1318] found that dietary cholesterol was an independent predictor of coronary heart disease. Gotto considered that it might be prudent to limit cholesterol intake,[1316] as about 30% of the population may be expected to be sensitive to dietary cholesterol.

Coffee

A number of studies have suggested that there is a relationship between coffee consumption and levels of serum cholesterol (Table 197) Changes in cholesterol levels have been related to the method of coffee preparation, with an increase in cholesterol in those drinking coffee made by using boiling water and ground coffee. Thelle et al. reviewed 22 published studies from a number of countries and noted that filtered or instant coffee had little effect.[1323] They concluded that there is a relationship between coffee consumption and cholesterol levels, but that there are other relevant factors, including the method of preparation — the effect of which is not clear. Not all studies showed an increase, but in those giving a positive response, it was about 5% or more.

Garlic

Serum cholesterol is lowered soon after administration of garlic. Experiments on five healthy subjects, by Bordia and Bansal,[1324a] found that there was a mean increase in serum cholesterol of 0.42 mmol/L 3 h after a meal containing 100 g of butter, but a mean decrease of 0.41 mmol/L 3 h after a meal containing 100 g of butter plus the juice of 50 g of garlic given in gelatin capsules.

Jain et al. studied 42 subjects with serum cholesterol more than 5.7 mmol/L who were given 900 mg of garlic powder per day in tablet form.[1325a] They found that after 6 weeks, serum cholesterol had fallen by about 6%. There was no further fall after another 3 months. References were given to seven other studies with serum cholesterol falling by up to 21% after ingesting garlic.

Nuts

Sabaté et al., in an experiment on 18 men 21 to 43 years old,[1326a] found that cholesterol was reduced when a diet was given in which 20% of the calories were supplied from walnuts. Mean serum cholesterol, estimated by an enzymic method, fell from a mean of 5.1 mmol/L (range of 3.54 to 6.47) to 4.1 ± 0.60 mmol/L on the walnut diet, compared with a fall to 4.7 ± 0.60 mmol/L on a reference cholesterol-lowering diet, after 4 weeks. Unpublished work was said to suggest that almonds and hazel nuts also had a cholesterol-lowering effect. It was thought that the cause was either due to the fatty acid composition, the type of fiber, or a lower lysine–arginine ratio.

EXERCISE

In the literature there is no clear consensus about the effect of exercise programs on serum cholesterol levels. Campbell[1324] found a significant decrease in the level of serum cholesterol in young male students undertaking vigorous sports, such as cross-country running and tennis, but little change in those participating in relatively static sports, such as wrestling or weightlifting. Carlson and Froberg noted a considerable reduction in conditions where calorific restriction and weight loss accompanied the exercise.[1325] In a review, Wood and Haskell referred to a number of studies giving different results.[1326] They concluded that this was not surprising, since serum cholesterol is the sum of cholesterol in different lipoprotein complexes; with exercise, HDL levels tend to rise, whereas LDL levels tend to fall.

POSTURE

There is a change in serum cholesterol of 10 to 15% when a subject changes from a supine position to a standing position (Table 198). This is related to the change in serum protein concentration.

SEASONAL VARIATION

A number of workers have found that serum cholesterol is lower during the summer months (Table 199). It has been suggested[1332] that seasonal swings appear to be light- or temperature-related, being most marked in those parts of the world showing the greatest differentiation, in these respects, between winter and summer.

STRESS

There have been several investigations of changes in serum cholesterol in stressful situations, such as examinations, occupations, or surgery (Table 200). Few reasons have been suggested for the higher levels found after periods of stress, apart from the speculation, without any supporting evidence, of Zarafanetis et al.[1335] when studying changes after surgery, that a lipid-mobilizing enzyme was released.

TABLE 197.
Some Reports of the Effect on Serum Cholesterol (in mmol/L) of Drinking Coffee

Reference		N	Method	Difference	Comment
1319	Men	7368	Those drinking nine cups daily compared with noncoffee drinkers	+14%	Men drank more coffee than women, and older subjects drank more coffee
	Women	7213			
1320		17	Group 1: At least six cups daily followed by none for 4 weeks Group 2: No coffee for 4 weeks followed by at least six cups daily for 4 weeks	−0.40	
1321			More than nine cups daily compared with noncoffee drinkers:	+0.56 Men +10% Women +8%	Mean 11% higher in men drinking boiled coffee
1322		107	4–6 cups boiled coffee daily for 9 weeks 4–6 cups filtered coffee daily for 9 weeks	+10% Little effect	

TABLE 198.
Change in Serum Cholesterol with Posture

Reference	Subjects	N	Change in posture	Change Mean	Range	Comment
1312	Normal cholesterol	13	Lying down to standing for 15 min	+12.9%	+7.7–+17.3%	
1153	Obese males 18–50 years old	7	Standing to lying down for 30 min	−10.4%	7–17%	Fall up to 5% at 5 min
			Standing to sitting for 30 min	−6.4%	1.3–9%	Fall up to 3% at 5 min
591	Male medical students	8	Lying down for 60 min followed by standing for 60 min	+15%		
	Female medical students	4				

TABLE 199.
Seasonal Variation in Serum Cholesterol (in mmol/L)

Reference	Subjects	N		Jan Mean	Feb Mean	Mar Mean	Apr Mean	May Mean	Jun Mean	Jul Mean	Aug Mean	Sep Mean	Oct Mean	Nov Mean	Dec Mean	Comment
1327	White prisoners 20–29 years old	25														Over one year highest in Nov, Dec, Jan; lowest in Jun, Jul, Aug
1328	Student nurses	7														Winter Mean 5.41 Summer Mean 5.28
	Postman	11														Winter Mean 6.60 Summer Mean 6.03
1329	Men 39–59 years old					7.23	7.23	7.23	6.97	6.97	6.97		7.07	7.07	7.07	
	Women 40–59 years old					7.36	7.36	7.36	8.13	8.13	8.13		6.89	6.89	6.89	
1330	Men 46–62 years old	52		5.85	6.03	5.83	5.88	5.62	5.57	5.46	5.85	5.88	6.01	6.03	5.80	
			SD	1.33	1.37	1.28	1.32	1.23	1.20	1.27	1.32	1.22	1.33	1.41	1.29	
1175	Healthy men 15–74 years old and healthy women of same age	3624 2840														Fall of 10% from May to July Rise to maximum in December
1331	Samples submitted to a routine laboratory over 2 years					6.73	6.73					5.96	5.96			Mean similar in each month in each year

TABLE 200.
Some Reports of the Effect of Stress on Serum Cholesterol (in mmol/L)

Reference	Subjects	N	Stress period	Time and level Mean		
1333	Tax accountants	39	Maximum stress in April	Jan	5.33	
				Feb	5.62	
				Apr	6.01	Mean increase 13%
				Jun	5.57	
	Corporate accountants		Maximum stress assessed from workload records	Minimum	5.44	
				Maximum	6.53	Mean increase 16%
1334	Male medical students	50	Winter term			
			Minimum midterm		5.52	
			Examination end of term		6.43	Mean increase 17%
		47	Spring term			
			Minimum midterm		5.59	
			Examination end of term		6.20	Mean increase 11%
1335	Patients before and after surgery		Surgery			Mean increase 25.4% Range 2.1–83.4

MENSTRUAL CYCLE

Changes in serum cholesterol during the menstrual cycle were first reported by Gonalonus in 1917.[1336] A number of workers have claimed that the changes have a definite pattern, but interpretation has been confused by the large day-to-day variation in levels, which is not always related to the cycle, and the difficulty of comparing results in cycles of different length. Table 201 shows the variation found by a number of workers. It seems likely that there is a peak in serum cholesterol a little before ovulation, after which levels fall and then rise slowly during menstruation.

RANGE IN HEALTHY SUBJECTS

BETWEEN- AND WITHIN-PERSON VARIATION

A wide range of levels of serum cholesterol in healthy subjects, both within and between, communities, is reported. A study of the literature is complicated by method differences, variations due to different life styles, and changes in diet in recent years. Serum cholesterol is found to vary with both the ethnic group and the location of the population. Lewis points out that levels range from a mean of 2.82 mmol/L in Pacific islanders to a mean of 6.97 mmol/L in the population of eastern Finland.[1341] Immigrants rapidly aquire the cholesterol levels of the host country, suggesting that the variation is not always genetic in origin. Lewis considered it likely that differences in diet, particularly fat consumption, were responsible for the differences. Studies of serum cholesterol in a local population usually show that the distribution is unimodal and near gaussian in form.

Most large series show that there is a difference between men and women and an increase with age, although it has been said that the level does not increase with age in communities with low incidence of ischemic heart disease.[1342] Change with age may relate to the cumulative effect of nutrition rather than to age alone. It is clearly impossible to give universally applicable ranges for serum cholesterol in healthy persons. If required, they must be based on data obtained from local populations.

Tables 202 and 203 give ranges found in several large series in different countries in men and nonhormone-using women. Cooper calculated serum values from plasma analysis, using published formulae. The figures can be taken as representing the "white" population of the United States. Values from Great Britain are higher than those found in American or French populations.

TABLE 201.

Reported Changes in Serum Cholesterol During the Menstrual Cycle

Reference	Method of determination of ovulation	Day of cycle	Change from mean for subject
1337	Ovulation determined by observing body temperature changes	Start of menstruation	–4%
		5 days	+5%
		8 days (6 days before ovulation)	+5%
		11 days (3 days before ovulation)	0
		14 days (ovulation)	–10%
		17 days (3 days after ovulation)	0
		20 days (6 days after ovulation)	+4%
		3 days before menstruation	0
1338	Ovulation calculated from length of cycle	Start of menstruation	–5%
		5 days	–0.5%
		8 days	+2%
		11 days	+3%
		Ovulation	+4%
		3 days after ovulation	–3.5%
		6 days after ovulation	+2%
		3 days before menstruation	–0.5%
1339		Mid-cycle fall of about 20% in an ovulatory cycle. No change in an anovulatory cycle	
1340	Ovulation calculated from length of cycle	Rise during menstruation, reaching a peak a day or two before ovulation, followed by a fall	

Populations are not necessarily composed of subjects with ideal or healthy values; there is a substantial incidence of cardiovascular disease in most populations studied. According to Stamler,[1345] serum cholesterol greater than that of the fortieth percentile of the male population of the United States gives an increased risk of cardiovascular disease.

There is some evidence that the mean cholesterol level in the United States population has altered over the years. Beaglehole et al. compared data from five epidemiologic surveys[1346] and estimated that from 1968 to 1976 there had been a mean fall of 0.13 mmol/L, which was consistent with observed changes in dietary intake. They suggested that this change had contributed to the known decline in death from coronary heart disease during this period.

The National Heart, Lung, and Blood Institute Collaborative Lipid Group[1347] compared a study of the United States noninstitutionalized population, 20 to 74 years old, in 1960–1962 with another survey in 1976–1980. Age-adjusted mean serum cholesterol fell by 3 to 4%. A significant fall was found in whites, but not in blacks, and there was a fall in all education subgroups (determined by the highest grade attended at school) for whites, except for those with less than 9 years of education.

Diurnal Variation

A large variation in serum cholesterol during the day in individuals has been known for many years (Table 204). Woodman, working in the author's laboratory,[1340] found that the highest mean value during the normal working day was at 9 am and that the value decreased slowly during the day (Figure 9). Keys said that the variation was much greater in healthy subjects with normal activity than in subjects confined to a metabolic ward with constant diet and activity.[1354] Consequently, it might be expected that within-day variation would be less in hospital patients than in the general population.

TABLE 202.
Serum Cholesterol (in mmol/L) in Healthy Males — Large Series from Several Countries

Reference	Statistic	20-24	25-29	30-34	35-39	40-44	45-49	50-54	55-59	60-64	65-69	>70
1343[a]	N	84		126			176		131		92	
	Mean	5.46		6.19			6.57		6.71		6.39	
	SD	0.43		0.57			0.57		0.58		0.48	
142[b]	Mean	4.58		5.39		5.94		6.13		6.02		
1180[c]	N	1925	3407	3198	1916	2052	5661	1958				
	Mean	4.53	4.84	5.18	5.46	5.70	5.80	5.75				
1181[d]	Mean	4.45	4.84	5.13	5.36	5.52	5.65	5.67	5.70	4.38	5.67	5.52
	Range	3.29-5.80	3.52-6.50	3.68-6.79	3.89-7.20	4.01-7.15	4.20-7.38	4.20-7.41	4.14-7.38	4.20-7.38	4.20-7.30	4.01-7.20
1344[e]	N											
	Mean					6.26	6.33	6.31	6.30			

a   1500 healthy subjects in London. Collected in afternoon into heparin. Analysis using a Technicon 12/60 analyzer.

b   500 male blood donors in London. Distribution reported to be log gaussian.

c   Study of French civil servants. Analysis using a continuous-flow analyzer.

d   Study from ten collaborating Lipid Research Clinics. Adults taken from 48,431 individuals of all ages. Range from fifth to ninety-fifth percentile.

e   Study of 7735 men in 24 towns in Britain. Analysis using a Technicon 12/60 analyzer.

TABLE 203.
Serum Cholesterol (in mmol/L) in Healthy Females — Large Series from London and United States

Reference	Statistic	20-24	25-29	30-34	35-39	40-44	45-49	50-54	55-59	60-64	65-69	>70	
1343[a]	N	118		191			215		144		93		Oral contraceptive takers excluded
	Mean	5.80		6.16			6.43		7.13		7.27		
	SD	0.51		0.55			0.53		0.60		0.65		
142	Mean	5.01		5.48		5.97		6.13		6.02			
1181	Mean	4.38	4.56	4.66	4.90	5.18	5.41	5.80	6.16	6.16	6.22	6.09	Nonhormone users
	Range	3.24-5.75	3.39-5.93	3.44-6.14	3.73-6.45	3.91-6.73	4.04-7.07	4.30-7.61	4.58-8.03	4.58-7.93	4.56-8.11	4.51-7.72	
	Mean	4.77	4.90	5.02	5.18	5.31	5.57	5.80	5.80	5.98	5.96	5.75	Hormone users
	Range	3.47-6.29	3.76-6.29	3.70-6.55	3.89-6.66	4.04-6.89	4.12-7.38	4.45-7.46	4.38-7.56	4.58-7.61	4.61-7.46	4.25-7.33	

a   No indication of hormone takers in paper from Leonard.

<h2 style="text-align:center">TABLE 204.
Variation of Cholesterol During the Day</h2>

Reference	Subjects	N	Change
1348	Unselected patients	9	Over 8 h, SD ± 8% of mean
1349			Over 24 h, 10% variation from individual mean
1350	Healthy persons Four samples taken during day	4	About 10% variation from individual mean (range 1.6–20%)
1351	Healthy soldiers Obese young men	22 13	SD about 10% of individual mean
1352	Healthy subjects	10	SD from mean 7.7% (range 5.1–10%)
1353	Healthy hospital workers 20–61 years old	53	Range of variation 0.5–4.3% About 60% attributed to biologic variation

Day-to-Day variation

The change in serum cholesterol in individuals from day to day appears to be little different from the within-day variation (Table 205). If conditions of collection are standardized and allowance is made for between-assay variation, within-individual variation probably has a coefficient of variation of about 5%.

RACIAL DIFFERENCES

Differences in mean serum cholesterol levels in various communities and differences between different races in the same community have been reported. It is frequently difficult to establish if the variations are genetic or due to different life styles.

In the United States Tyroler et al. studied approximately 90% of the residents of Evans County, a biracial community in the South, on two occasions.[1185] In 1960 mean serum cholesterol in males 30 to 60 years old was higher in the white population than in the black population. The difference was still present, but less, in another study in 1967. In a study of a biracial community in Louisiana by Fredrichs et al.,[1186] mean serum cholesterol of 1274 black children 5 to 14 years old was 4.40 mmol/L, whereas the mean of 2172 white children

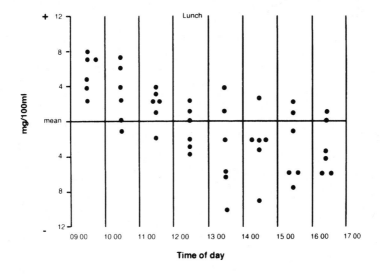

FIGURE 9. Change in serum cholesterol in healthy hospital staff during the working day. (From Woodman, D. D., Master's thesis, Council for National Academic Awards, 1974.)

TABLE 205.
Intraindividual Variation of Serum Cholesterol

Reference	Subjects	Method	N	Individual variation from mean
1349	Healthy males and females	Two to ten estimations over up to 28 months	25	Maximum variation up to 12.35%
1355	Males and females, 13–72 years old	Two samples taken 8–64 weeks apart (mean 35)	32	Mean difference 5.5% (range 0–19%)
163	Male and female white and black subjects 20–59 years old	Fasting specimen taken at 9 am once a week for 10–12 weeks	68	Mean cv 6.4% after allowing for analytic variation of 3.9%
164	White doctors	One fasting specimen taken once a week for 10 weeks. Stored frozen and analyzed on same day	9	Mean cv 5.3% after allowing for analytic variation
1356	Random sample of healthy adults and adolescents			Approximately 8%. (Between-assay variation SD 3.5%)
1353	Healthy staff 20–61 years old	Sampled monthly for a year	53	4–11% (about 60% attributed to biologic variation)

of the same age was 4.20 mmol/L. This was supported by a study by Christenson et al., who found that black males had a mean serum cholesterol level of 4.20 mmol/L, and black females had a mean level of 4.33, whereas white males had a mean level of 4.01, and white females had a mean level of 4.12.[1187] The level is higher in black children at all ages from 2 to 19 years.

In South Africa, Bronte-Stewart et al. found differences in the European, Bantu, and Colored adults in Cape Town.[1357] "Colored" subjects are of mixed European, Hottentot, and Malay origin. Mean serum cholesterol was 4.31 mmol/L in the Bantu population, 5.29 in the Colored population, and 6.06 in the European population.

NEONATES, INFANTS, AND CHILDREN

Harnung, in 1926, reported that cholesterol increases during the first day of life.[1358] Rafstadt found that the increase was before the first feed.[1359] Table 206 shows reported changes during the first week of life. Levels increase slowly during the first year of life. Darmady et al. noted that babies fed with an SMA formulation,[1360] which includes polyunsaturated fatty acids, showed lower levels of serum cholesterol. Throughout childhood serum cholesterol levels are higher in girls than in boys. There is a fall in the mean level in both sexes from the age of approximately 12 years (Table 207).

CORD BLOOD

Herrman and Neuman, in 1912, noted that serum cholesterol in cord blood is lower than in the blood of healthy adults.[1363] This has been confirmed by a number of studies, although varying levels have been reported (Table 208). Kaplan and Lee[1367] reviewed the literature and found that the mean level of serum cholesterol from a number of United States reports was higher than the mean reported from other countries. However, a report from Israel[1364] gave a mean level similar to that found in the United States. Differences may be due to method differences or to different life styles in different populations.

RANGE DURING PREGNANCY

A number of studies have shown that serum cholesterol almost doubles from conception to term. Probably the first report was from Herrman in 1912.[1363] Detailed findings from two groups are shown in Table 209. Peters et al. observed that at 8 to 12 weeks of pregnancy, mean serum cholesterol was lower than the accepted mean for healthy nonpregnant women.[1369] This fall during the first trimester was confirmed by the studies of Darmady and Postle.[1194]

OTHER CHANGES

BODY WEIGHT

A direct relationship with serum cholesterol has been found if obesity is based on weight in excess of standard body weight, rather than on body weight alone (Table 210). Classification according to somatotype, which takes into account body fat, muscle, and the height/weight ratio, also shows a relationship to serum cholesterol.

BLOOD PRESSURE

In a study of 4422 French civil servants by Lellough and Claude,[905] mean serum cholesterol was found to increase with increasing systolic pressure. Systolic bp was less than 110 mm Hg, serum cholesterol mean was 5.46 mmol/L; systolic bp was less than 150 mm Hg, serum cholesterol mean was 5.91 mmol/L; and systolic bp was more than 210 mm Hg, serum cholesterol mean was 6.40 mmol/L.

TABLE 206.
Mean Serum Cholesterol (in mmol/L) During the First Week of Life

Reference	N	Cord	Age (days)			
			0–1	2–3	4–5	6–7
1360	22	1.68	2.20	2.64	3.26	3.11
1361	Girls	2.10				4.20
	Boys	2.02				3.86

TABLE 207.
Serum Cholesterol in Infants and Children (in mmol/L)

Age	Ref. 1359	Ref. 1361		Ref. 1181		Ref. 1362			
		Boys Mean	Girls Mean	Boys Mean	Girls Mean	Boys		Girls	
						Mean	Range	Mean	Range
6 weeks		3.94	4.12						
1 month	3.40								
2 months									
3 months		4.71							
4 months			4.82						
5 months	3.11								
6 months					4.04				
8 months	3.47	4.87	5.26	2.64–4.92	2.93–5.21				
1 year	3.76	4.90	4.97						
2 year				4.12	4.14				
3 year				2.93–5.15	3.03–5.28				
4 year				4.20	4.22				
5 year				3.03–5.65	3.11–5.23	4.1	3.1–5.3	4.6	3.1–5.8
6 year				4.22	4.33	4.3	3.1–5.6	4.4	3.0–5.6
7 year				3.21–5.28	3.37–5.44	4.1	3.4–5.3	4.4	3.4–5.7
8 year				4.30	4.40	4.4	3.0–5.4	4.4	3.1–5.7
9 year				3.24–5.46	3.32–5.52	4.4	3.4–5.6	4.4	3.3–5.8
10 year				4.27	4.30	4.4	3.1–5.6	4.4	3.4–5.7
11 year				3.34–5.44	3.37–5.41	4.4	3.3–5.6	4.4	3.1–5.7
12 year				4.17	4.20	4.4	3.3–5.8	4.4	3.1–5.7
13 year				3.13–5.31	3.26–5.28	4.1	2.8–5.7	4.4	3.0–5.7
14 year				4.01	4.14	4.0	3.0–5.2	4.3	3.1–5.7
15 year				3.00–5.21	3.19–5.31	4.0	2.8–5.8	4.3	3.1–5.6
16 year				3.99	4.17	4.3	2.8–5.7	4.3	3.1–5.8
17 year				2.98–5.28	3.19–5.34	4.1	3.0–5.8	4.4	3.1–5.9
18 year				4.07	4.25				
19 year				3.03–5.28	3.19–5.52				

TABLE 208.
Serum Cholesterol (in mmol/L) in Cord Blood

Reference	Subjects	N	Mean	SD	Comment
1360			1.68		
1361			2.02		Boys
			2.10		Girls
1364	Normal births in Israel	129	1.71		
1365	Normal births in Cincinatti, OH	1800	1.68	0.50	No significant difference between black and white babies
1366	Normal babies	2927	1.82	0.44	Few black babies

TABLE 209.
Serum Cholesterol (in mmol/L) During Pregnancy

Reference	Before Mean	Stage of pregnancy (weeks)											
		4 Mean	8 Mean	12 Mean	16 Mean	20 Mean	24 Mean	28 Mean	32 Mean	36 Mean	40 Mean		
1368	5.48	5.43	4.56	4.79	5.59	5.57	6.32	6.45	6.92	6.94	7.15		
1194			4.78	5.28	6.00	6.54	7.11	7.58	7.86	8.02	8.25	About 36 weeks after delivery preconception level	

TABLE 210.
Serum Cholesterol (in mmol/L) and Body Bulk

Reference	Subjects	Type	N	Mean	Comment
1370	Young men 18–36 years old	In Minnesota	46		Serum cholesterol found to be related to endomorphic component
1371	White-collar workers	In Naples, Italy			No relationship to body weight
					Lower in underweight subjects
1372	Male soldiers	Ectomorph	476	5.02	Direct relationship with weight in excess of standard body weight
		Mesomorph		5.26	
		Endomorph		5.55	
905	French civil servants 46–52 years old	Less than 8 kg of fat body weight	206		1% more than 7.7
		More than 30 kg fat body weight	141		5.7% more than 7.7
1373	Men 50–59 years old from 24 towns in Britain	Body mass index (kg/m²)	7735		
		22.5		5.93	
		22.5–24.5		6.22	
		24.5–26.5		6.37	
		26.5–28.5		6.48	
		28.5		6.48	

1374   White men and women in Chicago

Relative body weight defined as observed body weight divided by desirable weight for age and sex

Men 19730
Women 13872

Age (years)		Men — Relative body weight %				Women — Relative body weight %				
		100	100–109	110–119	120–134	135	100	100–109	110–119	120–134	135
18–24		4.14	4.29	4.58	4.68	4.85	4.35	4.48	4.51	4.57	4.49
	SD	0.72	0.73	0.87	0.87	0.90	0.77	0.84	0.86	0.80	0.78
25–34		4.56	4.74	4.94	5.07	5.15	4.62	4.73	4.88	4.92	5.00
	SD	0.82	0.84	0.78	0.93	0.91	0.81	0.84	0.86	0.86	0.89
35–44		5.02	5.20	5.30	5.46	5.53	5.02	5.06	5.23	5.14	6.28
	SD	0.84	0.94	0.93	0.98	0.98	0.84	0.86	0.94	0.89	0.96
45–54		5.16	5.42	5.55	5.60	5.61	5.52	5.56	5.75	5.72	5.81
	SD	0.84	0.91	0.94	0.95	0.99	1.02	0.82	1.12	0.99	1.11
55–64		5.34	5.38	5.50	5.59	5.55	5.77	5.14	5.41	5.51	5.62
	SD	0.93	0.90	0.86	0.94	0.91	1.06	1.05	1.14	1.06	1.12

TABLE 211.
Serum Cholesterol in Blind
and Partially Sighted Persons[a]

Subjects	N	Mean	SD
Normal sight	50	5.01	0.89
Blind	220	6.32	1.43
Severely impaired (1/35 to 1/10 vision)	140	5.85	1.42

[a] From Hollwich, F. and Dieckhues, B., *German Med.*, 1, 122, 1971.

TABLE 212.
Relation Between Ethanol Intake
and Serum Cholesterol (in mmol/L)

Intake Drinks per month	Mean	SD
Nondrinkers	6.15	1.10
1–15	6.16	1.03
16–45	6.28	1.18
46–135	6.40	1.17
More than 135	7.14	1.32

[a] From Allen, J. K. and Adena, M. A., *Ann. Clin. Biochem.*, 22, 62, 1985.

The correlation was thought to be linked to the relationship between obesity and blood pressure.

SMOKING

Tobacco smoking is associated with an increase in serum cholesterol. In a study of a large number of subjects 15 to 74 years old,[1175] Carlson and Lindstedt found the level was higher in smoking males of all ages and in smoking women in the higher-age groups. Wynder et al. considered results from 15,892 participants in a screening program in Connecticut, of whom 12% smoked.[1375] An increase related to the number of cigarettes smoked was found, with a mean increase in serum cholesterol in men of 0.03 mmol/L per cigarette smoked, and in women, of 0.015 mmol/L per cigarette smoked.

BLINDNESS

Blind and partially sighted persons are reported to have higher serum cholesterol than normally sighted persons[329] (Table 211). Further work would be useful to confirm this, as it is not clear if the groups were matched for age, sex, diet, etc., and no similar studies appear to have been reported.

ALCOHOL

A correlation between increased serum cholesterol levels and increased alcohol intake was reported by Allen and Adena[1198] (Table 212). It is possible that the increase is linked to an increase in obesity, but this was not apparently investigated.

DRUGS AFFECTING SERUM CHOLESTEROL

CHOLESTEROL-LOWERING DRUGS

Atromid

Originally, a mixture of androsterone and ethyl chlorophenoxy isobutyrate (Atromid) was used. Later, Atromid-S (Clofibrate) containing ethyl chlorophenoxy isobutyrate alone was introduced. Reduction of serum cholesterol is probably by inhibition of hepatic synthesis. Other isobutyric acid derivatives used similarly are bezafibrate (Bezalip) and gemfibrozil (Lopid).

D-Thyroxine

Thyroid hormones reduce serum cholesterol by accelerating the breakdown to bile acids. The synthetic substance D-thyroxine was first reported to have little effect on serum cholesterol.[1376] However, Greene et al. later concluded, after giving the drug to 30 patients,[1377] that 5 to 15 mg daily reduces abnormal levels to the normal range, without affecting the ECG or the metabolic rate. No ill effects were found if not more than 5 mg daily was given.

Ion exchange resins

Ion exchange resins such as cholestyramine (Questran) and colestipol (Colestid) bind to bile acids in the gastrointestinal tract, leading to an increase in bile acid synthesis and a fall in serum cholesterol. Ion exchange resins differ from other lipid-lowering drugs in that they do not give rise to a fall in serum triglyceride.

Neomycin

Oral administration of neomycin reduces serum cholesterol, although other antibiotics, such as chloramphenicol, penicillin, streptomycin, and tetracyclines, have little effect.[1378] A mean fall in serum cholesterol of 21% (range of 14 to 29) in 30 patients given 1.5 to 2 g daily for 4 to 37 weeks was reported by Samuel and Waithe.[1379] The cholesterol level increased after the drug was discontinued. No change was observed after intramuscular administration. Eyssen et al. considered that as neomycin is poorly absorbed from the gut, the fall might be due to formation of salts with bile acids in the gut.[1380]

Nicotinic Acid

The reduction by nicotinic acid of serum cholesterol was first reported by Altschug[1202] in 1956 and was later confirmed by a number of groups.[1381,1382] A dose of 1 g given three times daily reduces serum cholesterol by 15 to 30%, with an average of 10% of the subjects showing no response.[1383] Side effects commonly reported are flushing of the skin and gastrointestinal irritation. The mechanism is uncertain, as there does not appear to be an increase in fecal excretion of fats, sterols, or bile acids.[1202]

OTHER DRUGS

Amioderone

An increase in serum cholesterol has been reported in patients taking amioderone for heart conditions. Wiersinga et al. studied 23 white patients and found that after treatment for 30 months,[1384] mean serum cholesterol had increased from 5.1 to 6.9 mmol/L. The patients remained euthyroid by the TRH test, and no increase in serum triglyceride was noted.

Anticonvulsants

Both phenobarbitone and phenytoin have been reported to increase serum cholesterol (Table 213). The change is considered to be due to the induction of enzymes of the endoplasmic reticulum, which includes the rate-limiting enzyme for cholesterol synthesis.

TABLE 213.
Effect of Anticonvulsants on Serum Cholesterol (in mmol/L)

Reference		N		Length of treatment	Mean	SD
1385	Male volunteers 17–23 years old	4	240 mg of phenobarbitone daily		+0–0.75	
1386	Previously untreated epileptic patients	11	Dose as required for control	Before	5.5	0.6
				3 month	6.5	0.8
				6 month	6.4	0.7
				9–12 month	6.8	0.9

TABLE 214.
Effect of Danazol on Serum Cholesterol (in mmol/L)

Reference	Subjects	Daily dose	N	Change in mean	
1392	Patients with recurrent endometriosis	600 mg	6	6 months	Approx +10%
1219	Healthy women 24–40 years old	800 mg	7	2 months	−0.67
1393	Healthy women and women with severe endometriosis	800 mg	7 25	6 months	−0.26
1220	Women 26–43 years old with endometriosis		12	Before	5.05 SD 1.0
				½ month	4.84 SD 1.01
				2 month	5.24 SD 1.47
				6 month	5.62 SD 2.16

Ascorbic Acid

Several groups have found no change in serum cholesterol in subjects after receiving up to 5 g ascorbic acid daily.[1387,1388] However, Spittle et al. reported a decrease in serum cholesterol in healthy young subjects given 1 g/day orally,[1389] from a mean of 5.02 to a mean of 4.58 mmol/L, but no fall in those 25 years old or older or in those with atherosclerosis. No explanation was suggested for the difference.

Asparaginase

Haskell et al. found that mean serum cholesterol fell from about 5 mmol/L to a little below 3 mmol/L in patients with neoplastic disease who were given 50 to 2000 IU of asparaginase per kilogram of body weight.[1390] Abnormal liver function was noted, and it was considered possible that the reduction was associated with interference with synthesis in the liver.

Beta-Blocking Drugs

Only a small, or no, change in serum cholesterol is found after treatment with beta blockers. Fogari found no change in the mean level after 6 months of treatment with atenolol, bisprolol, and propranolol; a fall of about 2% after mepadolol; and a fall of about 10% after celiprolol.[1214]

Corticosteroids

Stern et al. studied 12 patients with rheumatic disease who were given prednisolone[1391] and found a rise in serum cholesterol of about 45% from a mean of about 5.2 mmol/L.

Danazol

Different accounts have been given of the effect on serum cholesterol levels of danazol given to treat endometriosis (Table 214). No explanation has been suggested for the differences.

Diazepam

An increase in serum cholesterol, following treatment with diazepam, has been reported. Mazzaferri and Skillman gave 24 healthy euthyroid volunteers 12 mg daily[1394] and found mean serum cholesterol of 5.02 ± 0.82 mmol/L before treatment, 5.12 ± 0.77 after 6 weeks of treatment, and 5.67 ± 0.39 after 12 weeks.

Diuretics

Little change in serum cholesterol has been found in subjects following treatment with hydrochlorthiazide, but after chlorthalidone treatment, a small increase was reported (Table 215).

Estrogen

Subjects taking estrogen experience an increase in serum cholesterol, which is associated with an increase in carrier protein. A number of studies have been made of women taking oral contraceptives, and it has been shown that the estrogenic component is responsible for an increase in serum cholesterol and that the progesterogenic component has little effect and may, in fact, reduce the level slightly (Table 216).

L-Dopa

Sirtori et al. found an increase in serum cholesterol of approximately 10% in 12 male and 11 female patients who were given L-dopa for 1 year,[1397] but no figures were given.

Glutethimide

Bolton et al. found a rise in serum cholesterol from 4.80 ± 0.67 to 5.94 ± 1.73 mmol/L after 15 days, in a study of four healthy men and four healthy women, 20 to 23 years old, who were given 500 mg of glutethimide at bedtime.[1398] The change was considered to be due to the induction of enzymes concerned with cholesterol synthesis.

Isoniazid (INAH)

A fall in serum cholesterol after treatment with isoniazid was reported by Nanyam.[1399] In five men 28 to 65 years old who were given 600 mg and 100 mg of pyridoxine daily for 6 weeks, the mean level was 4.01 mmol/L compared with a mean of 5.59 when a placebo was given for the same time.

Para-amino Salicylic Acid

More than 6 g/day of para-amino salicylic acid given orally reduces serum cholesterol. Samuel and Waithe found a mean fall of 26% (range of 14 to 44) when 15 subjects were given 8 to 12 g/day for 5 to 23 weeks.[1379] Levene et al. found a fall from 4.51 ± 1.14 to 3.19 ± 0.93 mmol/L when 12 g/day was given to seven healthy volunteers,[1404] but no change in serum cholesterol was found with 6 g/day.

Spironolactone

A group of 11 mild hypertensives had their therapy changed from chlorthalidine to an equivalent amount of spironolactone by Ames and Peacock.[1405] The mean serum cholesterol was found to fall by about 9%. The reason for this fall was not identified. The possibility that it was a correction for a previous increase due to chlorthalidone was not excluded.

TABLE 215.
Effect of Diuretics on Serum Cholesterol in Groups of Hypertensive Patients

Reference		Treatment	N	Mean change
1221	Primary hypertensives	Diet only	31	−5%
		Diet + chlorthalidone	32	+6%
1222		Chlorthalidone	311	+4.8%
		Placebo	325	0.2%
1395	Black and white men and women	Chlorthalidone for one year	1012	Age 20–40y +10% 30–50y +5%
1396	Nonsmokers	100 mg daily hydroclorthiazide		+7%
		100 mg daily chlorthalidone		+9%
		Placebo		+1%
1397	Hypertensives	Hydrochlorthiazide for one year		Lttle change

TABLE 216.
Serum Cholesterol (in mmol/L)
in Subjects Taking Various Oral Contraceptives (OC)

Reference	Amount of OC	N	Time	Mean	SD	Comment
1400	2 mg of norethisterone + 0.1 mg of mestranol, for 21 days of 28 day cycle	55	Before 2 years	4.77 5.85		Steady increase over 2 years almost linear with time
	1 mg of norethisterone + 0.05 mg of mestranol, for 21 days of 28 day cycle	118	Before 6 months 2 years	5.26 4.87 5.57		Steady fall for 6 months followed by a steady increase almost linear with time
1401	1 mg of norethindrone + 0.05 mg of mestranol			5.18		
	1 mg of norethindrone + 0.08 mg of mestranol			5.13		
	0.05 mg of norgestrol + 0.05 mg of ethinyl estradiol			5.49		
	Non-OC users			4.90		
1402	50, 80, or 100 µg of mestranol, +1–2 mg of norethindrone	34		4.82	0.59	All results adjusted for age, obesity, alcohol intake, and smoking statistically by linear regression
	50 µg of ethinyl estradiol + 1–25 mg of norethindrone acetate	8		4.22	0.58	
	50 µg of ethinyl estradiol + 0.5 mg of norgestrol	20		4.69	0.63	
	100 µg mestranol + 1 mg of ethynodiol diacetate	9		5.39	1.23	
	100 mg of ethinyl estradiol 16 days followed by 25 mg of dinesthisterone 5 days			5.83	1.04	
	Control group	113		4.45	1.04	
1403	25 µg daily of norgestrol	37	Before During	5.67 5.13	0.92 0.94	Low-dose progesterogen only OC

Chapter 16

GLUCOSE

Glucose is quantitatively the most abundant carbohydrate in bodily circulation, control and maintenance of the level of glucose in blood involves a number of factors. Hormones affecting glucose homeostasis include insulin, glucagon, adrenalin, noradrenalin, cortisone, and growth hormone. Although the glucose level in blood varies according to the time since eating food, it is well maintained during periods of fasting. Glucose rarely falls below 2.5 mmol/L in healthy persons, although occasionally lower levels are found in premenopausal women and in children.[1406]

The response to glucose, as used in the oral glucose tolerance test, is often used to investigate patients with a suspected abnormality of carbohydrate metabolism. Originally, a test dose of 50 g of glucose was given, but some workers, particularly in the United States, used 100 grams. A procedure for the test has been recommended by the World Health Organization (WHO) Expert Committee on Diabetes Mellitus,[1407] and a dose of 75 g is recommended.

ANALYTIC CONSIDERATIONS

Methods for estimating blood glucose levels were described over 100 years ago and used large quantities of blood. Reid, in 1896, described one procedure that required 50 mL of blood.[1408] Since then, many procedures have been described, and satisfactory methods are now available that use 100 μL or less of sample. An excellent review of these methods is given by Burrin and Price.[1409]

For many years, relatively nonspecific methods that involved the reduction of picrate, copper salts, or ferricyanide were used, with workers in the field making considerable efforts to obtain better specificity by modifying the composition of the reagents. Levels obtained using reduction methods must be interpreted according to the degree of specificity obtained.

The Somogyi-Nelson procedure that uses zinc and barium salts as a protein precipitant[1410] excludes most nonglucose reducers and is said to give results "equivalent" to those obtained by specific methods. The procedure utilizing a change in color when yellow potassium ferricyanide is reduced, which has been adapted for use on continuous-flow analyzers, also gives results near to the true glucose content. This method has been used in several large series,[141,142,1343] to obtain the range in healthy people.

More-specific methods have been developed. Chemical methods using the reaction with phenols, such as naphthol or anthrone, and with aromatic amines, are more specific, although some sugars not usually found in blood, such as galactose, also react. The most successful method used o-toluidine[1411-1413] and has been adapted for use on continuous-flow analyzers.[1414] Results were near to the true glucose level,[1407] but the procedure is not now favored, due to worries about the possible carcinogenicity of the reagent.

Many laboratories now use enzymic methods for glucose estimation. The first attempt was probably by Hiller et al. in 1925,[1415] who measured the difference in reducing sugar before and after yeast fermentation. Later, glucose oxidase was used. Keilin and Hawtree, in 1948,[1416] used a manometric technique, and later, Froesch and Renold estimated reducing substances before and after action of the enzyme.[1417]

Better methods were devised that used photometric measurement. Sunderman and Sunderman used the reaction between the hydrogen peroxide formed and methanol to give formaldehyde[1418] and then used the reaction with chromotrophic acid to give a colored compound.

Others used an enzyme system in which hydrogen peroxide was coupled, via a peroxidase, to a chromogenic oxygen acceptor such as dianisidine, indophenol, or aminophenazone.[1419-1421] The procedure is almost specific for D-glucose, although desoxyglucose also reacts at about 12% the rate of D-glucose. Methods were developed using continuous-flow analyzers.[1421]

Trinder[1421] used phenol and 4-aminophenazone in a method in which, due to the high affinity of the reagent for oxygen, there was little interference from drugs. The use of reagents with less affinity for oxygen make it possible to obtain low results in the presence of tolazide, isoniazid, hydralazine, iproniazid,[1422] and paracetamol.[1423-1425] Richardson adapted Trinder's method to the Technicon AAII analyzer, using 2-4-dichlorophenol.[1426]

A number of commercial analyzers have been introduced that were based on the use of glucose oxidase and an oxygen electrode to give a direct determination of the glucose concentration in about 20 sec. Paper-strip methods based on glucose oxidase have been developed that are widely used by diabetic patients and in clinics, to monitor blood glucose (Visidex II, Ames; B.M. Test 1–44, Boehringer). The paper strip is impregnated with glucose oxidase, peroxidase, and chromogen, and a color change is obtained according to the glucose content of the blood, which can be measured photometrically to give a quantitative result. Another method based on hexokinase uses the reactions

$$\text{Glucose + ATP} \quad \overset{\text{hexokinase}}{=} \quad \text{glucose 6 phosphate + ADP}$$
$$\text{Glucose 6 phosphate + NAD + OH} \quad \overset{\text{G.6.P.D.}}{=} \quad \text{6 phosphogluconate + NADH}$$

A change in absorption at 340 nm or an increase in fluorescence is measured. A procedure based on this method has been proposed as a reference method.[1427]

The method using the dehydrogenase reaction is now considered to be the most specific for estimating blood glucose:

$$\text{D-Glucose + NAD} \quad \overset{\text{glucose}}{\underset{\text{dehydrogenase}}{=}} \quad \text{D-Gluconolactone + NADH}$$

Only xylose and mannose are reported as causing interference. It is essential to use satisfactory reagent enzymes, as errors have been reported that were due to the action of impurities, such as glutathione reductase on glutathione, and phosphoglucoisomerase on fructose.

ACCURACY AND PRECISION

Methods based on *o*-toluidine, glucose oxidase, hexokinase, and glucose dehydrogenase give results close to the true glucose content. Although the WHO Expert Committee stated that the Somogyi–Nelson copper method and continuous flow-analyzer methods using ferricyanide or neocuproine give results "equivalent" to those obtained by specific methods,[1407] most workers disagree. Sunderman and Sunderman found that the ferricyanide method using a continuous-flow analyzer gave results about 0.4 mmol/L higher than a glucose oxidase method,[1418] and the neocuproine method was said to give similar high results. This has been the author's experience, with results when using the Somogyi–Nelson procedure even higher.

Between-batch precision was investigated by Passey et al.,[1428] using lyophilized control serum. Ten methods using hexokinase, glucose oxidase, toluidine, neocuproine, and ferricyanide were considered, and the imprecision, expressed as the standard deviation from the mean, was generally less than 0.17 mmol/L at 4.4 mmol/L of glucose. At 8.9 mmol/L most methods showed a SD of less than 0.34 mmol/L, with the SD of the reference hexokinase method about

0.29 mmol/L. Gaspart found similar imprecision,[1429] using a glucose oxidase method with cv of 1.48 to 2.67%, depending on the glucose level.

Dry-chemical methods may be less precise. McLauchlan stated that the between-batch cv is better than 5%,[1430] whereas the WHO Expert Committee stated that the "bedside" estimation, using strips and a meter, will give results with a cv of less than 12%, with careful use.[1407]

SI UNITS

To convert blood or serum glucose from mass to molar units,

$$\text{mmol/L} = 0.0555 \times \text{mg/100 mL}$$

INTERFERENCE WITH ANALYSIS

COPPER REDUCTION METHODS

A number of nonglucose reducers, such as glutathione and urate, are found in blood. As already discussed, the copper reduction methods have been developed to obtain maximum specificity. The Somogyi–Nelson procedure probably gives results nearest to those of the enzymic procedures and is the most satisfactory reduction method.

O-TOLUIDINE METHODS

Hemoglobin of up to 3 g/L does not interfere with glucose estimation by the *o*-toluidine method.[1431] Interference by higher concentrations can be avoided by using a protein-free filtrate for analysis. Mannose, galactose, and L-dopa, in serum, can cause significant interference.[1427] Bilirubin above levels found in healthy subjects can result in falsely high results.[1431] Thus, analysis of icteric sera should use a protein-free filtrate.

Error due to turbidity was reported by Barash et al.[1432] when analyzing samples from patients who had been given dextran as a plasma volume expander. The precipitate was shown to be caused by the addition of acetic acid. For satisfactory analysis, other methods, such as hexokinase or reduction, should be used.

GLUCOSE OXIDASE

Contamination of glucose oxidase reagent with amylase or maltase may cause error due to the action on glycogen. Thus, a satisfactory quality of enzyme reagent should be used.

Chlorine from tap water, and ascorbic acid, have been reported to affect reagent strips based on glucose oxidase used for testing urine and may potentially affect methods for blood analysis. The effect of drugs on glucose oxidase methods has been discussed. Trinder's method is little affected by drugs. Pennock et al.[1433] found no significant effect of phenformin, tolbutamol, or chlorpromamide, compared with a GLC reference method. Some interference by mannose, xylose, galactose, ascorbic acid, and L-dopa has been reported, in Trinder's method.[1427,1434]

HEXOKINASE METHODS

Errors have been reported that were due to impurities in the reagent enzyme, such as glutathione reductase acting on glutathione, and phosphoglucomutase acting on fructose.[1435] Fructose, if present, may interfere due to the presence of phosphoglucomutase in blood. High levels of anticoagulant or of thiomersal found in some control sera and glucose standards may also interfere.[1430]

GLUCOSE DEHYDROGENASE METHODS

The only substances reported to interfere with glucose dehydrogenase methods are mannose and xylose.[1409] Xylose, not normally present in blood, will only be a problem if it is present due to being administered as part of a test for malabsorption.

WOODEN APPLICATOR STICKS

Joseph reported an increase in glucose in serum when wooden sticks were used to remove fibrin.[94] A mean increase of 0.4 mmol/L was found after 30 min of contact. The method used was not stated.

PREANALYTIC ERROR

COLLECTION OF THE SPECIMEN

Whole blood, usually preserved with fluoride, is often used for blood glucose estimation, although a number of laboratories use plasma or serum. Skin-puncture blood measured directly into diluent or protein precipitant is sometimes used, and with paper-strip methods, blood is placed directly onto the strip.

Glucose is freely diffusible. Thus, due to the different water content of cells and serum, analytic results will differ, with the serum level being about 15% higher than the blood level, in samples with a normal hematocrit. For each change in hematocrit of 10 units, blood glucose alters by about 0.2 mmol/L in the opposite direction.[1436]

There is little difference between skin-puncture and venous blood glucose concentration in fasting subjects. However, in nonfasting subjects, skin-puncture blood gives results about 7% higher than the corresponding venous blood, due to glucose uptake in the tissues.[1407] At the peak of the glucose tolerance test, the difference is 1.1 to 1.9 mmol/L.[1437] Serum glucose is said to be about 8% less than the plasma level, due to glycolysis during clotting.[1429]

SAMPLE STABILITY

Glucose is rapidly lost from blood after sampling, due to glycolysis with conversion to lactate. When serum remains in contact with cells at room temperature, less than 50% remains after 24 h, and there is complete absence after 48 h.[1438] Centrifugation of the specimen, with removal of serum, results in the glucose being stable for at least 24 h; this shows that the activity of glycolytic enzymes is low in serum.

It has long been believed that loss of glucose can be prevented by adding 20 mg of a mixture of 1 part sodium fluoride and 3 parts potassium oxalate, per 5 mL blood. Blood clotting is also prevented. Doubt has been expressed by several workers about the efficacy of this practice.[1439-1441] Loss of glucose has been demonstrated, with Meites and Saniel-Banrey unable to reduce glucose loss to below 4.9% after 4 h,[1440] and Clark et al. noting a fall in plasma glucose by a mean 10% after 48 h.[1442] Chan et al. studied the fall in blood glucose concentration with different concentrations of sodium fluoride[1443] (Table 217). They found that the effect was less with increased amounts of sodium fluoride, but that a fall could not be completely abolished.

Burrin and Alberti have concluded that if absolute accuracy is required, either blood should be analyzed immediately after sampling or plasma should be separated and stored at 4°C.[1444] There is some evidence that glucose is not stable even in frozen plasma. Giampitro et al. stored plasma for up to 1 year at –20°C and found, on average, a decrease of about 1% per month in the glucose level.[1445] Lloyd et al. found that perchloric acid extracts of blood were stable at –20°C for 1 year.[1446]

PAPER-STRIP METHODS

Special problems may occur with paper-strip methods. One must be certain that deterioration of the strip has not taken place. In an unpublished study of community screening in Tanzania,[1444] it was reported that although results were very precise, they were about 50% too high due to the exacting climatic conditions.

The hematocrit value has also been found to affect the result with paper-strip methods, with false low-blood-glucose results obtained with hematocrits above 50%, and false high results with hematocrits below 40%.[1447]

TABLE 217.
Decrease in Blood Glucose (in mmol/L) with Time,
at Different Sodium Fluoride Concentrations[a]

Naf (g/L)	Time (min)				
	0	**30**	**60**	**90**	**120**
0	8.17 ± 1.76	0.25 ± 0.07	0.48 ± 0.12	0.65 ± 0.22	0.86 ± 0.22
1	8.18 ± 1.79	0.23 ± 0.17	0.42 ± 0.07	0.53 ± 0.15	0.57 ± 0.15
2	8.18 ± 1.81	0.12 ± 0.10	0.37 ± 0.10	0.47 ± 0.17	0.53 ± 0.17
6	8.18 ± 1.79	0.13 ± 0.07	0.27 ± 0.07	0.38 ± 0.12	0.45 ± 0.07
12	8.23 ± 1.81	0.07 ± 0.10	0.07 ± 0.10	0.03 ± 0.12	0.32 ± 0.12

[a] From Chan, A. Y. W., et al., *J. Clin. Chem. Clin. Biochem.*, 28, 181, 1990. n = 6.
Values in columns 30 min or greater show difference from mean. With permission.

PLASMA SEPARATOR TUBES

In a study of samples collected into heparinized gel separator tubes (Becton Dickenson Co., NJ), Doumas et al. collected specimens and centrifuged them within 30 min.[1448] No change in plasma glucose was found after 2 h, but a fall of 6% was found after 4 h, a fall of 10% after 8 h, and a fall of 15% after 24 h.

PHYSIOLOGIC CHANGES

A study of the literature, by Peters and Van Slyke in 1932,[1449] suggested that most of the factors affecting blood glucose were already known, despite the methods available for measuring reducing substances, which included 10 to 20% nonglucose reducers. It was stated that the variation within a given individual is almost as great as the variation within a group.

THE GLUCOSE TOLERANCE TEST

Disorders of carbohydrate metabolism have been investigated using the change in blood glucose following a test dose, for many years. Peters and Van Slyke noted that when test doses were varied from 20 to 200 g,[1449] the different doses affected the duration of the increase in blood glucose, but not its height, except in diabetics. More recently, test doses of either 50 g (commonly used in Europe) or 100 g (more frequently given in the United States) have been used. Peters and Van Slyke also noted that exercise should be avoided before or during the test, as should emotional disturbances, and that an unrestricted diet should have been taken.

A WHO Committee has attempted to standardize the conditions for, and the interpretation of, the glucose tolerance test.[1407] They have recommended that 75 g of glucose should be given. There has been some discussion about whether 75 g of anhydrous glucose or 75 g of glucose monohydrate should be given, as frequently test doses issued from pharmacy departments are the less hydroscopic monohydrate.

I believe that "75 g of glucose" means that anhydrous glucose should be used, and if the monohydrate is given, the test dose should be 81.7 g of the monohydrate. Formal dietary preparation is not necessary unless the patient is taking a diet with less than 125 g of carbohydrate per day when a preparation period of 150 g of carbohydrate per day is advisable. Patients should fast overnight for 10 to 14 h, and the test should be performed during the morning. Smoking must be forbidden during the test.

FASTING

Peters and Van Slyke said that when a subject fasted for long periods,[1449] blood glucose fell after 48 h without food. After 7 to 14 days, blood sugar tended to rise, but not to the

TABLE 218.
Change in Plasma Glucose during Fasting[1406]

Fasting time (h)	Women (mmol/L)	Men (mmol/L)
24	3.202 ± 0.644	4.390 ± 0.716
48	2.753 ± 0.355	4.140 ± 0.683
72	2.292 ± 0.744	3.746 ± 0.477

prestarvation value. It was assumed that the effect was due to utilization of glycogen, followed later by catabolism of tissue protein.

Later experiments by Merimee and Tyson[1406] did not agree. They fasted subjects for up to 72 h, with water allowed as wanted, and estimated glucose, using a glucose oxidase method. Plasma glucose was found to fall steadily during the fasting period (Table 218).

DIET

Postprandial blood glucose levels can be affected by diet. Amounts of guar gum as low as 2.5 g in a 425-kcal meal given to healthy adults will reduce the postprandial rise.[1450,1451] Thirty minutes after the meal, there is a mean rise in blood glucose of about 2.4 mmol/L without guar gum, and a mean rise of only about 1.0 mmol/L with 2.5 to 12.5 g of guar gum added.

The effect of low- and high-sodium chloride diets on fasting blood glucose was reported by Iwaoka et al.[1452] On a diet containing 2 g/day of salt, the mean fasting glucose level was 5.07 mmol/L, compared with a mean of 5.34 in those taking 20 g/day of salt. A similar difference was noted after a 75-g glucose tolerance test. The absorption of glucose was considered to be facilitated by an increased sodium concentration in the intestinal lumen. Onions and garlic have been said to have hypoglycemic properties.[1453] Jain et al., investigating this claim,[1454] observed that ingestion of fried onions reduced blood sugar levels in diabetics, they also showed that extracts of onion and garlic had a hypoglycemic effect on glucose tolerance, when given to rabbits.

EXERCISE

Intense, predominantly aerobic exercise reduces blood glucose, and predominantly anaerobic exercise increases the level. This was noted by Rakestraw, in 1921,[1041] who found a decrease in blood glucose after a marathon run, but an increase after severe intense exertion. Klashko et al., studying 28 healthy subjects, found a decrease in blood glucose after a 1/2 mile walk on a treadmill.[1455] At a slope of 2.5°, the mean fall was 0.29 mmol/L, and at a slope of 5°, it was 0.65 mmol/L. Levels returned to resting levels within 60 min. These findings were confirmed by Galteau et al.,[120] who found a reduction of 2 to 6% after 12 min of moderate exercise, and by Udassin et al.,[1456] who found a reduction of 10 to 40% after 90 min of prolonged exercise.

SEASONAL VARIATION

In a study of 4541 men and women 20 to 79 years old in southern California, Suarez and Connor found that fasting blood glucose, estimated by a hexokinase method, was lower in the warmer months (Table 219).[1457] The level of fasting blood glucose found was considerably higher than that found by other workers in healthy people; this is difficult to explain. This was supported by work in Antarctica by Campbell et al.,[1458] who found lower fasting glucose levels in December, when the temperature was about 0°C, than at other times of the year, when temperatures were –20 to –45°C. Other factors, such as the amount of physical activity, may also contribute.

TABLE 219.
Seasonal Variation of Blood Glucose[a] (in mmol/L)

	Age	N	Dec–Feb	N	March–May	N	June–Aug	N	Sept–Nov
Men	20–39	83	6.09 ± 0.08	118	5.50 ± 0.06	58	5.65 ± 0.10	90	5.74 ± 0.08
	40–59	135	6.59 ± 0.11	149	5.97 ± 0.12	94	5.80 ± 0.12	164	5.97 ± 0.07
	60–79	301	6.36 ± 0.06	269	5.72 ± 0.05	169	5.93 ± 0.12	410	5.97 ± 0.04
Women	20–39	68	5.79 ± 0.11	110	5.33 ± 0.07	56	5.30 ± 0.12	93	5.32 ± 0.07
	40–59	100	6.09 ± 0.05	105	5.40 ± 0.08	71	5.84 ± 0.21	115	5.79 ± 0.08
	60–79	237	6.07 ± 0.06	201	5.60 ± 0.05	141	5.81 ± 0.11	297	5.80 ± 0.07
Women on	20–39	25	5.66 ± 0.14	28	5.08 ± 0.14	26	5.18 ± 0.22	31	5.27 ± 0.10
hormones	40–59	77	5.87 ± 0.10	86	5.43 ± 0.08	62	5.43 ± 0.14	128	5.56 ± 0.06
	60–79	101	6.17 ± 0.10	107	5.45 ± 0.06	66	5.50 ± 0.13	170	5.86 ± 0.17

[a] From Suarez, L. and Barrett-Connor, E., *Diabetologia*, 22, 250, 1982, mean ± SEM.

ALTITUDE

Blood glucose has been found to be higher in subjects living at sea level than in those living at an altitude. Picáon-Reátegui[1459] reported a mean fasting blood glucose of 4.11 mmol/L (range of 3.77 to 4.55) in 12 males 19 to 21 years old who lived at sea level, compared with a mean of 3.16 mmol/L (range of 2.33 to 4.83) in a similar group living at 14,900 ft. The difference was greater than could be explained by the change in hematocrit.

RANGE IN HEALTHY SUBJECTS

BETWEEN- AND WITHIN-INDIVIDUAL VARIATION

Surprisingly few accounts of blood or serum glucose in nonfasting or fasting subjects, using analytic methods giving "true" glucose, have been reported. Table 220 shows some published series. A small but statistical difference between levels in men and women has been noted.

Small abnormalities in glucose metabolism may be relatively common in the population. A working party of the British College of General Practitioners[1461] arranged for 345 oral glucose tolerance tests to be carried out on a sample of the general population, with no glucose detected in urine by stick tests after the largest meal of the day, and found only 191 completely normal curves.

Diurnal Variation

Blood glucose varies during the day in response to food intake. Mean blood glucose rises by about 13.5% after a standard 700-cal meal.[1429]

The response to a test dose of glucose has been reported to vary during the day. Peters and Van Slyke say that it is preferable to perform the glucose tolerance test during the morning, but do not discuss the matter further.[1449] Jarrett and Keen, giving a test dose of 50 g of glucose and analyzing using an alkaline ferricyanide method,[1462] found that blood glucose increased more in the afternoon than in the morning. Afternoon levels were a mean 1.77 mmol/L higher than in the morning, 60 min after glucose, a mean 2.77 mmol/L higher 90 min after glucose, and a mean 2.00 mmol/L higher 120 min after glucose. Grabner et al. obtained similar results.[1463] In some earlier work, Roberts gave 14 nondiabetic subjects with hypoglycemic symptoms 100 g of glucose and found a similar blood glucose response in the morning and the afternoon.[1464]

If these reports are correct and there is a different response according to the amount of glucose given, it is important to know the effect of giving 75 g, as in the WHO recommendations. Until this is documented, it would be wise to perform oral glucose tolerance tests only in the morning.

TABLE 220.
Blood and Serum Glucose (in mmol/L) in Some Large Series of Healthy Subjects

Reference		Age (years)												Comment
		21–25	26–30	31–35	36–40	41–45	46–50	51–55	56–60	61–65	66–70	71–75	76–80	
413	Range	3.77–5.72			3.61–6.11				3.44–6.49					Capillary blood; Ferricyanide method; 258 male and female fasting subjects
141	**Male**													Serum; Glucose oxidase method; Not fasting
	N		96	721		1268		1112			415		105	
	Mean		5.10	5.10		5.22		5.32			5.37		5.20	
	SD		0.81	0.80		0.92		0.90			1.01		1.16	
	Female													
	N		72	193		283		278			229		39	
	Mean		5.00	5.15		5.23		5.43			5.34		5.35	
	SD		0.85	0.76		0.82		0.83			0.89		1.07	
145	**Male**			Median 4.77	Range 3.50–5.83				Median 5.16		Range 4.05–8.82			Serum; Ferricyanide method on SMA 12/60 calibrated against toluidine method
	Female			4.61	3.22–6.22				5.05		3.77–7.22			
1460	**Male**													Plasma + fluoride; Fasting; Method not given
	N	2708	3261	3286	3422	3406	3115	2289	1920	1189	250			
	Mean	4.33	4.27	4.44	4.44	4.50	4.55	4.61	4.61	4.66	4.66			
	SD	0.56	0.56	0.56	0.61	0.67	0.72	0.72	0.78	0.78	0.78			
	Female													
	N	4662	3150	2506	2519	2665	2466	1520	1153	650	170			
	Mean	4.27	4.33	4.38	4.38	4.44	4.44	4.50	4.50	4.55	4.66			
	SD	0.50	0.50	0.50	0.50	0.55	0.55	0.61	0.67	0.78	0.83			
1429	**Male**													Plasma; Glucose oxidase method; Fasting subjects; Excluding obesity, recent alcohol or cigarettes, prolonged recent exercise, or family history of diabetes
	N	567	1485		743			335	172					
	50 percentile	4.94	5.11		5.22			5.27	5.27					
	2.5–95.5 percentile	4.11–5.88	4.22–6.16		4.22–6.22			4.27–6.22	4.27–6.27					
	Female													
	N	574	1173		574			297	86					
	50 percentile	4.72	4.77		4.83			4.88	4.94–6.16					
	2.5–95.5 percentile	4.11–5.72	4.11–5.88		4.11–5.88			4.22–6.05						

TABLE 221.
Blood or Plasma Glucose (in mmol/L) in Children[a]

Age	Male,[b] percentile				Female,[b] percentile			
	N	2.5	50	97.5	N	2.5	50	97.5
5	79	3.5	4.8	5.2	91	4.1	4.7	5.6
6	149	4.1	4.9	5.7	135	4.2	4.8	5.5
7	146	4.4	5.0	5.6	157	4.3	4.8	5.5
8	143	4.2	5.0	5.5	154	4.2	4.9	5.4
9	145	4.4	5.0	5.9	149	4.4	4.9	5.5
10	152	4.3	5.0	5.8	152	4.4	5.0	5.6
11	198	4.4	5.1	5.8	155	4.5	5.1	5.8
12	177	4.6	5.2	5.9	167	4.4	5.2	6.1
13	157	4.6	5.2	6.1	143	4.7	5.2	5.9
14	131	4.6	5.3	6.1	129	4.7	5.2	6.0
15	101	4.5	5.2	5.8	134	4.3	5.0	5.8
16	79	4.5	5.1	5.8	104	4.2	5.0	5.7
17	67	4.2	5.1	5.8	60	4.3	5.0	5.6

[a] From Haas, R. G., in *Paediatric Clinical Chemistry Reference (Normal Values),* Meites, S., Ed., AACC Press, Washington, DC, 1989, 135. With permission.[1467]

[b] Fasting about 12 h. Kept on ice. Analyzed same day by glucose oxidase/Trinder method.

THE ELDERLY

Mean fasting blood glucose levels increase with age by about 0.1 mmol/L per decade, and post prandial levels, by about 0.2 mmol/L.[1465] After a glucose load, the rise is about 0.4 to 0.7 mmol/L per decade.[1466] It is possible that part of the increase is pathologic rather than physiologic, because although the rise in glucose affects the whole distribution, it is greater at higher values. Hodkinson says that there is no case for adjusting standards of normality,[1465] as the changes appear to represent genuine impairment of carbohydrate tolerance.

CHILDREN

Fasting plasma glucose levels in children are shown in Table 221. Lockitch and Halstead[1468] found similar levels (3.9 to 5.9 mmol/L) in 400 children 7 to 19 years old, but a higher range (4.1 to 7.0 mmol/L) in 82 children 1 to 6 years old.

NEONATES AND INFANTS

Blood sugar was noted to be slightly lower in neonates than in adults, by Brown in 1925.[1469] Table 222 shows ranges found using modern methods of analysis. Collection is complicated by feeding times, the different feeds given, and the need to use capillary blood. It is generally agreed that levels are lower during the first days of life.

RANGE DURING PREGNANCY

Fasting blood glucose during pregnancy is 10 to 20% lower than the nonpregnant level (Table 223). The time taken to reach the maximum glucose concentration, after a test dose of glucose, is delayed as the pregnancy advances.[1473] It increases from a mean of 38 min at 10 weeks of pregnancy to a mean of 56 min at term.

OTHER CHANGES

SMOKING

There is a small but significant increase in blood glucose in smokers. Table 224 shows levels found by Dales et al.[47] 1 h after giving 75 g of glucose to a large series of subjects who had not smoked or taken food for at least 4 h.

TABLE 222.
Blood and Plasma Glucose (in mmol/L) in the First Days of Life

Reference	Subjects and method	Age (h)	N	95% limits		
1470	Healthy full-term infants.	Cord	52	2.72–10.1		
	Heelstick blood collected into	1	52	1.44–5.83		
	heparin.	2	51	2.33–10.2		
	Analysis on plasma.	3	51	2.55–5.66		
	Fed at age 3–4 h	4	49	2.44–5.55		
	and every 4 h after	6	69	2.39–5.11		
		12–24	40	2.44–5.44		
		25–48	55	2.94–5.16		
		49–72	55	2.78–5.55		
		73–96	35	3.44–6.11		
		97–168	26	3.16–5.94		
				5	**50**	**95 percentile**
1471	Healthy full-term infants.					
	Heelstick blood analyzed by	Cord	110	3.50	5.00	8.77
	Beckman glucose analyzer 2	1	113	2.00	3.11	5.50
	Fed at age 2 h, 5–6 h, and	2	107	2.16	3.22	4.94
	then at 4 h intervals	5–6	105	1.89	3.11	4.27
		10–14	102	1.83	3.11	4.11
		20–28	101	2.55	3.33	4.50
		44–52	92	2.66	3.61	4.39

TABLE 223.
Fasting Glucose (in mmol/L) During Pregnancy

Reference	Method	Subjects	N	Mean	SD	Range
1472	Somogyi-Nelson method	30–39 weeks pregnant	10	4.17		3.77–5.33
		Subjects at least 6 days after a normal delivery	10	5.30		4.33–5.72
1473	Glucose oxidase method	Subjects first and second trimester	5	3.69		
		third trimester		3.55		
		Nonpregnant white females	9	4.36		
1474	Glucose oxidase method	10 weeks gest.		4.16	0.46	
		20 weeks gest.		3.95	0.40	
		30 weeks gest.		4.12	0.40	
		38 weeks gest.		3.82	0.43	
		10–12 weeks postpartum		4.27	0.33	

BLINDNESS

Fasting glucose has been found to be lower in blind people than in those who are partially sighted or who have normal vision[329] (Table 225).

DRUGS AFFECTING BLOOD GLUCOSE

DRUGS USED IN THE TREATMENT OF DIABETES

Two groups of drugs are used in treating diabetes: insulin preparations, which may be short, intermediate, or long acting, and oral preparations, which are used in patients in whom dietary

TABLE 224.
Mean Blood Glucose (in mmol/L) in Smoking (S) and Nonsmoking (NS) Population of White and Black Subjects at Various Ages[a]

Age (years)	Male				Female			
	White		Black		White		Black	
	NS	S	NS	S	NS	S	NS	S
15–19	8.35	8.04	7.21	7.00	8.56	8.74	7.45	7.35
20–29	8.87	8.94	7.50	7.90	8.94	8.92	7.89	7.95
30–39	9.31	9.65	8.22	8.65	9.60	9.68	8.20	8.41
40–49	9.83	10.13	8.57	9.00	9.86	10.16	8.77	8.67
50–59	10.15	10.43	9.56	9.27	10.44	10.77	9.22	9.37
60–69	10.43	10.61	9.36	9.14	10.91	11.19	9.47	9.55
70–79	10.65	10.74			11.21	11.38		

[a] Dales et al.[47]

TABLE 225.
Fasting Serum Glucose (in mmol/L) in Blind and Partially Sighted Persons[a]

Subjects	N	Mean	SD
Normal sight	50	5.72	0.97
Blind	220	4.96	0.84
Severely impaired (1/35 to 1/10 vision)	140	5.70	1.78

[a] From Hollwich, F. and Dieckhues, B., Endrocrine systems and blindness, *Germ. Med.*, 1, 122, 1971.

treatment is appropriate, but who are not responding to a restriction of energy and carbohydrate intake.

Oral drugs are usually sulfonyl ureas and related drugs, such as acetohexamide, carbutamide, chlorpropamide, glycodiazine, metahexamide, tolbutamide, and tolazamide, which act by augmenting insulin secretion, or biguanidines, such as buformin, metformin, and phenformin, which act by decreasing gluconeogenesis and increasing peripheral utilization of glucose.

OTHER DRUGS AFFECTING BLOOD GLUCOSE

A number of compounds that induce hyperglycemia are listed by the National Diabetes Data Group.[1475] They are grouped into several categories.

Hormonally Active Agents

A number of substances are known to be concerned with glucose metabolism and to increase blood glucose, including ACTH, corticosteroids, glucagon, calcitonin, thyroid hormones, prolactin, catecholamines, and somatotrophin. Impairment of glucose tolerance is a common finding in women taking oral contraceptives. Approximately 30 to 40% show hyperglycemia 2 h after a test dose of glucose, and a number may have a diabetic tolerance curve.[1476-1479] The effect is due to the estrogen component, and progesteronic oral contraceptives do not alter carbohydrate tolerance.

Neurologically Active Drugs
Phenytoin

Large doses of phenytoin may increase blood glucose, but there is probably no increase if average doses are given to nondiabetics. Overdoses of phenytoin can mimic diabetic coma, with hyperglycemia, drowsiness, and neurologic signs, but without ketosis. Patients recover on withdrawal of the drug. Single cases have been reported by Klein,[1480] in a 20-month-old boy, and by Peters and Samaan,[1481] who demonstrated relative hypoinsulinism.

L-Dopa

Small changes in blood glucose are found in patients taking L-dopa. Brogden et al.[1482] and Langrall and Joseph[1483] found that 20% of their patients had transient hyperglycemia 2 h postprandially, with normal fasting levels.

Beta Blockers

Propranolol has been found to give a small rise in mean blood glucose from 5.6 to 6.0 mmol/L in 99 mildly hypertensive patients given 160 to 480 mg daily for 6 months.[1484] It has been shown that propranolol can produce severe hypoglycemia in healthy subjects and diabetics after insulin, exercise, or prolonged fasting,[1485] as the hypoglycemic response to insulin is potentiated, delaying recovery of the blood glucose concentration.

Other beta blockers have a different effect. Acebutolol potentiates initial hypoglycemia, but does not prevent or delay blood glucose recovery,[1486] whereas atenolol has no effect, and metoprolol has an effect similar to propranolol.[1487]

Diuretics

The interference of benzothiazine diuretics with carbohydrate metabolism was reported soon after the introduction of chlorothiazide.[1488-1490] It was suggested that the drugs brought to light latent diabetes mellitus in those with a family history of diabetes.[1491] Two studies suggested that the incidence of abnormal glucose tolerance in patients taking thiazides was about 30%.[1492,1493] Wilson, in a review of diuretic therapy, said that their use is not precluded in patients with diabetes, but the dose should be kept low, and diabetic control maintained.[1494]

Senior et al. noted in a study of 32 hypoglycemic neonates[1495] that almost half of the mothers had taken benzothiazines. It was speculated that thiazide-induced hyperglycemia in the mother may have caused fetal hypersecretion of insulin.

Other diuretics have less effect on carbohydrate metabolism. Anderson and Persson found that only 1 of 15 patients given ethacrynic acid and 3 of 16 given chlorthalidone showed a reduction in glucose tolerance.[1496] Frusemide has a similar effect. Spino et al. reported that 12 of 204 patients given frusemide had hyperglycemia.[1497]

Psychoactive Agents

The National Diabetes Data Group lists a number of psychoactive drugs that decrease glucose tolerance, including haloperidol, lithium carbonate, phenothiazines, and tricyclic antidepressants. Thonnard-Neuman found that the prevalence of diabetes in hospitalized psychotic females increased from 4.2% to 17.3% between 1955 and 1966 and that remission occurred in 25% on stopping drugs.[1498]

Other Drugs

Reports of hyperglycemia caused by morphine and ether were noted many years ago.[1499] Drug-induced diabetes, demonstrated in animal experiments with phlorizine, which affects tubular reabsorption of glucose, and alloxan, which destroys the islets of Langerhans, has also been reported.[1500]

L-Asparaginase has been shown to have a diabetogenic effect due to the resulting impaired insulin production with minimal islet cell damage.

Amioderone has a possible hyperglycemic effect, as noted by Politi et al.[1213] that two patients given the drug had impaired carbohydrate tolerance, with fasting blood glucose of 24 and 12.2 mmol/L. As they were unable to stop the drug, a return to normal could not be demonstrated.

There are conflicting reports about the effect of the calcium channel blocker nifedipine. Charles et al. gave six subjects 20 mg every 8 h for 3 days and found that mean blood glucose, 120 min after 100 g of glucose, increased from about 6 mmol/L to 9.89.[1501] Donnelly and Harrower, in a study of eight diabetic and eight nondiabetic subjects, found no significant effect on either glucose or insulin levels.[1502] Giugliano et al. gave 20 subjects 30 mg/day for 10 days.[1503] In those with normal carbohydrate tolerance, improved glucose tolerance was found, whereas in ten subjects with impaired tolerance, the peak blood glucose increased to 10 mmol/L or more.

A similarity between the physical and laboratory findings on salicylate intoxication and diabetic coma was recognized in 1906 by Langmead.[1504] Raised blood sugar levels were reported by Olmstead and Aldrich[1505] and Sevringhaus and Meyer,[1506] some years later. Morris and Graham[1507] stated that the fasting blood sugar of rheumatic children taking salicylates was increased by 15% above normal, but gave no figures. It was suggested by Segar and Holliday[1508] that salicylates have several separate effects on carbohydrate metabolism and that hyperglycemia may be due to increased glucose absorption, increased release of adrenocorticoids, and inhibition of some enzymes in the tricarboxylic acid cycle. The mechanism may be deficient in diabetic subjects, since Kaye et al.[1509] found some reduction in hyperglycemia in diabetic patients on moderate to high doses of salicylate.

A paradoxic response in carbohydrate-depleted children was noted by Limbeck et al.,[1510] who found hypoglycemia arising as a complication of a febrile viral illness. Mortimer and Lepour[1511] had earlier reported hypoglycemia, possibly due to salicylates, in cases of varicella, and Barnett et al.[1512] had found hypoglycemia with blood glucose of 1.4 mmol/L in 1 of 4 children with salicylate intoxication.

REFERENCES

1. **Rowe, A. H.,** The albumin and globulin content of human blood serum. *Arch. Int. Med.,* 18, 454, 1916.
2. **Zilva, J. F., Pannall, P. R., and Mayne, P. D.,** *Clinical Chemistry in Diagnosis and Treatment,* 5th ed., Lloyd Luke, London, 1988, 454. (Similar sentiments were first expressed in the 2nd edition, 1975, 469, in slightly different words.)
3. **Hawk, P. B. and Beirgeim, O.,** *Practical Physiological Chemistry,* 9th ed., Blaikston, Philadelphia, 1927.
4. **Martin, H. F., Gudzinowcz, E. J., and Fanger, H.,** *Normal Values in Clinical Chemistry — a Guide to Statistical Analysis of Laboratory Data,* Marcel Dekker, New York, 1975.
5. **Statland, B. E.,** *Clinical Decision Levels for Laboratory Tests,* 2nd ed., Medical Economics, Oradell, NJ, 1987, 8.
6. **Nabarro, J. D.,** *Biochemical Investigations in Diagnosis and Treatment,* H. K. Lewis, London, 1954, 260 and 261.
7. **King, E. J.,** *Microanalysis in Medical Biochemistry,* 1st ed., J. and A. Churchill, London, 1946, 1.
8. **Grasbeck, R. and Saris, N. E.,** Establishment and use of normal values. *Scand. J. Clin. Lab. Invest.,* 24 (Suppl.) 110, 26, 1969.
9. **Alström, T.,** in *Reference Values in Laboratory Medicine,* Gräsbeck, R. and Alström, T., Eds., John Wiley & Sons, Chichester, U.K., 1981, 7.
10. **Committee on Reference Values of the Scandinavian Society for Clinical Chemistry and Clinical Physiology,** Recommendations concerning the collection of reference values in clinical chemistry and activity report. *Scand. J. Clin. Lab. Invest.,* 35 (Suppl. 144), 39, 1975.
11. **International Federation of Clinical Chemistry Expert Panel on Theory of Reference Values, and International Committee for Standardization in Hematology, Standing Committee on Reference Values,** Approved recommendations (1986) on the theory of reference values. 1. The concept of reference values. *Clin. Chim. Acta,* 165, 111, 1987.
12. **International Federation of Clinical Chemistry Expert Panel on Theory of Reference Values,** Approved recommendations (1987) on the theory of reference values. 2. Selection of individuals for the production of reference values. *Clin. Chim. Acta,* 170, S1, 1987.
13. **International Federation of Clinical Chemistry Expert Panel on Theory of Reference Values,** Approved recommendations (1988) on the theory of reference values. 3. Preparation of individuals and collection of specimens for the production of reference values. *Clin. Chim. Acta,* 177, S1, 1988.
14. **International Federation of Clinical Chemistry, Scientific Division,** Approved recommendations on the theory of reference values. 4. Control of analytical variation in the production, transfer, and application of reference values. *Eur. J. Clin. Chem. Clin. Biochem.,* 29, 531, 1991.
15. **International Federation of Clinical Chemistry Expert Panel on Theory of Reference Values,** Approved recommendations (1987) on the theory of reference values. 5. Statistical treatment of collected reference values. Determination of reference limits. *Clin. Chim. Acta,* 170, S13, 1987.
16. **International Federation of Clinical Chemistry Expert Panel on Theory of Reference Values,** Approved recommendations (1987) on the theory of reference values. 6. Presentation of observed values related to reference values. *Clin. Chim. Acta,* 170, S33, 1987.
17. **Wooton, I. D. P. and King, E. J.,** Normal values for blood constituents. *Lancet,* i, 470, 1953.
18. **Herrara, L.,** The precision of percentiles in establishing normal limits in medicine. *J. Lab. Clin. Med.,* 52, 34, 1958.
19. **Dybkaer, R. and Jorgenson, K.,** *Quantities and Units in Clinical Chemistry,* Munksgaard, Copenhagen, 1967.
20. **International Federation of Clinical Chemistry Education Division Expert Panel on Quantities and Units,** A protocol for the conversion of clinical laboratory data. *Clin. Chim. Acta,* 190, S51, 1990.
21. **International Union of Biochemistry,** *International Union of Biochemistry Report of the Commission on Enzymes,* Pergamon Press, Oxford, 1961.
22. **International Federation of Clinical Chemistry Committee on Standards, Expert Committee on Enzymes,** Approved recommendations (1978) on IFCC methods for the measurement of catalytic concentration of enzymes. *Clin. Chim. Acta,* 98, 163F, 1979.
23. **Gowenlock, A. H.,** The influence of accuracy and precision on the normal range. *Ann. Clin. Biochem.,* 6, 3, 1969.
24. **Ballantyne, F. C., Morrison, B., and Ballantyne, D.,** Effect of storage on the estimation of protein concentration in human plasma. *Clin. Chim. Acta,* 87, 455, 1978.
25. **Wilding, P., Zilva, J. F., and Wilde, C. E.,** Transport of specimens for clinical chemistry analysis, Technical Bulletin No. 58. *Ann. Clin. Biochem.,* 14, 301, 1977.
26. **Pryce, J. D.,** The "normal" range. *JAMA,* 212, 884, 1970.

27. **Gräsbeck, R.,** Reference values, why and how. *Scand. J. Clin. Lab. Invest.,* 50 (Suppl. 201), 45, 1990.
28. **Berg, B., et al.,** in *Reference Values in Laboratory Medicine,* Gräsbeck, R. and Alström, T., Eds., John Wiley & Sons, Chichester, U.K., 1981, 55.
29. **Gräsbeck, R.,** Committee on Reference Values of the Scandinavian Society of Clinical Chemistry. *Scand. J. Clin. Lab. Invest.* 46 (Suppl. 185), 26, 1986.
30. **Flynn, F. V., et al.,** Some immediate effects of blood donation on plasma chemistry. *Clin. Chim. Acta,* 24, 51, 1969.
31. **Scott, E. L.,** What constitutes an adequate series of physiological observations. *J. Biol. Chem.,* 73, 81, 1927.
32. **Copeland, B. E.,** in *"Todd-Sanford" Clinical Diagnosis by Laboratory Methods,* 15th ed., Davidsohn, I. and Henry, J. B., Eds., W. B. Saunders, Philadelphia, 1974, 2.
33. **Reed, A. H., Henry, R. J., and Mason, W. B.,** Influence of statistical methods on the resulting estimate of normal range. *Clin. Chem.,* 17, 275, 1971.
34. **Lott, J. A., et al.,** Estimation of reference range: how many are needed. *Clin. Chem.,* 38, 648, 1992.
35. **Pickard, N. A.,** in *Clinical Chemistry — Theory Analysis and Correlation,* 2nd ed., Kaplan, L. A. and Pesce, A. J., Eds., C. V. Mosby, St. Louis, 1989, 41.
36. **Herbeth, B. and Bagel, H.,** in *Interpretation of Clinical Laboratory Tests,* Siest, G., et al., Eds., Biomedical Publishers, Foster City, CA, 1985, 393.
37. **Fawcett, J. K. and Wynn, V.,** Effects of posture on plasma volume and some blood constituents. *J. Clin. Pathol.,* 13, 304, 1960.
38. **Statland, B. E., Bokelund, H., and Winkel, P.,** Factors contributing to intraindividual variation of serum constituents. 4. Effects of posture and tourniquet application on variation of serum constituents in healthy subjects. *Clin. Chem.,* 20, 1513, 1974.
39. **Hesse, B., et al.,** Renin stimulation by passive tilting. *Scand. J. Clin. Invest.,* 38, 163, 1978.
40. **Stearns, E., Winter, J. S. D., and Faiman, C.,** The effect of coitus on gonadotrophins prolactin and sex steroid levels in man. *Clin. Res.,* 20, 923, 1972.
41. **Statland, B. E. and Winkel, P.,** in *Reference Values in Laboratory Medicine,* Gräsbeck, R. and Alström, T., Eds., John Wiley & Sons, Chichester, U.K., 1981, 127.
42. **Adlercreutz, H.,** Western diet and western diseases — some hormonal and biochemical mechanisms and associations. *Scand. J. Clin. Lab. Invest.,* 50 (Suppl 201), 3, 1990.
43. **McLaughlan, D. M. and Gowenlock, A. H.,** The normal range and reference values, in *"Varleys" Practical Clinical Biochemistry,* Gowenlock, A. H., Ed., Heinemann, London, 1988, 277.
44. **Ahlberg, B. and Brohult, J.,** Immediate and delayed metabolic reactions in well trained subjects after prolonged physical exercise. *Acta Med. Scand.,* 182, 41, 1967.
45. **Galteau, M. M. and Siest, G.,** Proc. *2nd Int. Coll. on Automatisation and Prospective Biology,* Karger, Basel, 1973, 223.
46. **Statland, B. E. and Winkel, P.,** Response of clinical chemistry quantity values to selected physical dietary and smoking activities. *Prog. Clin. Pathol.,* 8, 25, 1981.
47. **Dales, L. G., et al.,** Cigarette smoking and serum chemistry tests. *J. Chron. Dis.,* 27, 293, 1974.
48. **Freer, D. E. and Statland, B. E.,** Effects of ethanol (0.75 g/kg body weight) on the activities of selected enzymes in the sera of healthy young adults. Intermediate term effects. *Clin. Chem.,* 23, 830, 1977.
49. **Freer, D. E. and Statland, B. E.,** Effects of ethanol (0.75 g/kg body weight) on the activities of selected enzymes in the sera of healthy young adults. 2. Interindividual variations in response of glutamyl transferase to repeated ethanol challenge. *Clin. Chem.,* 23, 2099, 1977.
50. **Rollason, J., Pincherle, G., and Robinson, D.,** Serum gamma glutamyl transpeptidase in relation to alcohol consumption. *Clin. Chim. Acta,* 39, 75, 1972.
51. **Weitzman, E. D.,** Circadian rhythms and episodic hormone secretion in man. *Ann. Rev. Med.,* 27, 225, 1976.
52. **Varley, H., Gowenlock, A. H., and Bell, M.,** *Practical Clinical Biochemistry, Vol. 2, Hormones Vitamins Drugs Poisons,* Heinemann, London, 1976, 110.
53. **Guyda, H. J. and Friesen, H. G.,** Serum prolactin levels in humans from birth to adult life. *Pediatr. Res.,* 7, 534, 1973.
54. **Kallner, A. and Tryding, N.,** IFCC guidelines to the evaluation of drug effects in clinical chemistry based on the IFCC recommendations of the Expert Panel on Drug Effects in Clinical Chemistry. *Scand. J. Clin. Lab. Invest.,* 49 (Suppl.), 195, 1989.
55. **Young, D. S., Pestaner, L. C., and Gibberman, V.,** Effect of drugs on clinical laboratory tests. *Clin. Chem.,* 21, 1D, 1975.
56. **Young, D. S.,** *Effect of Drugs on Clinical Laboratory Tests,* 3rd ed., AACC, Washington, D.C., 1990. (Also supplement to 3rd ed. 1991.)
57. **Sherlock, S.,** in *Diseases of the Liver and Biliary System,* 8th ed., Blackwell Scientific, Oxford, 1989, 372.
58. **Briggs, M. H. and Briggs, M.,** Clinical and biochemical investigations of an ultra-low dose combined type oral contraceptive. *Curr. Med. Res. Opin.,* 3, 618, 1976.

59. **Tryding, N. and Linblad, C., Eds.,** *Drug Interference and Effects in Clinical Chemistry,* Apoteksbolaget and Socialstyrelsen, Uppsala, Sweden.
60. **Salway, J. G., Ed.,** *Drug-Test Interactions Handbook* Chapman and Hall, London, 1990.
61. **Alström, T., et al.,** Recommendations for collection of skin puncture blood from children, with special reference to production of reference values. *Scand. J. Clin. Lab. Invest.,* 47, 199, 1987.
62. **Meites, S. and Leveitt, M. J.,** Skin puncture and blood collection techniques for infants. *Clin. Chem.,* 25, 183, 1979.
63. **Meites, S. M.,** Skin puncture and blood collecting techniques for infants — update and problems, in *Paediatric Clinical Chemistry Reference (Normal Values),* 3rd ed., AACC, Washington, D.C., 1989, 5.
64. **Hammond, R. E. and Knight, J. A.,** Venous serum capillary serum and capillary plasma compared for use in determination of lactic dehydrogenase and aspartate amino transferase. *Clin. Chem.,* 21, 896, 1975.
65. **Henderson, M. J. and Dear, P. R. F.,** Role of the clinical biochemistry laboratory in the management of very low birth weight infants. *Ann. Clin. Biochem.,* 30, 341, 1993.
66. **Young, D. S.,** in *Chemical Diagnosis of Disease,* Brown, S., Mitchell, F. L., and Young, D. S., Eds., Elsevier, Amsterdam, 1971, 20.
67. **Lind, T.,** Clinical chemistry of pregnancy. *Adv. Clin. Chem.,* 21, 1, 1980.
68. **Walser, M.,** Ion association. 4. Interactions between calcium magnesium inorganic phosphate citrate and protein in normal human plasma. *J. Clin. Invest.,* 40, 723, 1961.
69. **Clark, E. P. and Collip, J. B.,** A study of the Tisdall method for the determination of blood serum calcium with a suggested modification. *J. Biol. Chem.,* 63, 461, 1925.
70. **MacIntyre, I.,** The flame-spectrophotometric determination of calcium in biological fluids and an isotopic analysis of errors in the Kramer Tisdall procedure. *Biochem. J.,* 67, 164, 1957.
71. **Bold, A. M.,** Determination of calcium in plasma: a review of some modern methods. *Ann. Clin. Biochem.,* 7, 131, 1970.
72. **Gosling, P.,** Analytical reviews in clinical biochemistry: calcium measurement. *Ann. Clin. Biochem.,* 23, 146, 1986.
73. **Cali, J. P., Bowers, G. N., and Young, D. S.,** A referee method for the determination of total calcium in serum. *Clin. Chem.,* 19, 1208, 1973.
74. **Henry, R. J.,** in *Clinical Chemistry. Principles and Technics,* 1st ed., Harper & Row, New York, 1964, 359.
75. **Alexander, R. L. J.,** Evaluation of an automatic calcium titrator. *Clin. Chem.,* 17, 1171, 1971.
76. **Meites, S.,** Calcium (fluorometric). *Stand. Methods Clin. Chem.,* 6, 207, 1970.
77. **Sonntag, O.,** Haemolysis as an interference factor in clinical chemistry. *J. Clin. Chem. Clin. Biochem.,* 24, 127, 1986.
78. **Corns, C. M.,** Interference by haemoglobin with the cresolphthalein complexone method for serum calcium measurement. *Ann. Clin. Biochem.,* 27, 152, 1990.
79. **Brett, E. M. and Hicks, J. M.,** Total calcium measurement in serum from neonates: limitations of current methods. *Clin. Chem.,* 27, 1733, 1981.
80. **Mann, S. W. and Green, A.,** A new colorimetric method for the measurement of serum calcium using a zinc zircon indicator. *Ann. Clin. Biochem.,* 25, 444, 1988.
81. **Olthuis, F. M. F. G., Kruisinga, K., and Soons, J. B. J.,** Interference of free fatty acids with the determination of calcium in serum. *Clin. Chim. Acta,* 49, 123, 1973.
82. **Singh, H. P., Herbert, M. A., and Gault, M. H.,** Effect of some drugs on clinical laboratory values as determined by the Technicon SMA 12/60. *Clin. Chem.,* 18, 137, 1972.
83. **Lacher, D. A. and Elsea, A. R.,** Effect of a lipid-clarifying reagent on results of Beckman ASTRA methods. *Clin. Chem.,* 32, 394, 1986.
84. **Radcliff, F. J., Baume, P. E., and Jones, W. O.,** Effect of venous stasis and muscular exercise on total serum calcium concentration. *Lancet,* ii, 1249, 1962.
85. **Broome, T. P. and Holt, J. M.,** Venous stasis and forearm exercise during venipuncture as sources of error in plasma electrolyte determinations. *Can. Med. Assoc. J.,* 90, 1105, 1964.
86. **Berry, E. M., et al.,** Variation in plasma calcium with induced changes in plasma specific gravity total protein and albumin. *Br. Med. J.,* 4, 640, 1973.
86a. **Pybus, J.,** Determination of calcium and magnesium in serum and urine by atomic absorption spectroscopy. *Clin. Chim. Acta,* 23, 309, 1969.
87. **Smith, F. E., Reinstein, H., and Braverman, L. E.,** Cork stoppers and hypercalcemia. *N. Engl. J. Med.,* 272, 787, 1965.
88. **Foster, L. B., et al.,** Presence of calcium contamination in vacuum tubes for blood collection. *Clin. Chem.,* 16, 546, 1970.
89. **Pragay, D. A., Howard, S. F., and Chilcote, M. E.,** Inorganic ion contamination in vacutainer tubes and micropipets used for blood collection. *Clin. Chem.,* 17, 350, 1971.
90. **Pragay, D. A., et al.,** Vacutainer contamination revisited. *Clin. Chem.,* 25, 2058, 1979.
91. **Helman, E. Z., Wallick, D. K., and Reingold, I. M.,** Vacutainer contamination in trace-element studies. *Clin. Chem.,* 17, 61, 1971.

92. **Hallworth, M. J., West, N. J., and Allen, A. R. G.,** Artifactual elevation of plasma calcium results due to contamination of lithium heparin tubes. *Ann. Clin. Biochem.,* 24, 525, 1987.

93. **Fitzpatrick, M. F., et al.,** Spurious increase in plasma potassium ion concentration and reduction in plasma calcium due to in vitro contamination with liquid potassium edetic acid at phlebotomy. *J. Clin. Pathol.,* 40, 588, 1987.

94. **Joseph, T. P.,** Interference from wooden applicator sticks used in serum. *Clin. Chem.,* 28, 544, 1982.

95. **Hanok, A. and Kuo, J.,** The stability of a reconstituted serum for the assay of fifteen chemical constituents of human serum. *Clin. Chem.,* 14, 58, 1968.

96. **Wilson, S. S., Guillan, R. A., and Hocker, E. V.,** Studies of the stability of 18 chemical constituents of human serum. *Clin. Chem.,* 18, 1498, 1972.

97. **Lester, E. and Wills, M. R.,** Longterm variations in serum calcium concentration in normal subjects. *Ann. Clin. Biochem.,* 11, 1974, 230.

98. **Omang, S. M. and Vellar, O. D.,** Analytical error due to concentration gradients in frozen and thawed samples. *Clin. Chim. Acta,* 49, 125, 1973.

99. **Hall, R. A. and Whitehead, T. P.,** Adsorption of serum calcium by plastic sample cups. *J. Clin. Pathol.,* 23, 323, 1970.

100. **Bailey, I. R.,** Effect on 16 analytes of overnight storage of specimens collected into heparinised evacuated tubes with plasma separator. *Ann. Clin. Biochem.,* 27, 56, 1990.

101. **Goldie, D. L., McConnell, A. A., and Cooke, P. R.,** Heat treatment of whole blood and serum before chemical analysis. *Lancet,* i, 1161, 1985.

102. **Houssain, I., Wilcox, H., and Barron, J.,** Effect of heat treatment on results for biochemical analysis of plasma and serum. *Clin. Chem.,* 31, 1028, 1985.

103. **Collinson, P. O., Stein, P. E., and Light, P. K.,** Effect on biochemical values of heat treatment of plasma for the safe handling of samples from AIDS patients. *Ann. Clin. Biochem.,* 23, 102, 1986.

104. **Savoury, D. J. and Grey, S. J.,** The use of heat treated plasma for biochemical analysis. *Ann. Clin. Biochem.,* 23, 701, 1986.

105. **Pollard, A. C.,** Technicon International Symposium 1964, quoted by J. R. Daly in *Scientific Foundations of Clinical Biochemistry,* Vol. 1, Williams, D., Nunn, R., and Marks, V., Eds., William Heinemann Medical Books, London, 1978, 448.

106. **Pederson, K. O.,** On the cause and degree of intraindividual serum calcium variables. *Scand. J. Clin. Lab. Invest.,* 30, 191, 1972.

107. **Felding, P., et al.,** Effect of posture on concentration of blood constituents in healthy adults; practical application of blood specimen collection procedure recommended by the Scandinavian Committee on Reference Values. *Scand. J. Clin. Lab. Invest.,* 40, 615, 1980.

108. **Stutzman, F. L. and Amatuzio, D. S.,** A study of serum and spinal fluid calcium and magnesium in normal humans. *Arch. Biochem. Biophys.,* 39, 271, 1952.

109. **Annino, J. S. and Relman, A. S.,** The effect of eating on some of·the clinically important chemical constituents of blood. *Am. J. Clin. Pathol.,* 31, 155, 1959.

110. **Wills, M. R.,** The effect of diurnal variation on total plasma calcium concentration in normal subjects. *J. Clin. Pathol.,* 23, 772, 1970.

111. **Seamonds, B., Towfighi, J., and Arvan, D. A.,** Determination of ionised calcium by use of an ion selective electrode. 1. Determination of normal values under physiological conditions with comments on the effects of food ingestion and hyperventilation. *Clin. Chem.,* 18, 155, 1972.

112. **McCance, R. A. and Walsham, C. H.,** The digestibility and absorption of the calories, proteins, purines, fat and calcium in wholemeal wheaten bread. *Br. J. Nutr.,* 2, 26, 1948.

113. **Anon.,** Dietary Fibre. *Lancet,* ii, 337, 1977.

114. **Heaton, K. H. and Pomere, E. W.,** Effect of bran on blood lipids and calcium. *Lancet,* i, 49, 1974.

115. **Reinhold, J. G., et al.,** Effects of purified phytate and phytate rich bread upon metabolism of zinc, calcium, phosphorous, and nitrogen in man. *Lancet,* i, 283, 1973.

116. **Dietrick, J. E., Whedon, G. D., and Shorr, E.,** Effect of immobilization upon various metabolic and physiologic functions of normal men. *Am. J. Med.,* 4, 3, 1948.

117. **Hulley, S. B., et al.,** The effect of supplemental oral phosphate on the bone mineral changes during prolonged bed rest. *J. Clin. Invest.,* 50, 2506, 1971.

118. **Heath, H., III, et al.,** Serum ionised calcium during bed rest in fracture patients and normal men. *Metabolism,* 21, 633, 1972.

119. **Keys, A. and Adelson, L.,** Calcium changes in the plasma resulting from brief severe work and the question as to the permeability of the capillaries to calcium. *Am. J. Physiol.,* 115, 539, 1936.

120. **Galteau, M. M., Siest, G., and Boura, M.,** Un effort limite peut-il modifier les valeurs de reference des parametres sanguins. *Clin. Chim. Acta,* 55, 353, 1974.

121. **Aloia, J. F., et al.,** Exercise-induced hypercalcemia and the calciotropic hormones. *J. Lab. Clin. Med.,* 106, 229, 1985.

122. **Mostellar, M. E. and Tuttle, E. P.,** Effects of alkalosis on plasma concentration and urinary excretion of inorganic phosphate in man *J. Clin. Invest.,* 43, 138, 1964.
123. **Bakwin, H. and Bakwin, R. M.,** Seasonal variation in the calcium content of infants serum. *Am. J. Dis. Child.,* 34, 994, 1927.
124. **Josephson, B. and Dahlburn, G.,** Variations in the cell content and chemical composition of the human blood due to age, sex, and season. *Scand. J. Clin. Lab. Invest.,* 4, 216, 1952.
125. **Frank, H. A. and Carr, M. H.,** "Normal" serum electrolytes with a note on seasonal and menstrual variation. *J. Clin. Lab. Med.,* 49, 246, 1957.
126. **Iwanani, M., et al.,** Seasonal variation in serum inorganic phosphate and calcium with special reference to parathyroid activity. *J. Physiol. (Lond.),* 149, 23, 1959.
127. **McLaughlan, M., et al.,** Seasonal variations and serum 25 hydroxycholecalciferol in healthy people. *Lancet,* i, 536, 1974.
128. **Ljundhall, S., et al.,** Calcium phosphate and albumin in serum. A population study with special reference to renal stone and the prevalence of hyperparathyroidism. *Acta Med. Scand.,* 210, 23, 1977.
129. **Broughton, P. R., Holder, R., and Ashby, D.,** Long-term trends in biochemical data obtained from two population surveys. *Ann. Clin. Biochem.,* 23, 475, 1986.
130. **Hodkinson, H. M., et al.,** Sunlight, vitamin D, and osteomalacia in the elderly. *Lancet,* i, 910, 1973.
131. **Dent, C. E.,** Some problems of hyperparathyroidism. *Br. Med. J.,* 2, 1419, 1962.
132. **Parfitt, A. M.,** Chlorthiazide-induced hypercalcemia in juvenile osteoporosis and hyperparathyroidism. *N. Engl. J. Med.,* 281, 55, 1969.
133. **Husdan, H., et al.,** Effect of venous occlusion of the arm on the concentration of calcium in serum and methods for its compensation. *Clin. Chem.,* 20, 529, 1974.
134. **Orrell, D. H.,** Albumin as an aid to the interpretation of serum calcium. *Clin. Chim. Acta,* 35, 483, 1973.
135. **Payne, R. B., et al.,** Interpretation of serum calcium in patients with abnormal serum proteins. *Br. Med. J.,* 4, 643, 1973.
136. **Moore, E. W.,** Ionized calcium in normal serum, ultrafiltrates and whole blood determined by ion-exchange electrodes. *J. Clin. Invest.,* 49, 318, 1970.
137. **Ashby, J. P., Wright, D. J., and Rinsler, M. G.,** The adjusted serum calcium concept — a reappraisal. *Ann. Clin. Biochem.,* 23, 533, 1986.
138. **Kanis, J. A. and Yates, A. J. P.,** Measuring serum calcium. *Br. Med. J.,* 270, 728, 1985.
139. **Walker, B. E. and Payne, R. B.,** Venepuncture for calcium assays: should we still avoid tourniquet. *Postgrad. Med. J.,* 67, 489, 1991.
140. **Keating, F. R., et al.,** The relation of age and sex to distribution of values in healthy adults of serum calcium, inorganic phosphate, magnesium, alkaline phosphatase, total protein albumin and blood urea. *J. Lab. Clin. Med.,* 73, 825, 1969.
141. **Wilding, P., Rollason, J. G., and Robinson, D.,** Patterns of change for various biochemical constituents detected on well population screening. *Clin. Chim. Acta,* 41, 375, 1972.
142. **McPherson, K., et al.,** The effect of age and sex and other factors on blood chemistry in health. *Clin. Chim. Acta,* 84, 373, 1978.
143. **Ballard, M.,** in *Interpretation of Clinical Laboratory Tests,* Siest, G., et al., Eds., Biomedical Publishers, Foster City, CA, 1985, 172.
144. **O'Kell, R. T. and Elliot, J. R.,** Development of normal values for use in multitest biochemical screening of sera, *Clin. Chem.,* 16, 161, 1970.
145. **Reed, A. H., et al.,** Estimation of normal ranges from a controlled sample survey. 1. Sex and age related influence on the SMA 12/60 screening group of tests. *Clin. Chem.,* 23, 829, 1985.
146. **Baadenhuijsen, H. and Smit, J. C.,** Indirect estimation of clinical chemical reference intervals from total hospital data: application of a modified Bhattacharya procedure. *J. Clin. Chem. Clin. Biochem.,* 23, 829, 1985.
147. **Sinton, T. J., Cowley, D. M., and Bryant, S. J.,** Reference intervals for calcium phosphate and alkaline phosphatase derived on the basis of multichannel analyser profiles. *Clin. Chem.,* 32, 76, 1986.
148. **Foweather, F. S.,** *A Handbook of Clinical Chemical Pathology,* J. and A. Churchill, London, 1929.
149. **Harrison, G. A.,** *Chemical Methods in Clinical Medicine,* 1st ed., J. and A. Churchill, London, 1930.
150. **Peters, J. P. and Van Slyke, D. D.,** *Quantitative Clinical Chemistry, Vol. 1, Interpretations,* Bailliere Tyndall, London, 1932.
151. **Canterow, A. and Trumper, M.,** *Clinical Biochemistry,* 4th ed., W. B. Saunders, Philadelphia, 1950.
152. **Varley, H.,** *Practical Clinical Biochemistry,* 1st ed., William Heinemann Medical Books, London, 1954.
153. **Varley, H.,** *Practical Clinical Biochemistry,* 3rd ed., William Heinemann Medical Books, London, 1954.
154. **Eastham, R. D.,** *Biochemical Values in Clinical Medicine,* 3rd ed., Wright, Bristol, UK, 1967.
155. **Grey, C. H.,** *Clinical Chemical Pathology,* 7th ed., Edward Arnold, London, 1974.
156. **Wooton, I. D. P.,** *Micro Methods in Clinical Chemistry,* 5th ed., J. and A. Churchill, London, 1974.
157. **Lafner, A. L., Ed.,** *"Canterow and Trumper" Clinical Chemistry in Practical Medicine,* 7th ed., W. B. Saunders, Philadelphia, 1975.

158. **Grey, C. H. and Howarth, P. J. N.,** *Clinical Chemical Pathology,* 8th ed., Edward Arnold, London, 1977.

159. **Varley, H., Gowenlock, A. H., and Bell, M.,** *Practical Clinical Biochemistry,* 5th ed., William Heinemann Medical Books, London, 1980.

160. **Bishop, M. L., Duben-Van Lauden, J. L., and Fody, E. P.,** *Clinical Chemistry Principles Procedures Correlations,* Lippincott, Philadelphia, 1985.

161. **Tietz, N. W.,** *Textbook of Clinical Chemistry,* W. B. Saunders, Philadelphia, 1986.

162. **Caplan, L. A. and Pesce, A. J.,** *Clinical Chemistry Theory Analysis and Correlation,* 2nd ed., C. V. Mosby, St. Louis, 1989.

163. **Harris, E. K., et al.,** Biological and analytic components of variation. Long-term studies of serum constituents in normal subjects. II. Estimating biological components of variation. *Clin. Chem.,* 16, 1022, 1970.

164. **Young, D. S., Harris, E. K., and Cotlove, E.,** Biological and analytic components of variation. Long-term studies of serum constituents in normal subjects. IV. Results of a study designed to eliminate long-term analytic deviation. *Clin. Chem.,* 17, 403, 1971.

165. **Winkel, P., Statland, B., and Bokelund, H.,** Factors contributing to intra-individual variation of serum constituents. V. Short-term day-to-day and within hour variation of serum constituents in healthy subjects. *Clin. Chem.,* 20, 1520, 1974.

166. **Leask, R. G. S., Andrews, G. R., and Caird, F. I.,** Normal values for sixteen blood constituents in the elderly. *Age Aging,* 2, 14, 1973.

167. **Jernigan, J. A., et al.,** Reference values for blood findings in relatively fit elderly persons. *J. Am. Germ. Soc.,* 28, 308, 1980.

168. **Hale, W. E., Stewart, R. B., and Marks, R. G.,** Haematological and biochemical values in an ambulatory elderly population: an analysis of the effect of age, sex and drugs. *Age Aging,* 12, 275, 1983.

169. **Gallagher, J. C., Young, M. M., and Nordin, B. E. C.,** Effects of artificial menopause on plasma and urine calcium and phosphate. *Clin. Endocrinol.,* 1, 57, 1972.

170. **Marshall, R. W., Francis, R. M., and Hodkinson, A.,** Plasma total and ionised calcium, albumin and globulin concentration in pre- and postmenopausal women and the effects of oestrogen administration. *Clin. Chim. Acta,* 122, 283, 1982.

171. **Cheng, M. H., et al.,** Microchemical analysis for 13 constituents of plasma from healthy children. *Clin. Chem.,* 25, 692, 1979.

172. **Widham, K. and Hötzel, M.,** Changes of alkaline phosphatase inorganic phosphorous and total calcium in sera of 11 to 17 year old healthy adolescents and their relationship to growth. *J. Clin. Chem. Clin. Biochem.,* 23, 711, 1985.

173. **Haas, R. G.,** in *Paediatric Clinical Chemistry Reference (Normal Values),* 3rd ed., Meites, S., Ed., American Association of Clinical Chemists, Washington, D.C., 1989, 82.

174. **Meites, S.,** Normal total plasma calcium in the newborn. *Crit. Rev. Clin. Lab. Sci.,* 6, 1, 1975.

175. **Bakwin, H.,** Pathogenesis of tetany of the newborn. *Am. J. Dis. Child.,* 54, 1211, 1937.

176. **Oppé, T. E. and Redsone, D.,** Calcium and phosphorous levels in healthy new born infants given various types of milk. *Lancet,* i, 1045, 1968.

177. **Harvey, D. R., Cooper, L. V., and Stevans, J. F.,** Plasma calcium and magnesium in newborn babies. *Arch. Dis. Child.,* 45, 506, 1970.

178. **Cockburn, F., et al.,** Neonatal convulsions associated with primary disturbance of calcium phosphorous and magnesium metabolism. *Arch. Dis. Child.,* 48, 99, 1973.

179. **Anon.,** Neonatal calcium magnesium and phosphorous homeostasis. *Lancet,* i, 155, 1974.

180. **Watney, P. J. M. and Rudd, B. T.,** Calcium Metabolism in Pregnancy and the Newborn *J. Obstet. Gynecol. Br. Common.,* 81, 210, 1974.

181. **DeBaare, L., Lewis, J., and Sing, H.,** Ultamicroscale determination of clinical chemical values for blood during the first four days of postnatal life. *Clin. Chem.,* 21, 746, 1975.

182. **Widdows, S. T.,** Calcium content of the blood during pregnancy. *Biochem. J.,* 17, 34, 1923.

183. **Newman, R. L.,** Blood calcium; normal curve for pregnancy. *Am. J. Obstet. Gynecol.,* 53, 817, 1947.

184. **Pitkin, R. M. and Gebhardt, M. P.,** Serum calcium concentration in normal pregnancy. *Am. J. Obstet. Gynecol.,* 127, 775, 1977.

185. **Tan, C. M., Ramen, A., and Sinnathyray, T. A.,** Serum ionic calcium during pregnancy. *J. Obstet. Gynecol. Br. Common.,* 79, 694, 1972.

186. **Pitkin, R. M., et al.,** Calcium metabolism in normal pregnancy: a longitudinal study. *Am. J. Obstet. Gynecol.,* 133, 781, 1979.

187. **Moniz, C. F., et al.,** Normal reference ranges for biochemical substances relating to renal hepatic and bone function in fetal and maternal plasma throughout pregnancy. *J. Clin. Pathol.,* 38, 468, 1985.

188. **Pitkin, R. M.,** Calcium metabolism in pregnancy. *Am. J. Obstet. Gynecol.,* 121, 724, 1975.

189. **Forfar, J. O.,** Normal and abnormal calcium phosphorous and magnesium metabolism in the perinatal period. *Clin. Endocrinol. Meta.,* 5, 123, 1976.

190. **Okonofua, F., et al.,** Calcium, vitamin D and parathyroid hormone relationships in pregnant Caucasian and Asian women and their neonates. *Ann. Clin. Biochem.,* 24, 22, 1987.

191. **Goldberg, D. M., Handyside, A. J., and Winfield, D. A.,** Influence of demographic factors on serum concentrations of seven chemical constituents in healthy human subjects. *Clin. Chem.,* 19, 395, 1973.

192. **Munan, L., et al.,** Associations with body weight of selected chemical constituents in blood: epidemiologic data. *Clin. Chem.,* 24, 772, 1978.

193. **Bulger, H. A., et al.,** The functional pathology of hyperparathyroidism. *J. Clin. Invest.,* 9, 143, 1930.

194. **Albright, F., et al.,** Studies in parathyroid physiology. III. The effect of phosphate ingestion in clinical hyperparathyroidism. *J. Clin. Invest.,* 11, 411, 1932.

195. **Dent, C. E.,** Some problems of hyperparathyroidism. *Br. Med. J.,* 2, 1495, 1962.

196. **Goldsmith, R. S. and Ingbar, S. H.,** Inorganic phosphate treatment of hypercalcemia of diverse etiologies. *N. Engl. J. Med.,* 274, 1, 1966.

197. **Kenny, F. M. and Holliday, M. A.,** Hypoparathyroidism, moniliasis Addisons and Hashimoto's disease: hypercalcemia treated with intravenously administered sodium sulfate. *N. Engl. J. Med.,* 271, 708, 1964.

198. **Chakmakjiam, Z. H. and Bethune, J. E.,** Sodium sulphate treatment of hypercalcemia. *N. Engl. J. Med.,* 275, 862, 1966.

199. **Holland, J. F., Danielson, E., and Sahagian-Edwards, A.,** Use of ethylene diamine tetra acetic acid in hypercalcemic patients *Proc. Soc. Exp. Biol. Med.,* 84, 359, 1953.

200. **Dudley, H. R., et al.,** Pathologic changes associated with the use of sodium ethylene diamine tetraacetate in the treatment of hypercalcemia. *N. Engl. J. Med.,* 252, 331, 1955.

201. **Galante, L., et al.,** The calcium lowering effect of synthetic human porcine and salmon calcitonin in patients with Paget's disease. *Clin. Sci.,* 44, 3P, 1973.

202. **Cochran, M., et al.,** Renal effects of calcitonin. *Br. Med. J.,* 1, 135, 1970.

203. **Binstock, M. L. and Munday, G. R.,** Effect of calcitonin and corticosteroids in combination on the hypercalcemia of malignancy. *Ann. Int. Med.,* 93, 269, 1980.

204. **Anon.,** Management of severe hypercalcemia. *Br. Med. J.,* 280, 304, 1980.

205. **Dent, C. E.,** Cortisone test for hyperparathyroidism. *Br. Med. J.,* 1, 230, 1956.

206. **Jung, A.,** Comparison of two parental diphosphonates in hypercalcemia of malignancy. *Am. J. Med.,* 72, 221, 1982.

207. **Ralston, S. H., et al.,** Comparison of three intravenous biphosphonates in cancer associated hypercalcemia. *Lancet,* ii, 1180, 1989.

208. **Khairi, M. R. A., et al.,** Treatment of Paget disease of bone (osteitis deformans). Results of a one-year study with sodium etidronate. *JAMA,* 230, 562, 1974.

209. **Canfield, R., et al.,** Diphosphonate therapy of Paget's disease of bone. *J. Clin. Endocrinol. Meta.,* 44, 96, 1977.

210. **Hosking, D. J., et al.,** Paget's bone disease treated with diphosphonate and calcitonin. *Lancet,* i, 615, 1976.

211. **Douglas, D. L., et al.,** The effect of dichloromethylene diphosphonate in Paget's disease of bone and in hypercalcemia due to primary hyperparathyroidism or malignant disease. *Lancet,* i, 1043, 1980.

212. **Warrell, R. P., Jr., et al.,** Gallium nitrate for acute treatment of cancer-related hypercalcemia. A randomised double-blind comparison with calcitonin. *Ann. Int. Med.,* 108, 669, 1988.

213. **Richens, A. and Roe, D. J. F.,** Disturbance of calcium metabolism by anticonvulsant drugs. *Br. Med. J.,* 4, 73, 1970.

214. **Hahn, T. J., et al.,** Effect of chronic anticonvulsant therapy on serum 25-hydroxy calciferol in adults. *N. Engl. J. Med.,* 287, 900, 1972.

215. **O'Hare, J. A., et al.,** Biochemical evidence for osteomalacia with carbamazepine therapy. *Acta Neurol. Scand.,* 62, 282, 1980.

216. **Dent, C. E., et al.,** Osteomalacia with long-term anticonvulsant therapy in epilepsy. *Br. Med. J.,* 4, 69, 1970.

217. **Oettgen, H. F., et al.,** Toxicity of E. coli L-asparaginase in man. *Cancer,* 25, 253, 1970.

218. **Young, R. E., Ramsey, L. E., and Murray, T. S.,** Barbiturate and serum calcium in the elderly. *Postgrad. Med. J.,* 53, 212, 1977.

219. **Sherwood, J. K., Ackroyd, F. W., and Garcia, M.,** Effect of cimetidine on circulating parathyroid hormone in primary hyperparathyroidism. *Lancet,* i, 616, 1980.

220. **Heath, H.,** III, Cimetidine in hyperparathyroidism. *Lancet,* i, 980, 1980.

221. **Palmer, F. J., Sawyer, T. M., and Wierzbin, S. J.,** Cimetidine and hyperparathyroidism. *N. Engl. J. Med.,* 302, 692, 1980.

222. **Fisken, R. A., Wilkinson, R., and Heath, D. A.,** The effects of cimetidine on serum calcium and parathyroid hormone levels in primary hyperparathyroidism. *Br. J. Clin. Pharmacol.,* 14, 701, 1982.

223. **Schilsky, R. L. and Anderson, T.,** Hypomagnesaemia and renal magnesium wasting in patients receiving cisplatin. *Ann. Int. Med.,* 90, 929, 1979.

224. **Tishler, M., Creter, D., and Djaldetti, M.,** Decreased calcium content in patients with digoxin intoxication. *Biomedicine,* 31, 12, 1979.

225. **Egilmez, A. and Dobkin, A. B.,** Enfluane (Ethrane, compound 347) in man, *Anaesthesia,* 27, 171, 1972.
226. **Vale, J. A., Widdop, B., and Bluett, N. H.,** Ethylene glycol poisoning. *Postgrad. Med. J.,* 52, 598, 1976.
227. **Abukurah, A. B., et al.,** Acute sodium fluoride poisoning. *JAMA,* 222, 816, 1972.
228. **Larsen, M. J., et al.,** Effect of a single dose of fluoride on calcium metabolism. *Calcif. Tissue Res.,* 26, 199, 1978.
229. **McQuire, A., Cohen, S., and Brooks, F. P.,** Serum gastrin and calcium levels in man during infusion of synthetic human gastrin. *Clin. Res.,* 20, 734, 1972.
230. **Holmes, A. M., Hesling, C. M., and Wilson, T. M.,** Drug-induced secondary hyperaldosteronism in patients with pulmonary tuberculosis. *Q. J. Med.,* 39, 299, 1970.
231. **Holmes, A. M., Hesling, C. M., and Wilson, T. M.,** Capreomicin-induced serum electrolyte abnormalities. *Thorax,* 25, 608, 1970.
232. **Birge, S. J. and Avioli, L. V.,** Glucagon-induced hypocalcemia in man. *J. Clin. Endocrinol. Meta.,* 29, 213, 1969.
233. **Londono, J. H. and Rosenbloom, A. L.,** Serum calcium and magnesium levels after glucagon in children with diabetes. *Diabetes,* 20, 365, 1971.
234. **Londono, J. H., McGee, J. H., Sobel, R. E., Rosenbloom, A. C., and Savory, J.,** Variation in serum calcium and phosphorus concentration during glucose tolerance tests. Clin. Chem., 17, 648, 1971.
235. **Textor, S. C., et al.,** Renal, volume and hormonal changes during therapeutic administration of recombinant interleukin-2 in man. *Am. J. Med.,* 1978, 83, 1055.
236. **Strong, J. A.,** Serum potassium deficiency during treatment with sodium PAS and liquorice extract. *Br. Med. J.,* 2, 998, 1951.
237. **Roussak, N. J.,** Fatal hypokalaemic alkalosis with tetany during liquorice and PAS therapy. *Br. Med. J.,* 1, 360, 1952.
238. **Muir, A., Laithwaite, J. A., and Wood, W.,** Hypokalaemia complicating carbenoxolone (Duogastrone) therapy. *Br. Med. J.,* 2, 512, 1969.
239. **Mitchell, A. B. S.,** Duogastrone-induced hypokalaemia nephropathy and myopathy with myoglobinuria. *Postgrad. Med. J.,* 47, 807, 1971.
240. **Gross, E. G., Dexter, J. D., and Roth, R. C.,** Hypokalaemic myopathy with myoglobinuria associated with liquorice ingestion. *N. Engl. J. Med.,* 274, 602, 1966.
241. **Holmes, A. N., et al.,** Pseudohyperaldosteronism induced by habitual ingestion of liquorice. *Postgrad. Med. J.,* 46, 625, 1970.
242. **Shneerson, J. M. and Gazzard, B. G.,** Reversible malabsorption caused by methyl dopa. *Br. Med. J.,* 4, 1456, 1977.
243. **Brown, J. H. and Kennedy, B. J.,** Mithramycin in the treatment of disseminated testicular neoplasm. *N. Engl. J. Med.,* 272, 111, 1965.
244. **Parsons, V., Baum, M., and Self, M.,** Effect of mithramycin on calcium and hydroxyproline metabolism in patients with malignant disease. *Br. Med. J.,* 1, 474, 1967.
245. **Perlia, C. P., et al.,** Mithramycin in the treatment of hypercalcemia. *Cancer,* 25, 389, 1970.
246. **Young, M. M., et al.,** Some effects of ethininyl oestradiol on calcium and phosphorous metabolism in osteoporosis. *Clin. Sci.,* 34, 411, 1968.
247. **Stevenson, J. C., et al.,** Calcitonin and the calcium-regulating hormones in postmenopausal women. Effect of oestrogen. *Lancet,* i, 693, 1981.
248. **Aitkin, J. M., McKay-Hart, D., and Smith, D. A.,** The effect of long term mestranol administration on calcium and phosphorous homeostasis in oophorectomised women. *Clin. Sci.,* 41, 233, 1971.
249. **Kennedy, B. J., et al.,** Hypercalcemia a complication of hormone therapy of advanced breast cancer. *Cancer Res.,* 13, 445, 1953.
250. **Kennedy, B. J., et al.,** Biochemical alterations during steroid hormone therapy of advanced breast cancer. *Am. J. Med.,* 19, 337, 1955.
251. **Swaroof, S. and Krant, M. J.,** Rapid estrogen-induced hypercalcemia. *JAMA,* 223, 913, 1973.
252. **Cornbleet, M., Bondy, P. K., and Powles, T. J.,** Fatal irreversible hypercalcemia in breast cancer. *Br. Med. J.,* 1, 145, 1977.
253. **Danowski, T. S., et al.,** Endocrine and metabolic indices during administration of a lipophilic bis-phenol probucol. *Clin. Pharmacol.,* 12, 928, 1971.
254. **Sladen, G. E.,** Effects of chronic purgative abuse. *Proc. R. Soc. Med.,* 65, 288, 1972.
255. **Phillips, P. J., et al.,** Metabolic and cardiovascular side effects of the B_2-adrenocepter agonists salbutamol and romiterol. *Br. J. Clin. Pharmacol.,* 9, 483, 1980.
256. **Routh, J. I. and Paul, W. D.,** Assessment of interference by aspirin with some assays commonly done in the clinical laboratory. *Clin. Chem.,* 22, 837, 1976.
257. **Stanley, N. N., et al.,** Streptozotocin treatment of malignant islet cell tumour. *Br. Med. J.,* 3, 562, 1970.
258. **Laryea, E. A., Brodrick, R., and Hidvegi, R.,** Hypercalcemia and streptozocin. *Ann. Int. Med.,* 80, 276, 1974.
259. **Röjdmark, S., et al.,** Serum calcium after intravenous administration of thyrotropin-releasing hormone in man. *Horm. Metab. Res.,* 15, 290, 1983.

260. **Cam, J. M., et al.,** The effect of aluminium hydroxide orally on calcium phosphorous and aluminium metabolism in normal subjects. *Clin. Sci. Mol. Med.,* 51, 407, 1976.
261. **Pac, C. Y. C., Delea, C. S., and Bartter, F. C.,** Successful treatment of recurrent nephrolithiasis (calcium stones) with cellulose phosphate. *N. Engl. J. Med.,* 290, 175, 1974.
262. **Christensson, T. A. T.,** Lithium, hypercalcemia and hyperparathyroidism. *Lancet,* ii, 144, 1976.
263. **Mellerup, E. T., et al.,** Lithium effects on diurnal rhythm of calcium magnesium and phosphate metabolism in manic-melancholic disorder. *Acta Psychiatr. Scand.,* 53, 360, 1976.
264. **Christianson, C., Baastrup, P. C., and Transbøl, I.,** Lithium hypercalcemia hypermagnesaemia and hyperparathyroidism. *Lancet,* ii, 969, 1976.
265. **Odigwe, C. O., et al.,** A trial of the calcium antagonist nisolpine in hypertensive non-insulin-dependent diabetic patients. *Diabetic Med.,* 3, 463, 1986.
266. **Veterans Administration Cooperative Study Group on Antihypertensive Agents,** Comparison of propanolol and hydrochlorthiazide for the initial treatment of hypertension. Results of short-term titration with emphasis on racial differences in response. *JAMA,* 248, 1996, 1982.
267. **Brickman, A. S. and Isenberg, J. I.,** Secretin increase in serum calcium levels in man. *Clin. Res.,* 20, 236, 1972.
268. **Henningsen, B. and Amberger, M.,** Antiöestrogene Therapie des Metastaierenden Mammakarzinoms. Vier Jahre Erfahrung mit Tamoxifen. *Desch. Med. Wochenschr.,* 102, 713, 1977.
269. **Veldhuis, J. D.,** Tamoxifen and hypercalcemia. *Ann. Int. Med.,* 88, 574, 1978.
270. **Kiang, D. J. and Kennedy, B. J.,** Tamoxifen (antiestrogen) therapy in advanced breast cancer. *Ann. Int. Med.,* 87, 687, 1977.
271. **McPherson, M. L., et al.,** Theophylinne induced hypercalcemia. *Ann. Int. Med.,* 105, 52, 1986.
272. **Anderson, J. L. and Kincaid-Smith, P.,** Diuretics: II clinical considerations. *Drugs,* 1, 141, 1971.
273. **Seitz, H. and Jaworski, J. F.,** Effect of hydrochlorothiazide on serum and urinary calcium and urinary citrate. *Can. Med. Assoc. J.,* 90, 414, 1964.
274. **Lindy, S. and Tarssanen, L.,** Serum calcium and phosphorous in patients treated with thiazides and furosemide. *Acta Med. Scand.,* 194, 319, 1973.
275. **Harrop, J. S., Bailey, J. E., and Woodhead, J. S.,** Incidence of hypercalcemia and primary hyperparathyroidism in relation to the biochemical profile. *J. Clin. Pathol.,* 35, 395, 1982.
276. **Palmer, F. J.,** Incidence of chlorthalidone-induced hypercalcemia. *JAMA,* 239, 2449, 1978.
277. **Katz, C. and Tzagoumis, M.,** Chronic adult hypervitaminosis A with hypercalcemia. *Metabolism,* 21, 1171, 1972.
278. **Frame, B., et al.,** Hypercalcemia and skeletal effect in chronic hypervitaminosis A. *Ann. Int. Med.,* 80, 44, 1974.
279. **Dalderup, C. B. M.,** Vitamins, in *Side Effect of Drugs,* Meyler, L. and Herxheimer, A., Eds., Excerpta-Medica, Amsterdam, 1968, 377.
280. **Danowski, T. S., Winkler, A. W., and Peters, J. P.,** Tissue calcification and vitamin D therapy of arthritis. *Ann. Int. Med.,* 23, 22, 1945.
281. **Kanis, J. A. and Russell, R. G. G.,** Rate of reversal of hypercalcemia and hypocalciuria induced by vitamin D and its 1 a-hydroxylated derivatives. *Br. Med. J.,* 1, 78, 1977.
282. **Bell, R. D. and Doisey, E. A.,** Rapid colorimetric methods for the determination of phosphorus in urine and blood. *J. Biol. Chem.,* 44, 55, 1920.
283. **Henry, R. J.,** in *Clinical Chemistry. Principles and Technics,* 1st ed., Harper & Row, New York, 1964, 410.
284. **Fiske, C. H. and Subbarow, Y.,** The colorimetric determination of phosphorus. *J. Biol. Chem.,* 66, 375, 1925.
285. **Kuttner, T. and Cohen, H. R.,** Micro colorimetric studies. A molybdic acid stannous chloride reagent for the micro estimation of phosphate and calcium in pus plasma and spinal fluid. *J. Biol. Chem.,* 75, 517, 1927.
286. **Gomorri, G.,** A modification of the colorimetric phosphorus determination for use with the photoelectric colorimeter. *J. Biol. Chem.,* 27, 955, 1942.
287. **Power, M. H.,** Inorganic phosphate. *Stand. Methods Clin. Chem.,* 1, 84, 1953.
288. **Lawrence, R.,** Assay of serum inorganic phosphate without deproteinisation: automated and manual micro-methods. *Ann. Clin. Biochem.,* 11, 234, 1974.
289. **Weissman, N. and Pileggi, V. J.,** in *Clinical Chemistry. Principles and Technics,* Henry, R. J., Cannon, D. C., and Winkelman, J. W., Eds., 2nd ed., Harper & Row, New York, 1974, 723.
290. **Wiener, K.,** in *"Varleys" Practical Clinical Chemistry,* 6th ed., Gowenlock, A. H., Ed., William Heinemann Medical Books, London, 617.
291. **Mather, A. and Mackie, N. R.,** Effect of haemolysis on serum electrolyte values. *Clin. Chem.,* 6, 223, 1960.
292. **Bryden, W. G. and Roberts, L. B.,** The effect of haemolysis on the determination of plasma constituents. *Clin. Chim. Acta,* 41, 435, 1972.
293. **Pesce, M. A. and Bodourian, S. S.,** Bilirubin interference with ultraviolet determination of inorganic phosphate with the "centrifichem". *Clin. Chem.,* 19, 436, 1973.

294. **Cook, B. S. and Simmons, D. H.,** Mannitol interference in phosphate determination: method of correction. *J. Lab. Clin. Med.,* 60, 160, 1962.

295. **O'Kell, R. T., et al.,** Effect of drugs on results of laboratory tests. *Clin. Chem.,* 18, 1039, 1972.

296. **Donhowe, J. M., et al.,** Factitious hypophosphataemia related to mannitol therapy. *Clin. Chem.,* 27, 1755, 1981.

297. **Landesman, P. W., Lott, J. A., and Zager, R. A.,** Mannitol interferes with the DuPont ACA method for inorganic phosphorus. *Clin. Chem.,* 28, 1994, 1982.

298. **Eisenbrey, A. B., Mathew, R., and Kiechle, F. L.,** Mannitol interference in an automated serum phosphate assay. *Clin. Chem.,* 33, 2308, 1987.

299. **El-Dorry, H. F. A., Medina, H., and Bacila, M.,** Interference of phenothiazine compounds in the colorimetric determination of inorganic phosphate. *Anal. Biochem.,* 47, 329, 1972.

300. **Young, D. S. and Panek, E.,** in *Drug Interference and Drug Measurement in Clinical Chemistry. Proc. 3rd Int. Coll. on Prospective Biology 1975,* S. Karger, Basel, 1976, 10.

301. **Tokmakjian, S., Moses, G., and Haines, M.,** Excessive sample blanking in two analysers generate reports of apparent hypoglycaemia and hypophosphataemia in patients with macroglobulinaemia. *Clin. Chem.,* 36, 1261, 1990.

302. **Carothers, J. E., Kurtz, N. M., and Lemann, J., Jr.,** Error introduced by specimen handling before determination of inorganic phosphate concentration in plasma and serum. *Clin. Chem.,* 22, 1909, 1976.

303. **McGeown, M. G., Martin, E., and Neill, D. W.,** Phosphate contamination of commercial heparin. *J. Clin. Pathol.,* 8, 247, 1955.

304. **Vreman, H. J. and Jöbsis, F. F.,** Interference by mannitol and other compounds with phosphate determination. *Anal. Biochem.,* 17, 108, 1966.

305. **Caraway, W. T. and Kammeyer, C. W.,** Chemical interference by drugs and other substances with clinical laboratory test procedures. *Clin. Chim. Acta,* 41, 305, 1972.

306. **Howland, J. and Kramer, B.,** Calcium and phosphorus in relation to rickets. *Am. J. Dis. Child.,* 22, 105, 1921.

307. **Taussky, H. H. and Shorr, E.,** A microcolorimetric method for the determination of inorganic phosphorus. *J. Biol. Chem.,* 202, 675, 1953.

308. **Winsten, S.,** Collection and preservation of specimens. *Stand. Methods Clin. Chem.,* 5, 1, 1965.

309. **Desaty, D. and Green, R.,** Stability of constituents in human serum during storage. *Clin. Chem.,* 21, 953, 1975.

310. **Henry, R. J.,** *Clinical Chemistry. Principles and Technics,* 1st ed., Harper & Row, New York, 1964, 414.

311. **Lai, L., et al.,** Effect of heat treatment of plasma and serum on biochemical indices. *Lancet,* i, 1457, 1985.

312. **Ball, M. D.,** Effect of two disinfectant treatments on laboratory analyses. *J. R. Soc. Med.,* 80, 482, 1987.

313. **Harrop, G. A. and Benedict, E. H.,** The participation of inorganic substances in carbohydrate metabolism. *J. Biol. Chem.,* 59, 683, 1924.

314. **Hartman, F. W. and Bolliger, A.,** Curve of inorganic blood phosphate during the sugar tolerance test. *JAMA,* 85, 653, 1925.

315. **Baginski, E. S. and Marie, S. S.,** Phosphate, inorganic. *Sel. Methods Clin. Chem.,* 9, 316, 1982.

316. **Robertson, W. G.,** Plasma phosphate homeostasis, in *Calcium Phosphate and Magnesium Metabolism,* Nordin, B. E. C., Eds., Churchill Livingstone, Edinburgh, 1976, 217.

317. **Riley, W. J., et al.,** The effect of long-distance running on some biochemical variables. *Clin. Chim. Acta,* 65, 83, 1975.

318. **Pulkkinen, M. O. and Willman, K.,** Serum inorganic phosphate during oral contraceptive therapy and in maternal and foetal sera. *Ann. Chir. Gynaecol.,* 57, 172, 1968.

319. **Haldane, J. B. S., Wigglesworth, V. B., and Woodrow, C. E.,** The effect of reaction changes on human inorganic metabolism. *Proc. R. Soc.,* 96 (Series B), 1, 1924.

320. **Mostellar, M. E. and Tuttle, E. P.,** Effects of alkalosis on plasma concentration and urinary excretion of inorganic phosphate in man. *J. Clin. Invest.,* 43, 138, 1964.

321. **Hitz, J.,** in *Interpretations of Clinical Laboratory Tests,* Siest, G., et al., Eds., Biomedical Publishers, Foster City, CA 1985, 346.

322. **Stanbury, S. W.,** Some aspects of disordered renal tubular function. *Ann. Int. Med.,* 9, 231, 1958.

323. **Wesson, L. G.,** Electrolyte excretion in relation to diurnal cycles in renal function. Plasma electrolyte concentration and aldosterone secretion before and during salt and water balance. Changes in normotensive subjects. *Medicine,* 43, 547, 1964.

324. **Kemp, G. J., Blumsohn, A., and Morris, B. W.,** Circadian changes in plasma phosphate concentration, urinary phosphate excretion and cellular phosphate shifts. *Clin. Chem.,* 38, 400, 1992.

325. **Round, J. M.,** Plasma calcium, magnesium, phosphorus and alkaline phosphatase levels in normal British school children. *Br. Med. J.,* 3, 137, 1973.

326. **Cherian, A. G. and Hill, J. G.,** Percentile estimates of reference values for fourteen chemical constituents in sera of children and adolescents. *Am. J. Clin. Pathol.,* 69, 24, 1978.

327. **Haas, R. G.,** in *Pediatric Clinical Chemistry Reference (Normal) Values,* 3rd ed., Meites, S. Ed., AACC, Washington, D.C., 1989, 213.

328. **Ljundhall, S. and Hedstrand, H.,** Serum phosphate inversely related to blood pressure. *Br. Med. J.,* 1, 553, 1977.

329. **Hollwich, F. and Dieckhues, B.,** Endocrine systems and blindness. *Germ. Med.,* 1, 122, 1971.

330. **Bloom, W. L. and Flinchum, D.,** Osteomalacia and pseudofractures caused by the ingestion of aluminium hydroxide. *JAMA,* 174, 1327, 1960.

331. **Shields, H. M.,** Rapid fall of serum phosphate secondary to antacid therapy. *Gastroenterology,* 75, 1137, 1978.

332. **Lotz, M., Zisman, E., and Bartter, F. C.,** Evidence for a phosphorus-depletion syndrome in man. *N. Engl. J. Med.,* 278, 409, 1968.

333. **Spencer, H. and Lender, M.,** Adverse effects of aluminium-containing antacids on mineral metabolism. *Gastroenterology,* 76, 603, 1979.

334. **Goodman, L. S. and Gilman, G.,** in *The Pharmacological Basis of Therapeutics,* 2nd ed., MacMillan, New York, 1965, 481.

335. **Betro, M. G. and Pain, R. W.,** Hypophosphataemia and hyperphosphataemia in a hospital population. *Br. Med. J.,* 1, 273, 1972.

336. **Body, J., Jr., et al.,** Epinephrine is a hypophosphataemic hormone in man. *J. Clin. Invest.,* 71, 572, 1983.

337. **Hunter, J., et al.,** Altered calcium metabolism in epileptic children on anticonvulsants. *Br. Med. J.,* 4, 202, 1971.

338. **Adreasen, P. B., Lyngbye, J., and Trolle, E.,** Abnormalities in liver function tests during long-term diphenylhydantoin therapy in epileptic outpatients. *Acta Med. Scand.,* 194, 261, 1973.

339. **Siest, G., Batt, A. M., and Galteau, M. M.,** *Lab. Pharmacol.,* 233, 535, 1974, quoted by Hitz, J., in *Interpretations of Clinical Laboratory Tests,* Siest, G., et al., Eds., Biomedical Publishers, Foster City, CA, 1985.

340. **Scott, R., et al.,** Clinical and biochemical abnormalities in coppersmiths exposed to cadmium. *Lancet,* ii, 396, 1976.

341. **Wisnecki, L. A., et al.,** Salmon calcitonin in hypercalcaemia. *Clin. Pharmacol. Ther.,* 24, 219, 1978.

342. **Recker, R. R., et al.,** The hyperphosphataemic effect of sodium ethane-1-hydroxy-1,1-diphosphonate (EHDP): renal handling of phosphorus and the renal response to parathyroid hormone. *J. Lab. Clin. Med.,* 81, 258, 1973.

343. **Smith, L. H., Jr., Ettinger, R. H., and Seligson, D. A.,** A comparison of the metabolism of fructose and glucose in hepatic disease and diabetes mellitus. *J. Clin. Invest.,* 32, 273, 1953.

344. **Ingbar, S. H., et al.,** The effects of ACTH and cortisone on the renal tubular transport of uric acid phosphorus and electrolytes in patients with normal renal and adrenal function. *J. Lab. Clin. Med.,* 38, 533, 1951.

345. **Marcus, R., et al.,** Effects of short term administration of recombinant human growth hormone to elderly people. *J. Clin. Endocrinol. Meta.,* 70, 519, 1990.

346. **Wirth, W. A. and Thompson, R. L.,** The effect of various conditions and substances on the results of laboratory procedures. *Am. J. Clin. Pathol.,* 43, 579, 1965.

347. **Christian, D. G.,** Drug interference with laboratory blood chemistry determinations. *Am. J. Clin. Pathol.,* 54, 118, 1970.

348. **Okada, M., et al.,** Hypophosphataemia induced by intravenous administration of saccharated iron oxide. *Klin. Wochenschr.,* 61, 99, 1983.

349. **Brodie, M. J., et al.,** Effect of isoniazid on vitamin D metabolism and monooxygenase activity. *Clin. Pharmacol. Ther.,* 30, 363, 1981.

350. **Edwards, C. R. W. and Besser, G. M.,** Mithramycin treatment of malignant hypercalcaemia. *Br. Med. J.,* 3, 167, 1968.

351. **Slayton, R. E., et al.,** New approach to the treatment of hypercalcaemia. The effect of short term treatment with mithramycin. *Clin. Pharmacol. Ther.,* 12, 833, 1971.

352. **Refenstein, E. C. and Albright, F.,** The metabolic effect of steroid hormone in osteoporosis. *J. Clin. Invest.,* 26, 24, 1947.

353. **Parfitt, A. M.,** Changes in serum calcium and phosphorus during stilboestrol treatment of osteoporosis. *J. Bone Joint Surg.,* 47B, 137, 1965.

354. **Simpson, G. R. and Dale, E.,** Serum levels of phosphorus magnesium and calcium in women utilising combination oral or long acting injectable progestational contraceptives. *Fertil. Steril.,* 23, 326, 1972.

355. **Jones, A. F., Harvey, J. M., and Vale, J. A.,** Hypophosphataemia and phosphaturia in paracetamol poisoning. *Lancet,* ii, 608, 1989.

356. **Smith, D. A. and Nordin, B. E. C.,** The effect of a high phosphorus intake on total and ultra filtratable plasma calcium and on phosphate clearance. *Clin. Sci.,* 26, 479, 1964.

357. **Carrera, A. E.,** Effect of oral administration of fleet phospho-soda on serum phosphorus concentration. *Am. J. Clin. Pathol.,* 49, 739, 1968.

358. **Travis, S. F., et al.,** Alteration of red-cell glycolytic intermediates and oxygen transport as a consequence of hypophosphataemia in patients receiving intravenous hyperalimentation. *New. Engl. J. Med.,* 285, 763, 1976.

359. **Murchison, L. E., How, J., and Bewsher, P. D.,** Comparison of propanolol and metaprolol in the management of hyperthyroidism. *Br. J. Clin. Pharmacol.,* 8, 581, 1979.
360. **Phillips, P. J., et al.,** Metabolic and cardiovascular side effects of the B$_2$-adrenocepter agonists salbutamol and rimiterol. *Br. J. Clin. Pharmacol.,* 9, 483, 1980.
361. **Zantvoort, F. A., et al.,** Theophylline and serum electrolytes. *Ann. Int. Med.,* 104, 134, 1986.
362. **Duarte, C. G. and Bland, J. H.,** Changes in metabolism of calcium, phosphorus and uric acid after oral administration of chlorthiazide. *Metabolism,* 14, 899, 1965.
363. **Condon, J. R. and Nassim, R.,** Hypophosphataemia and hypokalaemia. *Br. Med. J.,* 1, 110, 1970.
364. **Brickman, A. S., et al.,** Effect of hydrochlorthiazide on calcium metabolism. *J. Clin. Invest.,* 50, 13a, 1971.
365. **Mohamadi, M., Bivins, L., and Becker, K. L.,** Effect of thiazides on serum calcium. *Clin. Pharmacol. Ther.,* 26, 390, 1979.
366. **Henry, R. J.,** in *Clinical Chemistry. Principles and Technics,* 1st ed., Harper and Row, New York, 1964, 345 and 350.
367. **Schwartz, M. K., et al.,** Chemical and clinical evaluation of the continuous flow analyser "SMAC". *Clin. Chem.,* 20, 1062, 1974.
368. **Lustgarten, J. A., et al.,** Evaluation of an automated selective-ion electrolyte analyser for measuring Na$^+$ K$^+$ and Cl$^+$ in serum. *Clin. Chem.,* 20, 1217, 1974.
369. **Annan, W., Kirwan, N. A., and Robertson, W. S.,** Normal range for serum sodium by ion-selective electrode analysis exceeds that by flame photometry. *Clin. Chem.,* 25, 643, 1979.
370. **Ladenson, J. H., et al.,** Sodium measurements in multiple myeloma: two techniques compared. *Clin. Chem.,* 29, 2383, 1982.
371. **Levy, G. B.,** Determination of sodium with ion-selective electrodes. *Clin. Chem.,* 20, 1435, 1981.
372. **Maas, A. H. J., et al.,** Ion selective electrodes for sodium and potassium: a new problem of what is measured and what should be reported. *Clin. Chem.,* 31, 482, 1985.
373. **Broughton, P. M. G., Smith, S. C. H., and Buckley, B. M.,** Calibration of direct ion-selective electrodes for plasma Na$^+$ to allow for the influence of protein concentration. *Clin. Chem.,* 31, 1765, 1985.
374. **Maas, A. H. J., et al.,** Ion-selective electrodes for sodium and potassium: a new problem of what should be measured. *IFCC News,* 31, 5, 1982.
375. **Russell, L. J., Smith, S. C. H., and Buckley, B. M.,** Plasma sodium and potassium measurement: minimising ISE-flame difference using specimens from patients. *Ann. Clin. Biochem.,* 25, 96, 1988.
376. **Broughton, P. M. G. and Maas, A. H. J.,** Recent developments with ion selective electrodes, *IFCC News,* 38, 4, 1984.
377. **Gunaratna, P. C., et al.,** Frozen human serum reference material for standardisation of sodium and potassium measurements in serum or plasma by ion-selective electrode analysers. *Clin. Chem.,* 38, 1459, 1992.
378. **Ng, R. H., Sparks, K. M., and Statland, B. E.,** Colorimetric determination of potassium in plasma and serum by reflectance photometry with a dry-chemistry reagent. *Clin. Chem.,* 38, 1371, 1992.
379. **Fiet, J., Barbe, M., and Dreux, C.,** Study of reference values of plasma electrolytes, in *Reference Values in Human Biochemistry,* Siest, G., Ed., S. Karger, Basel, 1973, 127.
380. **Weissman, N. and Pileggi, V. J.,** in *Clinical Chemistry. Principles and Technics,* 2nd ed., Henry, R. J., Cannon, D. C., and Winkleman, J. W., Eds., Harper and Row, New York, 1974, 643 and 646.
381. **Stevans, J. F. and Cresswell, M. A.,** *Assoc. Clin. Biochem. Newssheet,* 227, 5, 1982.
382. **Hawks, A. M.,** in *"Varleys" Practical Clinical Biochemistry,* 6th ed., Gowenlock, A. L., Ed., William Heinemann Medical Books, London, 1988, 561.
383. **Fraser, C. G.,** Desirable performance standards for clinical chemistry tests. *Adv. Clin. Chem.,* 23, 299, 1983.
384. **Mather, A. and Mackie, N. R.,** Effects of haemolysis on serum electrolyte values. *Clin. Chem.,* 6, 223, 1960.
385. **Mann, S. W. and Green, A.,** Interference from heparin in commercial heparinised tubes in the measurement of plasma sodium by ion selective electrode: a note of caution. *Ann. Clin. Biochem.,* 23, 354, 1986.
386. **Baer, D. M., et al.,** Protocol for the study of drug interferences in laboratory tests: cefotaxime interference in 24 chemical tests. *Clin. Chem.,* 29, 1736, 1983.
387. **Mullins, R. E., Sutton, P. S., and Conn, R. B.,** Effects of Flurosol-D A (artificial blood) on clinical chemistry tests and instruments. *Am. J. Clin. Pathol.,* 80, 478, 1983.
388. **Sonntag, O.,** quoted by Young, D. S. in *Effect of Drugs on Laboratory Tests,* 3rd ed., American Association of Clinical Chemists, Washington, D.C., 1990.
389. **Berliner, R. W., Kennedy, T. J., Jr., and Hilton, J. G.,** Renal mechanism for excretion of potassium. *Am. J. Physiol.,* 162, 348, 1950.
390. **Funder, J. and Wieth, J. O.,** Potassium, sodium, and water in normal human red cells. *Scand. J. Lab. Clin. Invest.,* 18, 167, 1966.
391. **Lum, G. and Gambino, S. R.,** Serum vs. plasma determination in routine chemistry. *Clin. Chem.,* 18, 710, 1972.
392. **Ladenson, J. H., et al.,** Serum versus heparinised plasma for eighteen common chemistry tests. *Am. J. Clin. Pathol.,* 62, 545, 1974.

393. **Kalsheker, N. and Jones, N.,** Inaccurate in vivo plasma potassium measurement due to in vitro changes in unseparated blood. *Clin. Chem.,* 30, 1582, 1984.

394. **Bailey, I. R.,** Effect on 16 analytes of overnight storage of specimens collected into heparinised evaporated tubes with plasma separator. *Ann. Clin. Biochem.,* 27, 56, 1990.

395. **McCormick, P. G., Burke, R. W., and Doumas, B. T.,** Precautions in use of soft-glass disposable pipets in clinical analysis. *Clin. Chem.,* 18, 854, 1972.

396. **Cook, J. D., Koch, T. R., and Knoblock, E. C.,** Erroneous electrolyte results caused by catheter. *Clin. Chem.,* 34, 211, 1988.

397. **Danowski, T. S.,** The transfer of potassium across the human blood cell membrane. *J. Biol. Chem.,* 139, 693, 1941.

398. **Webster, J. H., et al.,** Evaluation of serum potassium levels. *Am. J. Clin. Pathol.,* 22, 833, 1952.

399. **Goodman, J. R., Vincent, J., and Rosen, I.,** Serum potassium changes in blood clots. *Am. J. Clin. Pathol.,* 24, 111, 1954.

400. **Salzmann, M. B. and Male, I. A.,** Keep the lid on it: artifactual hypernatraemia in samples from paediatric patients. *Ann. Clin. Biochem.,* 30, 211, 1993.

401. **Ball, M. J. and Griffiths, D.,** Effect on chemical analysis of Beta-propriolactone treatment of whole blood and plasma. *Lancet,* i, 1160, 1985.

402. **McKechnie, J. K., Leary, W. P., and Joubert, S. M.,** Some electrocardiographic and biochemical changes recorded on marathon runners. *S. Afr. Med. J.,* 41, 722, 1967.

403. **Olivier, L. R., et al.,** Electrocardiographic and biochemical studies on marathon runners. *S. Afr. Med. J.,* 53, 783, 1978.

404. **Rose, L. I., et al.,** Serum electrolyte changes after marathon running. *J. Appl. Physiol.,* 29, 449, 1970.

405. **Statland, B. E., Winkel, P., and Bokeland, H.,** Factors contributing to intra-individual variation of serum constituents. 2. Effects of exercise and diet on variation of serum constituents in healthy subjects. *Clin. Chem.,* 19, 1380, 1973.

406. **Priest, J. B., Oei, T. O., and Moorehead, W. R.,** Exercise induced changes in common laboratory tests. *Am. J. Clin. Pathol.,* 77, 285, 1982.

407. **Faber, S. J., et al.,** Observations on the plasma potassium level in man. *Am. J. Med. Sci.,* 221, 678, 1951.

408. **Skinner, S. L.,** A cause of erroneous potassium levels. *Lancet,* i, 478, 1961.

409. **Pocock, S. J., et al.,** Diurnal variations in serum biochemical and haematological measurements. *J. Clin. Pathol.,* 42, 172, 1989.

410. **Hitz, J.,** in *Interpretation of Clinical Laboratory Tests,* Siest, G., et al., Eds., Biochemical Publishers, Foster City, CA 1985, 366.

411. **Mira, M., et al.,** Changes in sodium and uric acid concentration in plasma during the menstrual cycle. *Clin. Chem.,* 30, 380, 1984.

412. **Roberts, L. B.,** The normal range with statistical analysis for seventeen blood constituents. *Clin. Chim. Acta,* 16, 69, 1967.

413. **Mohun, A. F. and Cook, I. J. Y.,** A reassessment of normal plasma sodium levels. *Lancet,* i, 778, 1962.

414. **Owen, J. A. and Campbell, D. G. A.,** A comparison of plasma electrolyte and urea values in healthy persons and in hospital patients. *Clin. Chim. Acta,* 22, 611, 1968.

415. **Li, A. K., Wills, M. R., and Hanson, G. L.,** in *Fluid Electrolytes Acid-Base and Nutrition,* Academic Press, New York, 1980.

416. **Reidenberg, M. M., et al.,** Differences in serum potassium concentrations in normal men in different geographic locations. *Clin. Chem.,* 39, 72, 1993.

417. **King, E. J., Wooton, I. D. P., and MacLean-Smith, J.,** The quantitative approach to hospital biochemistry. *Br. Med. Bull.,* 7, 307, 1950.

418. **Clayton, B. E., Jenkins, P., and Round, J. M.,** in *Paediatric Chemical Pathology,* Blackwell Scientific, Oxford, 1980, 129 and 139.

419. **Handa, N.,** in *Paediatric Clinical Chemistry Reference (Normal) Values,* 3rd ed., Meites, S. Ed., American Association of Clinical Chemists, Washington, D.C., 1989, pages 222 and 238.

420. **Belton, N. R., et al.,** Clinical and biochemical assessment of a modified evaporated milk for infant feeding. *Arch. Dis. Child.,* 52, 167, 1977.

421. **Berger, H. M., et al.,** Milk pH, acid-base status, and growth in babies. *Arch. Dis. Child.,* 53, 926, 1978.

422. **Roy, R. N., et al.,** Late hypernatraemia in very low birth weight infants (<1.3 kilograms). *Paediatr. Res.,* 10, 526, 1976.

423. **Meites, S.,** in *Paediatric Clinical Chemistry. A Survey of Normal, Method and Instrumentation with Commentary,* Meites, S. Ed., AACC, Washington, D.C., 1977, 93.

424. **Lind, T., Billewitz, W. Z., and Cheyne, G. A.,** Composition of amniotic fluid and maternal blood through pregnancy. *J. Obstet. Gynaecol. Br. Common.,* 78, 505, 1971.

425. **MacDonald, H. N. and Good, W.,** Changes in plasma sodium, potassium and chloride concentration in pregnancy and the puerperum with plasma and serum osmolarity. *J. Obstet. Gynaecol. Br. Common.,* 78, 798, 1971.

426. **Hussain, M. K., et al.,** Nicotine-stimulated release of neurophysin and vasopressin in humans. *J. Clin. Endocrinol. Meta.,* 41, 1113, 1975.

427. **Blum, A.,** The possible role of tobacco cigarette smoking in hyponatraemia of long-term psychiatric patients. *JAMA,* 252, 2864, 198.

428. **Leppänen, E. A. and Gräsbeck, R.,** Experimental basis of standardised specimen collection: the effect of moderate ethanol consumption on some serum components (K Na ASAT ALAT CK LDH total protein). *Scand. J. Clin. Lab. Invest.,* 47, 337, 1987.

429. **Robertson, J. D. and Fraser, S. C.,** Biochemical disturbances associated with anaesthesia. *Br. Med. Bull.,* 14, 8, 1958.

430. **Grey, T. C., Nunn, J. F., and Utting, J. E.,** in *General Anaesthesia,* Vol. 1, 4th ed., Butterworths, London, 1980, 472.

431. **Naperstek, Y. and Gutman, A.,** Case report: spurious hypokalaemia in myeloproliferative disorders. *Am. J. Med. Sci.,* 288, 175, 1984.

432. **Anon.,** Intravenous feeding with amino acids and fats. *Drug Ther. Bull.,* 10, 49, 1972.

433. **Alberti, K. G. M. M., et al.,** Effect of arginine on electrolyte metabolism in man. *Clin. Res.,* 15, 467, 1967.

434. **Bennett, J. E.,** Chemotherapy of systemic mycoses (first of two parts). *N. Engl. J. Med.,* 290, 30, 1974.

435. **Atlas, S. A., et al.,** Interruption of the renin-angiotensin system in hypertensive patients by captopril induces sustained reduction in aldosterone secretion, potassium retention and natriuresis. *Hypertension,* 1, 274, 1979.

436. **Ikram, H., et al.,** Haemodynamics and hormonal effects of captopril in primary pulmonary hypertension. *Br. Heart J.,* 48, 541, 1982.

437. **Veterans Administration Co-Operative Study Group on Anti-hypertensive Agents,** Low-dose captopril for the treatment of mild to moderate hypertension. *Arch., Int. Med.,* 144, 1947, 1984.

438. **Ponce, S. B., et al.,** Drug-induced hyperkalaemia. *Medicine,* 64, 357, 1985.

439. **Tattersall, M. H. N., Spiers, A. S. D., and Darrell, J. H.,** Initial therapy with combinations of five antibiotics in febrile patients with leukaemia and neutropenia. *Lancet,* i, 62, 1972.

440. **Stapleton, F. B., et al.,** Hypokalaemia associated with antibiotic treatment. *Am. J. Dis. Child.,* 130, 1104, 1976.

441. **Sunderman, F. W., Jr.,** Drug interference in clinical biochemistry. *Crit. Rev. Clin. Lab. Sci.,* 1, 427, 1970.

442. **Brunner, F. P. and Frick, P. G.,** Hyperkalaemia, metabolic alkalosis, and hypernatraemia due to "massive" sodium penicillin therapy. *Br. Med. J.,* 4, 550, 1968.

443. **Rodriquez, V., Green, S., and Bodey, G. P.,** Serum electrolyte abnormalities associated with the administration of polymyxin B in febrile leukaemic patients. *Clin. Pharmacol. Ther.,* 11, 106, 1970.

444. **Martin, E. W.,** in *Hazards of Medication,* Lippincott, Philadelphia, 1971, 183.

445. **Bühler, F. R., et al.,** Propanolol inhibition of renin secretion. *N. Engl. J. Med.,* 287, 1209, 1972.

446. **Drayer, J. I. M., et al.,** Intrapatient comparison of treatment with chlorthalidone spironolactone and propanolol in normoreninaemic essential hypertension. *Am. J. Cardiol.,* 36, 716, 1975.

447. **Berglund, G., et al.,** Antihypertensive Effect and Side-effects of Bendroflumethiazide and Propanolol *Acta Med. Scand.,* 199, 499, 1976.

448. **Nordrehaug, J. E., et al.,** Effect of timolol on changes in serum potassium concentration during acute myocardial infarction. *Br. Heart J.,* 53, 388, 1985.

449. **Swenson, E. W.,** Severe hyperkalaemia as a complication of timolol, a topically applied B-adrenergic antagonist. *Arch. Int. Med.,* 146, 1220, 1986.

450. **Haalboom, J. R. E., Deenstra, M., and Struyvenburg, A.,** Hypokalaemia induced by inhalation of fenoterol. *Lancet,* i, 1125, 1985.

451. **Phillips, P. J., et al.,** Metabolic and cardiovascular side effects of the B_2 adrenorecepter agonists salbutamol and rimiterol. *Br. J. Clin. Pharmacol.,* 9, 483, 1980.

452. **Güngoḡdu, A. S., et al.,** Comparison of hormonal and metabolic effects of salbutamol infusion in normal subjects and insulin-requiring diabetics. *Lancet,* ii, 1317, 1979.

453. **O'Brian, I. A. D. O., et al.,** Hyperkalaemia due to salbutamol overdosage. *Br. Med. J.,* 282, 2055, 1981.

454. **Ind, P. W.,** New drugs. Salmeterol. *Br. J. Hosp. Med.,* 44, 343, 1990.

455. **Bengtssen, B.,** Plasma concentration and side-effects of terbutaline. *Eur. J. Resp. Dis.,* 65 (Suppl. 134), 231, 1984.

456. **Radó, J. P.,** Water intoxication during carbamazepine treatment. *Br. Med. J.,* 3, 479, 1973.

457. **Henry, D. A., et al.,** Hyponatraemia during carbamazepine treatment. *Br. Med. J.,* 1, 83, 1977.

458. **Perucca, E., et al.,** Water intoxication in epileptic patients receiving carbamazepine. *J. Neurol. Neurosurg. Psychiatr.,* 41, 713, 1978.

459. **Helin, I., et al.,** Serum sodium and osmolarity during carbamazepine treatment in children, *Br. Med. J.,* 2, 558, 1977.

460. **Weissman, P. N., Shenkman, L., and Gregerman, R. I.,** Chlorpromamide hyponatraemia. Drug-induced antidiuretic-hormone activity. *New. Engl. J. Med.,* 284, 65, 1971.

461. **Nisbet, P.,** Chlorpromamide-induced hyponatraemia. *Br. Med. J.,* 1, 904, 1977.

462. **Epstein, S., et al.,** Chlorpromamide hyponatraemia. *N. Engl. J. Med.,* 286, 785, 1972.

463. **Zalin, A. M., et al.,** Hyponatraemia during treatment with chlorpromamide and moduretic (amiloride plus hydrochlorthiazide). *Br. Med. J.,* 289, 659, 1984.

464. **Primack, W. A., et al.,** Hypernatreamia associated with cholestyramine therapy. *J. Paediatr.,* 90, 1024, 1977.

465. **Hill, J. B., Blachley, J. D., and Tootte, N.,** Hypomagnesaemia, hypocalcaemia and hypokalaeamia with cisplatin therapy. *Clin. Res.,* 26, 780A, 1978.

466. **Bethone, J. E.,** in *The Adrenal Cortex,* Upjohn, Kalamazoo, MI, 1974.

467. **Anon.,** *AMA Council on Drugs. New Drugs, 1967* ed., American Medical Association, Chicago.

468. **Goodman, L. S. and Gilman, A.,** *The Pharmacological Basis of Therapeutics,* 4th ed., MacMillan, New York, 1970, 665 and 1541.

469. **Davies, D. M.,** in *Textbook of Adverse Drug Reactions,* Davies, D. S., Ed., Oxford University Press, New York, 1981.

470. **DeFronzo, R. A., et al.,** Water intoxication in man after cyclophosphamide therapy. Time course and relation to drug activation. *Ann. Int. Med.,* 78, 861, 1973.

471. **Arseneau, J. C., et al.,** Hyperkalaemia a sequel to chemotherapy of Burkitts lymphoma. *Lancet,* i, 10, 1973.

472. **Adu, D., et al.,** Hyperkalaemia in cyclosporin treated renal allograft patients. *Lancet,* ii, 370, 1983.

473. **Foley, R. J., Hamner, R. W., and Weinman, E. J.,** Serum potassium concentration in cyclosporine and azothiaprine treated renal transplant patients. *Nephron,* 40, 280, 1985.

474. **Gordon, R. D., et al.,** Use of home-blood-pressure measurements to compare the efficacy of two diuretics. Effect of methylclothiazide and frusemide on blood pressure and plasma renin activity and electrolytes. *Med. J. Aust.,* i, 565, 1971.

475. **Morgan, D. B. and Davidson, C.,** Hypokalaemia and diuretics: an analysis of publications. *Br. Med. J.,* 280, 905, 1980.

476. **Knockel, J. P.,** Hypokalaemia. *Adv. Int. Med.,* 30, 317, 1985.

477. **Fishman, M. P., et al.,** Diuretic-induced hyponatraemia. *Ann. Int. Med.,* 75, 853, 1971.

478. **Spino, M., et al.,** Adverse biochemical and clinical consequences of furosemide administration. *Can. Med. Assoc. J.,* 118, 1513, 1978.

479. **Olesen, K. H., et al.,** Bumetanide, a new potent diuretic. *Acta Med. Scand.,* 193, 119, 1973.

480. **Kuzuya, F., et al.,** Clinical investigations on the pharmacology of azosemide (SK-110) in comparison with furosemide in healthy volunteers. *Int. J. Clin. Pharmacol. Ther. Toxicol.,* 22, 291, 1984.

481. **Millar, J. A., et al.,** Metabolic effects of high dose amiloride and spironolactone: a comparative study in normal subjects. *Br. J. Clin. Pharmacol.,* 18, 369, 1984.

482. **Chrysant, S. G. and Luu, T. M.,** Effects of amiloride on arterial pressure and renal function. *J. Clin. Pharmacol.,* 20, 322, 1980.

483. **Tarssanen, L., Huiko, K., and Rossi, M.,** Amiloride-induced hyponatraemia. *Acta Med. Scand.,* 208, 491, 1980.

484. **Forland, M. and Pullman, T. N.,** Electrolyte complications of drug therapy. *Med. Clin. N. Am.,* 47, 113, 1963.

485. **Greenblatt, D. J.,** Adverse reaction to spironolactone. A report from the Boston collaborative drug surveillance program. *JAMA,* 225, 40, 1973.

486. **Miller, K. P., Lazar, E. J., and Fotino, S.,** Severe hyperkalaemia during piroxican therapy. *Arch. Int. Med.,* 144, 2414, 1984.

487. **Wise, P. H., et al.,** Clopamide and carbohydrate metabolism. *Med. J. Aust.,* 2, 795, 1969.

488. **Jenson, O. B., Mosdal, C., and Reske-Nielson, E.,** Hypokalaemic myopathy during treatment with diuretics. *Acta Neurol. Scand.,* 55, 465, 1977.

489. **Osei, K., Holland, G., and Falks, J. M.,** Indapamide. Effects on apoprotein lipoprotein and glucose regulation in ambulatory diabetic patients. *Arch. Int. Med.,* 146, 1973, 1986.

490. **Pilewski, R. M., et al.,** Technique of drug assay in hypertension. V. Comparison of hydrochlorthiazide with a new quinethiazine diuretic metolazone. *Clin. Pharmacol. Ther.,* 12, 843, 1974.

491. **Bayer, A. J., et al.,** Plasma electrolytes in elderly patients taking fixed combination diuretics. *Postgrad. Med. J.,* 62, 159, 1986.

492. **Carlström, K., Döberl, A., and Rannevik, G.,** Peripheral androgen levels in danazol treated premenopausal women. *Fertil. Steril.,* 39, 499, 1983.

493. **Tomecki, K. J. and Catalano, C. J.,** Dapsone hypersensivity. The sulphone syndrome revisited. *Arch. Dermatol.,* 117, 38, 1981.

494. **Cowan, R. E. and Wright, J. T.,** Dapsone and severe hypoalbuminaemia in dermatitis herpetiformis. *Br. J. Dermatol.,* 104, 201, 1981.

495. **Bartorelli, C., et al.,** Hypotensive and renal effects of diazoxide, a sodium-retaining benzothiadiazine compound. *Circulation,* 27, 895, 1963.

496. **Johnson, B. F.,** Diazoxide and renal function in man. *Clin. Pharmacol. Ther.,* 12, 815, 1971.

497. **Smith, T. W., et al.,** Treatment of life threatening digitalis intoxication with digoxin-specific Fab antibody fragments. *N. Engl. J. Med.,* 307, 1357, 1982.
498. **Bailey, R. E. and Ford, H. C.,** The effect of heparin on sodium conservation and on the plasma concentration, the metabolic clearance and the secretion and excretion rates of aldosterone on normal subjects. *Acta Endocrinol.,* 60, 249, 1969.
499. **Wilson, I. D. and Goetz, F. C.,** Selective hypoaldosteronism after prolonged heparin administration. A case report with postmortem findings. *Am. J. Med.,* 36, 635, 1964.
500. **Phelps, K. R., Oh, M. S., and Carroll, H. J.,** Heparin-induced hyperkalaemia: report of a case. *Nephron,* 25, 254, 1980.
501. **Brohee, D. and Neve, P.,** Heparin side effects. *Arch. Int. Med.,* 144, 1693, 1984.
502. **Pearce, C. J. and Cox, J. G. C.,** Heroin and hyperkalaemia. *Lancet,* ii, 923, 19??.
503. **Trewby, P. N., Kalfayan, P. Y., and Elkeles, R. S.,** Heroin and hyperkalaemia. *Lancet,* i, 327, 1981.
504. **Silva, J. K.,** The action of adrenaline on serum potassium. *J. Physiol. (Lond.),* 82, 393, 1934.
505. **Moreno, M., Murphy, C., and Goldsmith, C.,** Increase in serum potassium resulting from administration of hypertonic mannitol and other solutions. *J. Lab. Clin. Med.,* 73, 291, 1969.
506. **Tractenburg, J. and Pont, A.,** Ketoconazole-therapy for advanced prostate cancer. *Lancet,* ii, 433, 1984.
507. **White, M. C. and Kendall-Taylor, P.,** Adrenal hypofunction in patients taking ketoconazole. *Lancet,* i, 44, 1985.
508. **Pillans, P. J., Cowan, P., and Whitelaw, D.,** Hyponatraemia and confusion in a patient taking ketoconazole. *Lancet,* i, 821, 1985.
509. **Murphy, D. L., Goodwin, F. K., and Bunney, W. E., Jr.,** Aldosterone and sodium response to lithium administration in man. *Lancet,* ii, 458, 1969.
510. **Coggins, F. C.,** Acute hyperkalaemia during lithium treatment of manic illness. *Am. J. Psychiatry,* 137, 860, 1980.
511. **Nelson, D. C., McGrew, W. R. G., and Hoyumpa, A. M.,** Hypernatraemia and lactulose therapy. *JAMA,* 249, 1295, 1983.
512. **Somani, P., et al.,** Hyponatraemia on patients treated with lorcainamide, a new antiarrhythmic drug. *Am. Heart J.,* 108, 1443, 1984.
513. **Buckell, M.,** Blood changes on intravenous administration of mannitol or urea for reduction of intracranial pressure in neurosurgical patients. *Clin. Sci.,* 27, 223, 1964.
514. **Crandell, W. B., Pappas, S. G., and MacDonald, A.,** Nephrotoxicity associated methoxyflurane anaesthesia. *Anaesthesia,* 27, 591, 1966.
515. **Stevens, D. A.,** Miconazole in the treatment of coccidioidomycoses. *Drugs,* 26, 347, 1983.
516. **Clive, D. M. and Stoff, J. S.,** Renal syndromes associated with nonsteroidal anti-inflammatory drugs. *N. Engl. J. Med.,* 310, 563, 1984.
517. **Kimberly, R. P., et al.,** Reduction of renal function by newer nonsteroidal anti-inflammatory drugs. *Am. J. Med.,* 64, 804, 1978.
518. **Kutyrina, I. M., Androsova, S. O., and Tareyeva, I. E.,** Indomethacin-induced hyporeninaemic hypoaldosteronism. *Lancet,* i, 785, 1979.
519. **Zimran, A., et al.,** Incidence of hypokalaemia induced by indomethacin in a hospital population. *Br. Med. J.,* 291, 107, 1985.
520. **De Jong, P. E.,** Incidence of hyperkalaemia induced by indomethacin. *Br. Med. J.,* 291, 1047, 1985.
521. **Frais, M. A., Burgess, E. D., and Mitchell, L. B.,** Piroxican-induced renal failure and hyperkalaemia. *Ann. Int. Med.,* 99, 129, 1983.
522. **Mitnick, P. D. and Klein, W. J., Jr.,** Piroxican-induced renal disease. *Arch. Int. Med.,* 144, 63, 1984.
523. **Singhi, S., et al.,** Iatrogenic neonatal and maternal hyponatraemia following oxytocin and aqueous glucose infusion during labour. *Br. J. Obstet. Gynaecol.,* 92, 356, 1985.
524. **Aron, N. B.,** Phenoxybenzamine-induced hyponatraemia simulating the syndrome of inappropriate antidiuretic hormone secretion. *Ann. Int. Med.,* 107, 119, 1987.
525. **Schwartz, W. B.,** Potassium and the kidney. *N. Engl. J. Med.,* 253, 601, 1955.
526. **Keith, N. M., and Osterberg, A. E.,** Human intolerance for potassium. *Proc. Staff Meet. Mayo Clin.,* 21, 385, 1946.
527. **Shapiro, S., et al.,** Fatal drug reactions among medical inpatients. *JAMA,* 216, 467, 1977.
528. **Soulillou, J. P., et al.,** Acute hyperkalaemic risks in recipients of kidney graft cooled with collins solution. *Nephron,* 19, 301, 1977.
529. **Horrobin, D. F., et al.,** Action of prolactin on human renal function. *Lancet,* ii, 352, 1971.
529a. **Chakmakjian, Z. H. and Bethune, J. E.,** Sodium sulphate treatment of hypercalcaemia. *N. Engl. J. Med.,* 296, 1082, 1967.
530. **Sherwood, L. M.,** Hypernatraemia during sodium sulphate therapy. *N. Engl. J. Med.,* 277, 314, 1967.
531. **Heckman, B. A. and Walsh, J. H.,** Hypernatraemia complicating sodium sulphate therapy for hypercalcaemic crisis. *N. Engl. J. Med.,* 276, 1082, 1967.

532. **Halma, C., et al.,** Life threatening water intoxication during somatostatin therapy. *Ann. Int. Med.,* 107, 518, 1987.

533. **Murray-Lyon, I. M., et al.,** Further studies on streptozotocin therapy for a multiple-hormone-producing islet cell carcinoma. *Gut,* 12, 717, 1971.

534. **Weintraub, H. D., Heisterkamp, D. V., and Cooperman, L. H.,** Changes in plasma potassium concentration after depolarising blockers in anaesthetised man. *Anaesthesia,* 36, 138, 1972.

535. **Miller, R. D., et al.,** Succinylcholine-induced hypokalaemia in patients with renal failure? *Anaesthesia,* 36, 142, 1972.

536. **Koide, M. and Waud, B. E.,** Serum potassium concentration after succinylcholine in patients with renal failure. *Anaesthesia,* 36, 142, 1972.

537. **Birch, A. A., et al.,** Changes in serum potassium response to succinylcholine following treatment, *JAMA,* 210, 490, 1969.

538. **Zantvoort, F. A., et al.,** Theophylline and serum electrolytes. *Ann. Int. Med.,* 104, 134, 1986.

539. **Rothanthal, S. and Kaukman, S.,** Vinchristine neurotoxicity. *Ann. Int. Med.,* 80, 733, 1974.

540. **McLauchlan, D. M.,** in *"Varleys" Practical Clinical Biochemistry* 6th ed., Gowenlock, A. H., Ed., William Heinemann Medical Books, London, 1988.

541. **Martland, M., Hansman, F. S., and Robison, R.,** C. The phosphoric-esterase of blood. *Biochem. J.,* 18, 1152, 1924.

542. **Lawaczeck, H.,** Uber die Dynamik der Phosphorsäure des Blutes. *Biochem. Z.,* 145, 351, 1924.

543. **Martland, M. and Robison, R.,** XCI, The possible significance of hexose-phosphoric esters in ossification. VII. The bone phosphatase. *Biochem. J.,* 21, 665, 1927.

544. **Bodansky, A.,** Phosphatase studies. II. Determination of serum phosphatase. Factors influencing the accuracy of the determination. *J. Biol. Chem.,* 101, 93, 1933.

545. **Kay, H. D.,** Plasma phosphatase. I. Method of determination. Some properties of the enzyme. *J. Biol. Chem.,* 89, 235, 1930.

546. **McComb, R. B., Bowers, G. N., Jr., and Posen, S.,** *"Alkaline Phosphatase"* Plenum Press, New York, 1979, 346.

547. **King, E. J. and Armstrong, A. R.,** Convenient method for determining serum and bile phosphatase activity. *Can. Med. Assoc. J.,* 31, 376, 1934.

548. **Kind, P. R. N. and King, E. J.,** Estimation of plasma phosphatase by determination of hydrolysed phenol with amino pyrine. *J. Clin. Pathol.,* 7, 322, 1954.

549. **Seligman, A. M., et al.,** The colorimetric determination of phosphatases in human serum. *J. Biol. Chem.,* 190, 7, 1951.

550. **Comfort, D. and Campbell, D. J.,** One-step automated alkaline phosphatase analysis. *Clin. Chim. Acta,* 14, 263, 1966.

551. **Babson, A. L.,** Phenolphthalein monophosphate, a new substrate for alkaline phosphatase. *Clin. Chem.,* 11, 789, 1965.

552. **Coleman, C. M.,** The synthesis of thymolphthalein monophosphate, a new substrate for alkaline phosphatase. *Clin. Chim. Acta,* 13, 401, 1966.

553. **Neuman, H.,** Some new substrates for determination of phosphatase. *Experientia,* 4, 74, 1948.

554. **Bessey, O. A., Lowry, O. H., and Brock, M. J.,** A method for the rapid determination of alkaline phosphatase with five cubic millimetres of serum. *J. Biol. Chem.,* 164, 321, 1946.

555. **Moss, D. W., Baron, D. N., and Wilkinson, J. H.,** Standardisation of clinical enzyme assays. *J. Clin. Pathol.,* 74, 740, 1971.

556. **Bowers, G. N., Jr. and McComb, R. B.,** A, Continuous spectrophotometric method for measuring the activity of serum alkaline phosphatase. *Clin. Chem.,* 12, 70, 1966.

557. **Anon.,** German Society for Clinical Chemistry recommendation. Standard method for determination of alkaline phosphatase (AP) activity. *Z. Klin. Chem. Klin. Biochem.,* 10, 290, 1972.

558. **Anon.,** The Committee on Enzymes of the Scandinavian Society for Clinical Chemistry and Clinical Physiology, Recommended methods for the determination of four enzymes in blood. *Scand. J. Clin. Lab. Invest.,* 33, 291, 1974.

559. **Bowers, G. N., Jr. and McComb, R. B.,** Selected method. Measurement of total alkaline phosphatase activity in human serum. *Clin. Chem.,* 21, 1988, 1975.

560. International Federation of Clinical Chemistry. Scientific Committee Analytical Section Expert Panel on Enzymes, IFCC methods for the measurement of catalytic concentration of enzymes. V. IFCC method for alkaline phosphatase (ortho-phosphoric-monoester phosphohydrolase alkaline optimum EC 3.1.3.1.). *Clin. Chim. Acta,* 135, 339F, 1983.

561. **Bowers, G. N., Jr. and McComb, R. B.,** Alkaline phosphatase. Total activity in human serum. *Sel. Methods Clin. Chem.,* 9, 79, 1982.

562. **Posen, S. and Doherty, E.,** The measurement of serum alkaline phosphatase in clinical medicine *Adv. Clin. Chem.,* 22, 163, 1981.

563. **Tietz, N. W., Woodrow, D., and Woodrow, B.,** A comparative study of the Bodansky and the Bessey, Lowry, and Brock method for alkaline phosphatase in serum *Clin. Chim. Acta,* 15, 365, 1967.

564. **Pentillä, I. M., et al.,** Activities of Aspartate and Alanine Aminotransferases and Alkaline Phosphatase in Sera of Healthy Subjects *Scand. J. Clin. Lab. Invest.,* 35, 275, 1975.

565. **Burnett, R. W.,** Accurate estimation of standard deviations for quantitative methods used in clinical chemistry. *Clin. Chem.,* 21, 1935, 1975.

566. **Sterling, R. E., et al.,** An automated determination of alkaline phosphatase utilising *p*-nitrophenol phosphate. *Clin. Chem.,* 10, 1112, 1964.

567. **Lohff, M. R., et al.,** Analytic clinical laboratory precision. State of the art for selected enzymes. *Am. J. Clin. Pathol.,* 78, 634, 1983.

568. **Whitehead, T. P., Browning, D. M., and Gregory, A.,** A comparative survey of the results of analysis of blood serum in clinical laboratories. *J. Clin. Pathol.,* 26, 435, 1973.

568a. **Proksch, G. J., Bonderman, D. P., and Griep, J. A.,** Auto analyser assay for serum alkaline phosphatase activity with sodium thymolphthalein monophosphate as substrate. *Clin. Chem.,* 19, 103, 1973.

569. **Strömme, J. H., Björnstad, P., and Eldjarn, L.,** Improvement in the quality of enzyme determinations by Scandinavian laboratories upon introduction of Scandinavian recommended methods. *Scand. J. Clin. Lab. Invest.,* 36, 505, 1976.

569a. **Grosset, A., Knapp, M. L., and Mayne, P. D.,** The effect of haemolysis on the measurement of plasma alkaline phosphatase activity. *Ann. Clin. Biochem.,* 24, 513, 1987.

570. **Vinet, B. and Letellier, G.,** The in vitro effect of drugs on biochemical parameters determined by a SMAC system. *Clin. Biochem.,* 10, 47, 1977.

571. **Raab, W. and Mörth, C.,** Inhibition of alkaline phosphatase activity by D-penicillamine. *Z. Klin. Chem. Klin. Biochem.,* 12, 309, 1974.

572. **Bailey, I. R.,** Effect on 16 analytes of overnight storage of specimen collected into heparinized evacuated tubes with plasma separator. *Ann. Clin. Biochem.,* 27, 56, 1990.

573. **Fleisher, G. A., Eickelberg, E. S., and Elveback, L. R.,** Alkaline phosphatase activity in the plasma of children and adolescents. *Clin. Chem.,* 23, 469, 1977.

574. **Bowers, G. N., Jr., McComb, R. B., and Kelley, M.,** Measurement of total alkaline phosphatase activity in human serum. *Sel. Methods Clin. Chem.,* 8, 31, 1977.

575. **Tietz, N. W., et al.,** A reference method for measurement of alkaline phosphatase activity in human serum. *Clin. Chem.,* 29, 751, 1983.

576. **Evered, D. F. and Steenson, T. I.,** Citrate inhibition of alkaline phosphatase. *Nature,* 202, 491, 1964.

577. **Belfanti, S., Contardi, A., and Ercoli, A.,** Researches on the phosphatases. III. On the mechanism of the inactivative action of sodium oxalate and of phosphates on the "alkaline" phosphatases of animal tissue. *Biochem. J.,* 29, 1491, 1935.

578. **Henny, J. and Schiele, F.,** in *Interpretation of Clinical Laboratory Tests,* Siest, G., et al., Biomedical Publishers, Foster City, CA, 1985, 96.

579. **Saloman, L. L., James, J., and Weaver, P. R.,** Assay of phosphatase activity by direct spectrophotometric determination of the phenolate ion. *Anal. Chem.,* 36, 1162, 1964.

580. **Bowers, G. N., Jr., et al.,** High purity 4-nitrophenol. Purification, characterisation, and specification for use as a spectrophotometric reference material. *Clin. Chem.,* 26, 724, 1980.

581. **Bergmeyer, H. U.,** Standardisation of enzyme assays. *Clin. Chem.,* 18, 1305, 1972.

582. **Bodansky, A.,** Paradoxical increase of phosphatase activity in preserved serum. *Proc. Soc. Exp. Biol. Med.,* 29, 1292, 1932.

583. **Kaplan, A. and Narahara, A.,** The determination of serum alkaline phosphatase activity. *J. Lab. Clin. Med.,* 41, 819, 1953.

584. **Tietz, N. W. and Green, A.,** An automated procedure for the determination of phosphorus and alkaline phosphatase in serum. *Clin. Chem. Acta,* 9, 392, 1964.

585. **Massion, C. G. and Frakenfeld, J. K.,** Alkaline phosphatase: lability in fresh and frozen human serum and in lyophilised control material. *Clin. Chem.,* 18, 366, 1972.

586. **Notrica, S., et al.,** Effect on chemical values of using polystyrene beads for serum separation. *Clin. Chem.,* 19, 792, 1973.

587. **Brojer, B. and Moss, D. W.,** Changes in the alkaline phosphatase activity of serum samples after thawing and after reconstitution from the lyophilised state. *Clin. Chim. Acta,* 35, 511, 1971.

588. **Czarnetzy, E. M., Richael, R. J., and O'Malley, J. A.,** Temperature-dependent changes with time in the alkaline phosphatase activity of commercial control serum. *Clin. Chem.,* 16, 521, 1970.

589. **Szasz, G.,** Increase of alkaline phosphatase activity in commercial reference sera after reconstitution. *Scand. J. Clin. Lab. Invest.,* 29 (Suppl 126), 12.7, 1972.

590. **Szasz, G.,** Influence of lyophilisation on the alkaline phosphatase activity. *Scand. J. Clin. Lab. Invest.* 29 (Suppl. 126), 12.8, 1972.

591. **Dixon, M. and Paterson, C. R.,** Posture and the composition of plasma. *Clin. Chem.,* 24, 824, 1978.

592. **Statland, B. A., Winkel, P., and Bokelund, H.,** Serum alkaline phosphatase after fatty meals: the effect of substrate on the assay procedure. *Clin. Chim. Acta,* 49, 299, 1973.

593. **Kleerekoper, M., et al.,** Serum alkaline phosphatase after fat ingestion: an immunological study. *Clin. Sci.,* 38, 339, 1970.

594. **Langman, M. J. S., et al.,** Influence of diet on the "intestinal" component of serum alkaline phosphatase in people of different ABO blood groups and secretor states. *Nature,* 212, 41, 1966.

595. **Walker, B. A., et al.,** The influence of ABO blood groups, secretor status and fat ingestion on serum alkaline phosphatase. *Clin. Chim. Acta,* 35, 433, 1971.

596. **Irwin, M. I. and Staton, A. J.,** Dietary wheat starch and sucrose. Effect on levels of five enzymes in blood serum of young adults. *Am. J. Clin. Nutr.,* 22, 701, 1969.

597. **King, S. W., Statland, B. E., and Savory, J.,** The effect of a short burst of exercise on activity values of enzymes in the sera of healthy young men. *Clin. Chim. Acta,* 72, 211, 1976.

598. **Stearns, G. and Warweg, E.,** Studies of phosphorus in blood. I. The partition of phosphorus in whole blood and serum. The serum calcium and plasma phosphatase from birth to maturity. *J. Biol. Chem.,* 102, 749, 1933.

599. **Bodansky, A. and Jaffe, H. L.,** Phosphatase studies. III. Serum phosphatase in diseases of bone: interpretation and significance. *Arch. Int. Med.,* 54, 88, 1934.

600. **Dent, C. E. and Harper, C. M.,** Plasma-alkaline-phosphatase in normal adults and in patients with hyperparathyroidism. *Lancet,* i, 559, 1962.

601. **Munan, L., Kelly, A., and Petitclerc, C.,** quoted in *Alkaline Phosphatase,* McComb, R. B., Bowers, G. N., Jr., and Posen, S., Eds., Plenum Press, New York, 1979, 528.

602. **Sharland, D. E.,** Alkaline phosphatase: the isoenzyme pattern in the elderly and changes in total serum levels with age. *Clin. Chim. Acta,* 56, 187, 1974.

603. **Carroll, D. O., et al.,** Chemical inhibition method for alkaline phosphatase isoenzymes in human serum. *Am. J. Clin. Pathol.,* 63, 564, 1975.

604. **Hodkinson, H. M. and McPherson, C. K.,** Alkaline phosphatase in a geriatric inpatient population. *Age Aging,* 2, 28, 1973.

605. **Bennett, D. L., Ward, M. S., and Daniel, W. A., Jr.,** The relationship of serum alkaline phosphatase concentration to sex maturity ratings in adolescents. *J. Paediatr.,* 88, 633, 1976.

606. **Fleisher, G. A., Eickelberg, E. S., and Elveback, L. R.,** Alkaline phosphatase activity in the plasma of children and adolescents. *Clin. Chem.,* 23, 469, 1977.

607. **Clark, L. C. and Beck, E.,** Plasma "alkaline" phosphatase activity. I. Normative data for growing children. *J. Paediatr.* 36, 335, 1950.

608. **Kantero, R. L., Wide, L., and Widholm, O.,** Endocrine changes before and after the menarche. II. Serum levels of growth hormone and alkaline phosphatase and urinary excretion of 17-ketosteroids and 17-hydroxycorticoids. *Acta Obstet. Gynecol. Scand.,* 54, 1, 1975.

609. **Stevens, J. M. L. and Stevenson, P.,** Alkaline phosphatase in normal infants. *Arch. Dis. Child.,* 46, 185, 1971.

610. **Posen, S., et al.,** Transient hyperphosphatasaemia of infancy — an insufficiently recognised syndrome. *Clin. Chem.,* 23, 292, 1977.

611. **Wieme, R. J.,** More on transient hyperphosphatasaemia in infancy — an insufficiently recognised syndrome. *Clin. Chem.,* 24, 520, 1978.

612. **Rosalki, S. B. and Foo, Y.,** Transient hyperphosphatasaemia of infancy: four new cases, and a suggested etiology. *Clin. Chem.,* 26, 1109, 1980.

613. **Rosalki, S. B. and Foo, A. Y.,** More on transient hyperphosphatasaemia of infancy. *Clin. Chem.,* 29, 723, 1983.

614. **Barnes, D. J. and Munks, B.,** Serum phosphatase, calcium and phosphorus values in infancy. *Proc. Soc. Exp. Biol. Med.,* 44, 327, 1940.

615. **Fomen, S. J., et al.,** Growth and serum chemical values of normal breast fed infants. *Acta Paediatr.* 202 (Suppl.), 1, 1970.

616. **Izquierdo, J. M., et al.,** Capillary blood potassium chloride sodium calcium phosphorus and alkaline phosphatase in the new born. *Clin. Chim. Acta,* 30, 343, 1970.

617. **Speert, H., Graff, S., and Graff, A. M.,** Serum phosphatase relation in mother and fetus. *Am. J. Obstet. Gynecol.,* 59, 148, 1950.

618. **Van Sydow, G.,** A study of development of rickets in premature infants. *Acta Paediatr.* 33 (Suppl.), 17, 1946.

619. **Kitchener, P. N., et al.,** Alkaline phosphatase in maternal and fetal sera at term and during the puerperium. *Am. J. Clin. Pathol.,* 44, 654, 1965.

620. **Kristensen, S. R., Hørder, M., and Pederson, G. T.,** Reference values for six enzymes in plasma from newborns and women at delivery. *Scand. J. Clin. Lab. Invest.,* 39, 777, 1977.

621. **Freer, D. E., et al.,** Reference values for selected enzyme activities and protein concentration in serum and plasma derived from cord-blood specimens. *Clin. Chem.,* 25, 565, 1979.

622. **Hilderbrand, D. C., et al.,** Caeruloplasmin and alkaline phosphatase levels in cord serum of term preterm and physiologically jaundiced neonates. *Am. J. Obstet. Gynecol.,* 118, 950, 1974.

623. **Coryn, G.,** *J. Chir. (Paris),* 33, 213, 1934, quoted by McMaster Y., et al., in *J. Obstet. Gynecol. Br. Common.,* 71, 737, 1964.

624. **Beck, E. and Clark, L. C., Jr.,** Plasma alkaline phosphatase. II. Normative data for pregnancy. *Am. J. Obstet. Gynecol.,* 60, 731, 1950.

625. **McMaster, Y., et al.,** The mechanism of the elevation of serum alkaline phosphatase in pregnancy. *J. Obstet. Gynecol. Br. Common.,* 71, 737, 1964.

626. **Neale, F. C., et al.,** Heat stability of human placental alkaline phosphatase. *J. Clin. Pathol.,* 18, 359, 1965.

627. **Fishman, W. H., et al.,** The exponential growth curve for the placental isoenzyme of alkaline phosphatase in sera of normal and diabetic pregnancies. *Am. J. Clin. Pathol.,* 60, 353, 1973.

628. **Fishman, W. H.,** in discussion on a paper on placental alkaline phosphatase of pregnancy. *Ann. N.Y. Acad. Sci.,* 166, 741, 1966.

629. **Vermehren, E.,** Plasmaphosphatase während der Gravidität und der Lactation. *Acta Med. Scand.,* 100, 254, 1939.

630. **Young, J., et al.,** Nutritional survey among pregnant women. *J. Obstet. Gynecol. Br. Emp.,* 53, 251, 1946.

631. **Ebbs, J. H. and Scott, W. A.,** Blood phosphatase in pregnancy an indication of twins. *Am. J. Obstet. Gynecol.,* 39, 1043, 1940.

632. **Neale, F. C., Clubb, J. S., and Posen, S.,** Artificial elevation of the serum alkaline phosphatase concentration. *Med. J. Austr.,* 2, 684, 1963.

633. **Bark, C. J.,** Artifactual elevations of serum alkaline phosphatase following albumin infusions. *Am. J. Clin. Pathol.,* 52, 466, 1969.

634. **Bamford, K. F., et al.,** Serum alkaline phosphatase and the ABO blood groups. *Lancet,* i, 530, 1965.

635. **Ferguson, D. B.,** Effects of low doses of fluoride on serum proteins and a serum enzyme in man. *Nature New Biol.,* 231, 159, 1971.

636. **Belfanti, S., Contardi, A., and Ercoli, A.,** Studies on the phosphatases: the influence of some electrolytes on the phosphatases of animal tissue. Phosphatases of the liver, kidney, serum and bones of the rabbit. *Biochem J.,* 29, 517, 1935.

637. **Nagamine, M. and Ohkuma, S.,** Serum alkaline phosphatase isoenzymes linked to immunoglobulin G. *Clin. Chim. Acta,* 65, 39, 1975.

638. **Dingjan, P. G., Postma, T., and Stroes, J. A. P.,** The diagnostic value of certain alkaline phosphatase isoenzyme patterns in human serum, fractions obtained by polyacrilamide disc electrophoresis. *Clin. Chim. Acta,* 60, 169, 1975.

639. **Crofton, P. M. and Smith, A. F.,** The properties and clinical significance of some electrophoretically slow forms of alkaline phosphatase. *Clin. Chim. Acta,* 83, 235, 1978.

640. **DeBroe, M. E., Borges-Wieme, R. J.,** The separation and characterization of liver plasma membrane fragments circulating in the blood of patients with cholestasis. *Clin. Chim. Acta,* 59, 369, 1975.

641. **Kolenda, K. D. and Hosenfeld, D.,** Leberbeschädigung und alkalische Phosphatase bei der Behandlung mit thyreostatika. *Therapiewoche,* 28, 972, 1978.

642. **Gutman, A. B.,** Drug reactions characterised by cholestasis associated with intrahepatic biliary tract obstruction. *Am. J. Med.,* 23, 841, 1957.

643. **Broulik, P. D., et al.,** Alterations in human serum alkaline phosphatase and its bone isoenzyme by chronic administration of lithium. *Clin. Chim. Acta,* 140, 151, 1984.

644. **Herbeth, B., et al.,** Influence of oral contraceptives of different doses on -1-antitrypsin-glutamyl transferase and alkaline phosphatase. *Clin. Chim. Acta,* 112, 293, 1981.

645. **Schade, R. W. B., Demacker, P. N. M., and Laar, A. V.,** Reduction of serum alkaline phosphatase by clofibrate. *Lancet,* i, 862, 1975.

646. **Ferrari, C., et al.,** Reduction of serum alkaline phosphatase and gamma glutamyl transpeptidase activity by short-term clofibrate. *N. Engl. J. Med.,* 295, 449, 1976.

647. **Wilkinson, J. H.,** The transaminases, in *An Introduction to Diagnostic Enzymology,* Edward Arnold, London, 1962, 107.

648. **Braunstein, A. E. and Kritzsman, M. G.,** *Biochemia (Moscow),* 2, 242, 1937.

649. **Karmen, A., Wróblewski, F., and LaDue, J. S.,** Transaminase activity in human blood. *J. Clin. Invest.,* 34, 126, 1965.

650. **Wróblewski, F. and LaDue, J. S.,** Serum glutamic pyruvic transaminase in cardiac and hepatic disease. *Proc. Soc. Exp. Biol. Med.,* 91, 569, 1956.

651. **Reitman, S. and Frankel, S.,** A colorimetric method for the determination of serum glutamic oxalacetic and glutamic pyruvic transaminases. *Am. J. Clin. Pathol.,* 28, 56, 1957.

652. **King, J.,** Routine methods for the estimation of serum transaminases. *J. Med. Lab. Technol.,* 15, 17, 1958.

653. **Babson, A. L., et al.,** The use of a diazonium salt for the determination of glutamic-oxalacetic transaminase in serum. *Clin. Chim. Acta,* 7, 199, 1962.

654. **Demetriou, J. A. and Drewes, P. A.,** in *Clinical Chemistry. Principles and Technics,* 2nd ed., Henry, R. J., Cannon, D. C., and Winkleman, J. W., Eds., Harper & Row, New York, 1974, 873 and 884.

655. **Rej, R., Fasce, C. F., Jr., and Vanderlinde, R. E.,** Increased aspartate aminotransferase activity of serum after in vitro supplementation with pyridoxyl phosphate. *Clin. Chem.,* 19, 92, 1973.

656. **Cheung, T. and Briggs, M. H.,** Pyridoxyl phosphate and the measurement of aminotransferase activity. *Clin. Chim. Acta,* 54, 127, 1974.

657. **Committee on Enzymes of the Scandinavian Society for Clinical Chemistry and Clinical Physiology,** Recommended methods for the determination of four enzymes in blood. *Scand. J. Clin. Lab. Invest.,* 33, 291, 1974.

658. **International Federation of Clinical Chemistry Committee on Standards, Expert Panel on Enzymes,** Provisional recommendations on IFCC methods for the measurement of catalytic concentrations of enzymes. II. IFCC method for aspartate amino transferase. *Clin. Chim. Acta,* 70, F19, 1976.

659. **International Federation of Clinical Chemistry Committee on Standards, Expert Panel on Enzymes,** Provisional recommendations on IFCC methods for the measurement of catalytic concentrations of enzymes. III. Revised IFCC method for aspartate aminotransferase (L-aspartate: 2-oxo glutarate aminotransferase. EC 2.6.1.1.). *Clin. Chim. Acta,* 80, F21, 1977.

660. **International Federation of Clinical Chemistry Committee on Standards, Expert Panel on Enzymes.** IFCC methods for the measurement of catalytic concentration of enzymes. III. IFCC method for alanine aminotransferase (L-alanine 2-oxoglutarate aminotransferase EC 2.6.1.2). *Clin. Chim. Acta,* 105, F147, 1980.

661. **Scandinavian Committee on Enzymes (SCE).** Experiences with the Scandinavian recommended method for determination of enzymes in blood. *Scand. J. Clin. Lab. Invest.,* 41, 107, 1981.

662. **Vincent-Viry, M., Schiele, F., and Galteau, M. M.,** Alanine aminotransferases, in *Interpretation of Clinical Laboratory Tests,* Siest, G., et al., Eds., Biomedical Publishers, Foster City, CA, 1985, 69.

663. **Friedman, M. M. and Taylor, J. H.,** Transaminase. *Stand. Methods Clin. Chem.,* 3, 207, 1961.

664. **Henry, R. J.,** in *Clinical Chemistry Principles and Technics,* 1st ed., Harper and Row, New York, 1964, 516.

665. **Sax, S. M. and Moore, J. J.,** Glutamic oxalacetic transaminase (Colorimetric), *Stand. Methods Clin. Chem.,* 6, 152, 1970.

666. **Miyada, D., et al.,** The effect of hyperlipidaemia on Technicon SMAC measurements. *Clin. Biochem.,* 15, 185, 1982.

667. **Cryer, P. E. and Daughaday, W. H.,** Diabetic ketosis: elevated serum glutamic-oxalacetic transaminase (SGOT) and other findings determined by multichannel analysis. *Diabetes,* 18, 781, 1969.

668. **Moore, J. J. and Sax, S. M.,** Serum glutamic oxalacetic transaminase assays using the sequential multiple analyser (SMA 12/30). *Clin. Chem.,* 15, 730, 1969.

669. **Chen, J. C. and Marsteers-Wirland, R. G.,** Diabetic ketosis. Interpretation of elevated serum glutamic-oxalacetic transaminase (SGOT) by multichannel chemical analysis. *Diabetes,* 18, 730, 1970.

670. **Wolf, P. L., et al.,** Ketosis causing spurious elevation of SGOT values. *Clin. Chem.,* 17, 341, 1971.

671. **Glynn, K. P., et al.,** False elevation of serum glutamic-oxalacetic transaminase due to para amino salicylic acid. *Ann. Int. Med.,* 72, 525, 1970.

672. **Rodgerson, D. O. and Osberg, I. M.,** Sources of error in spectrophotometric measurement of aspartate aminotransferase and alanine aminotransferase in serum. *Clin. Chem.,* 20, 43, 1974.

673. **McLauchlan, D. M.,** in *"Varleys" Practical Clinical Biochemistry,* Gowenlock, A. H., Ed., William Heinemann Medical Books, London, 1988, 502.

674. **Berg, J. D., et al.,** Heparin interferes with aspartate aminotransferase activity determinations on the Ektochem 700. *Clin. Chem.,* 34, 174, 1988.

675. **Hafkenscheid, J. C. M. and Hectors, M. P. C.,** Serum versus heparinised plasma for alanine aminotransferase and aspartate aminotransferase of normal individuals. *Clin. Chim. Acta,* 78, 23, 1977.

676. **Bergmeyer, H. H., Schiele, P., and Wahlefeld, A. W.,** Optimization of methods for aspartate aminotransferase and alanine aminotransferase. *Clin. Chem.,* 24, 58, 1978.

677. **Hafkenscheid, J. C. M. and Dijt, C. C. M.,** Is serum or heparinised plasma better for assay of aminotransferases? *Clin. Chem.,* 26, 354, 1980.

678. **Statland, B. E. and Winkel, P.,** Effects of preanalytical factors on the intraindividual variation of analytes in the blood of healthy subjects: consideration of preparation of the subject and time of venipuncture. *Crit. Rev. Clin. Lab. Sci.,* 8, 105, 1977.

679. **Fawcett, C. P., Ciotti, M. M., and Kaplan, N. O.,** Inhibition of dehydrogenase reactions by a substance formed from reduced diphosphopyridine nucleotidase. *Biochem. Biophys. Acta,* 54, 210, 1961.

680. **Henry, R. J., et al.,** Revised spectrophotometric method for the determination of glutamic-oxalacetic transaminase, glutamic-pyruvic transaminase and lactic dehydrogenase. *Am. J. Clin. Pathol.,* 34, 381, 1960.

681. **Schmidt, E. and Schmidt, F. W.,** in *Brief Guide to Practical Enzyme Diagnosis,* 2nd revised ed., Boehringer, Mannheim, 1976, 11.

682. **Bodansky, O., et al.,** Infectious hepatitis. *Am. J. Dis. Child.,* 98, 166, 1958.

683. **Steinmetz, J., Panek, E., and Siest, G.,** Influence of food intake on biological parameters, in *Reference Values in Human Chemistry,* Siest, G., Ed., S. Karger, Basel, 1973, 191.

684. **Henley, K. S., et al.,** Serum enzymes. *JAMA,* 174, 977, 1960.

685. **Schlang, H. A.,** The effect of physical exercise on human transaminase. *Am. J. Med. Sci.,* 242, 338, 1961.

686. **Ahlborg, B. and Brohult, J.,** Immediate and delayed metabolic reactions in well-trained subjects after prolonged physical exercise. *Acta Med. Scand.,* 182, 41, 1967.

687. **McKechnie, J. K., Leary, W. P., and Joubers, S. M.,** Some electrocardiographic and biochemical changes recorded in marathon runners. *S. Afr. Med. J.,* 41, 722, 1967.

688. **Remmers, A. R. and Kaljet, V.,** Serum transaminase levels. Effect of strenuous and prolonged physical exercise in healthy young subjects. *JAMA,* 185, 968, 1963.

689. **Röcker, L., et al.,** Jahreszeitliche Veränderungen Dianrstisch Wichtiger Blutbestandteile. *Klin. Wochenschr.,* 58, 769, 1980.

690. **Gidlow, D. A., Church, J. F., and Clayton, B. E.,** Haematological and biochemical parameters in an industrial workforce. *Ann. Clin. Biochem.,* 20, 341, 1983.

691. **Gidlow, D. A., Church, J. F., and Clayton, B. E.,** Seasonal variation in haematological and biochemical parameters. *Ann. Clin. Biochem.,* 23, 310, 1986.

692. **Donayre, J. and Pincus, G.,** Serum enzymes in the menstrual cycle. *J. Clin. Endocrinol. Meta.,* 25, 432, 1965.

693. **Sweetin, J. C. and Thomson, W. H. S.,** revised normal ranges for six serum enzymes: further statistical analysis and the effects of different treatments of blood specimens. *Clin. Chim. Acta,* 48, 49, 1973.

694. **Antebi, R. and King, J.,** Serum transaminase activity. *Lancet,* i, 1133, 1958.

695. **Siest, G., et al.,** Aspartate aminotransferase and alanine aminotransferase activity in plasma: statistical distribution, individual variation, and reference values. *Clin. Chem.,* 21, 1077, 1975.

696. **Järvisalo, J., et al.,** Health-base reference values of the Mini-Finland Health Survey. I. Serum gamma-glutamyl transferase aspartate aminotransferase and alkaline phosphatase. *Scand. J. Clin. Lab. Invest.,* 49, 623, 1989.

697. **Hetland, G., Holme, I., and Strømme, J. H.,** Co-variation of alanine aminotransferase levels with relative weight in blood donors. *Scand. J. Clin. Lab. Invest.,* 52, 51, 1992.

698. **Emanuel, B., West, M., and Zimmerman, H. J.,** Serum enzymes in disease. XII. Transaminases glycolytic and oxidative enzymes in normal infants and children. *Am. J. Dis. Child.,* 105, 261, 1963.

699. **Deschamps, J. P. and Lahrichi, M.,** Biological values in the child and adolescent, in *Reference Values in Human Chemistry,* Siest, G., Ed., S. Karger, Basel, 1973, 109.

700. **Haas, R. G.,** in *Paediatric Clinical Chemistry. Reference (Normal) Values,* 3rd ed., Meites, S., Ed., AACC, Washington, D.C., 1989, 61.

701. **Handa, N.,** in *Paediatric Clinical Chemistry. Reference (Normal) Values,* 3rd ed., Meites, S., Ed., AACC, Washington, D.C., 1989, 33.

702. **Kove, S., Goldstein, S., and Wróblewski, F.,** Serum transaminase activity in neonatal period. Valuable aid in differential diagnosis of jaundice in the newborn infant. *JAMA,* 168, 860, 1958.

703. **Stanton, R. E. and Joos, H. A.,** Glutamic-oxalacetic transaminase of serum in infancy and childhood. *Paediatrics,* 24, 362, 1959.

704. **Kessel, I. and Politzer, W. M.,** Neonatal and maternal serum transaminase activity at birth. *Arch. Dis. Child.,* 36, 217, 1961.

705. **Kristensen, S. R., Hørder, M., and Pedersen, G. T.,** Reference values for six enzymes in plasma from newborns and women at delivery. *Scand. J. Clin. Lab. Invest.,* 39, 777, 1979.

706. **Knutson, R. G., et al.,** Serum lactic dehydrogenase and glutamic oxalacetic transaminase activity in normal pregnancy. *J. Lab. Clin. Med.,* 51, 773, 1958.

707. **Borglin, N. E.,** Serum transaminase activity in uncomplicated pregnancy and the new born. *J. Clin. Endocrinol. Metab.,* 18, 872, 1958.

708. **Siest, G., et al.,** Aspartate aminotransferase and alanine aminotransferase activity in plasma: statistical distribution, individual variation, and reference values. *Clin. Chem.,* 21, 1077, 1975.

709. **Konttinen, A., Härtel, G., and Louhija, A.,** Multiple serum enzyme analyses in chronic alcoholics. *Acta Med. Scand.,* 188, 257, 1970.

710. **Lieberman, J., et al.,** Serum glutamic-oxalacetic transaminase activity in conditions associated with myocardial infarction. I. Bodily trauma. *Ann. Int. Med.,* 46, 485, 1957.

711. **Blodgett, R. C., et al.,** Glutamic oxalacetic transaminase activity in serum after transurethral prostatic resection. *Arch. Int. Med.,* 114, 344, 1964.

712. **Wolf, P. L., et al.,** Low aspartate transaminase activity in serum of patients undergoing chronic haemodialysis. *Clin. Chem.,* 18, 567, 1972.

713. **Kottinen, A., et al.,** A new cause of increased serum aspartate aminotransferase activity. *Clin. Chim. Acta,* 84, 145, 1978.

714. **Rajita, Y., et al.,** Demonstration of antibodies for glutamic pyruvic transaminase (GPT) in chronic hepatic disorders. *Clin. Chim. Acta,* 89, 485, 1978.

715. **Knirsch, A. K. and Gralla, E. J.,** Abnormal serum transaminase levels after parenteral ampicillin and carbenicillin administration. *N. Engl. J. Med.,* 282, 1081, 1971.

716. **Peters, T., Jr.,** Proposals for standardisation of total protein assays. *Clin. Chem.,* 14, 1147, 1968.

717. **Brand, E., Kassell, B., and Saidel, I. J.,** Chemical, clinical and immunologic studies on the product of human plasma fractionation. III. Amino acid composition of plasma protein. *J. Clin. Invest.,* 23, 437, 1944.

718. **Sunderman, F. W., Jr., et al.,** Studies of the serum proteins. II. The nitrogen content of purified serum proteins separated by continuous flow electrophoresis. *Am. J. Clin. Pathol.,* 30, 113, 1958.

719. **Chiaraviglio, E., Wolf, A. V., and Prentiss, P. G.,** Total protein/protein nitrogen ratio of human serum. *Am. J. Clin. Pathol.,* 39, 42, 1963.

720. **Watson, D.,** Albumin and "total globulin" fractions of blood. *Adv. Clin. Chem.,* 8, 265, 1965.

721. **Reigler, E.,** Eine Kolorimetrische Bestimmungsmethode des Eiweisses. *Z. Anal. Chem.,* 53, 242, 1914, quoted by Watson, D., *Adv. Clin. Chem.,* 8, 265, 1965.

722. **Doumas, B. T.,** Standards for total serum protein assays — a collaborative study. *Clin. Chem.,* 21, 1159, 1975.

723. **Doumas, B. T., et al.,** A candidate reference method for determination of total protein in serum. I. Development and valuation. *Clin. Chem.,* 27, 1642, 1981.

724. **Lowry, O. H., et al.,** Protein measurement with the folin phenol reagent. *J. Biol. Chem.,* 193, 263, 1952.

725. **Rej, R. and Richards, A. H.,** Interference by tris buffer in the estimation of protein by the Lowry procedure. *Anal. Biochem.,* 62, 240, 1974.

726. **Hunter, M. J. A.,** A method for the determination of protein partial specific volume. *J. Phys. Chem.,* 70, 3285, 1966.

727. **Varley, H., Gowenlock, A. H., and Bell, M.,** in *Practical Clinical Biochemistry,* Vol. 1, William Heinemann Medical Books, London, 1980, 547.

728. **Henry, R. J., Sobel, C., and Berkman, S.,** Interference with biuret methods for serum protein. Use of Benedict qualitative glucose reagent as a biuret reagent. *Anal. Chem.,* 29, 1491, 1957.

729. **Kingsley, G. R.,** Procedure for serum protein determination with a triphosphate biuret reagent. *Stand. Methods Clin. Chem.,* 7, 199, 1972.

730. **Peters, T., Jr. and Biamonte, G. T.,** Protein (total protein) in serum, urine and cerebrospinal fluid: albumin in serum. *Sel. Methods Clin. Chem.,* 9, 317, 1978.

731. **Panek, E., Young, D. S., and Bente, J.,** Analytical interference of drugs in clinical chemistry. *Am. J. Med. Technol.,* 44, 217, 1978.

732. **Moriaty, A. T., Moorhead, W. R., and Ryder, K. W.,** Sulfasalazine interference in total protein measurement with the Du Pont aca. *Clin. Chem.,* 29, 592, 1983.

733. **Böhme, A.,** Deutsch. *Arch. Klin. Med.,* 103, 522, 1911, quoted by Rowe, A. H., The albumin and globulin content of human blood serum. *Arch. Int. Med.,* 19, 499, 1917.

734. **Peters, J. P., Kydd, D. M., and Bulger, H. A.,** *J. Exp. Med.,* 1, 435, 1924/25, quoted by Lange, H. F., The normal plasma protein values and their relative variation. *Acta Med. Scand.,* 176 (Suppl.), 162, 1946.

735. **Young, D. S.,** in *Chemical Diagnosis of Disease,* Brown, S. S., Mitchell, F. L., and Young, D. S., Eds., Elsevier, Amsterdam, 1979, 63.

736. **Thompson, W. O., Thompson, P. K., and Daly, M. E.,** The effect of posture upon the composition and volume of blood in man. *J. Clin. Invest.,* 5, 573, 1928.

737. **Perera, G. A. and Berliner, R. W.,** The relation of postural hemodilution to paroxysmal dyspnoea. *J. Clin. Invest.,* 22, 25, 1943.

738. **Lange, H. F.,** The normal plasma protein values and their relative variation, *Acta Med. Scand. Suppl.,* 176, 162, 1946.

739. **Whitehead, T. P., Prior, A. P., and Barrowcliff, D. F.,** Effect of rest and activity on the serum protein fractions. *Am. J. Clin. Pathol.,* 27, 52, 1957.

740. **Aull, J. C. and McCord, W. M.,** Effects of posture and activity on the major fractions of serum protein. *Am. J. Clin. Pathol.,* 27, 52, 1957.

741. **McMurry, J. R.,** in *"Varleys" Practical Clinical Biochemistry,* 5th ed., Gowenlock, A. H., Ed., William Heinemann Medical Books, London, 1988, 419.

742. **Covian, F. G. and Krugh, A.,** The change in osmotic pressure and total concentration of the blood on man during and after muscular work. *Scand. Arch. Physiol.,* 71, 251, 1934.

743. **Poortmans, J. R.,** Serum protein determination during short exhaustive physical activity. *J. Appl. Physiol.,* 30, 190, 1971.

744. **Senay, L. C., Jr. and Christensen, M. L.,** Changes in blood plasma during progressive dehydration. *J. Appl. Physiol.,* 20, 1136, 1965.

745. **Dugue, B., et al.,** Preanalytical factors and standardised specimen collection: influence of psychological stress. *Scand J. Clin. Lab. Invest.,* 52, 43, 1992.

746. **Lelloch, J. and Claude, J. R.,** in *Reference Values in Clinical Chemistry,* Siest, G., Ed., S. Karger, Basel, 1973, 100.

747. **Salveson, H. A.,** Plasma proteins in normal individuals. *Acta Med. Scand.,* 65, 147, 1926.

748. **Sherbrooke Data,** quoted in *Reference Values in Clinical Chemistry,* Siest, G., Ed., S. Karger, Basel, 1973.

749. **Rawnsley, H. M., Yonah, V. L., and Reinhold, J. G.,** Serum protein concentration in the American negroid. *Science,* 123, 991, 1956.

750. **Buckley, C. E. and Dorsey, F. C.,** Serum immunoglobulin levels throughout the life span of healthy man. *Ann. Int. Med.,* 75, 673, 1971.

751. **Milam, D. F.,** Plasma protein levels in normal individuals. *J. Lab. Clin. Med.,* 31, 285, 1946.

752. **Bronte-Stewart, B., et al.,** An interracial study on the serum protein pattern of adult man in Southern Africa. *Am. J. Clin. Nutr.,* 9, 596, 1961.

753. **Luzzio, A. L.,** Comparison of serum proteins in Americans and Eskimos. *J. Appl. Physiol.,* 21, 685, 1966.

754. **Rennie, J. B.,** A note on the serum proteins in normal infants and children. *Arch. Dis. Child.,* 10, 415, 1935.

755. **Josephson, B. and Gyllenswürd, C.,** The development of the protein fractions and of cholesterol concentration in the serum of normal infants and children. *Scand. J. Clin. Lab. Invest.,* 9, 29, 1957.

756. **Haas, R. G.,** in *Paediatric Clinical Chemistry Reference (Normal Values),* 3rd ed., Meites, S., Ed., 1989, 228.

757. **Darrow, D. C. and Cary, M. K.,** The serum albumin and globulin of new born, premature and normal infants. *J. Paediatr.,* 3, 573, 1933.

758. **Hickmans, E. M., Finch, E., and Tonks, E.,** Plasma protein values in infants. *Arch. Dis. Child.,* 18, 96, 1943.

759. **Stürmer, K., Grell, A., and Prokop, O.,** *Klin. Wochenschr.,* 32, 425, 1954, quoted by Sternberg, J., Dagenais-Perusse, P., and Dreyfuss, M., *Can. Med. Assoc. J.,* 74, 49, 1956.

759a. **Brown, T.,** Electrophoretic analysis of serum proteins in pregnancy. II. Effect of labour and lactation. *J. Obstet. Gynaecol. Br. Emp.,* 63, 100, 1956.

760. **Sternberg, J., Dagenais-Perusse, P., and Dreyfuss, M.,** Serum proteins in parturient mothers and neonates: an electrophoretic study. *Can. Med. Assoc. J.,* 74, 49, 1956.

760a. **McGillvray, I. and Tovey, J. E.,** A study of the serum protein change in pregnancy and toxaemia using paper strip electrophoresis. *J. Obstet. Gynaecol. Br. Emp.,* 64, 361, 1957.

761. **Paaby, P.,** Changes in serum proteins during pregnancy. *J. Obstet. Gynaecol. Br. Emp.,* 67, 43, 1960.

762. **Hock, H. and Marrack, J. R.,** Composition of blood of women during pregnancy and after delivery. *J. Obstet. Gynaecol. Br. Emp.,* 55, 1, 1948.

763. **DeAlvarez, R. R., Afonso, J. I., and Sherrard, D. J.,** Serum protein fractionation in normal pregnancy. *Am. J. Gynecol.,* 82, 1096, 1961.

764. **Collins, R. D.,** in *Illustrated Manual of Laboratory Diagnosis,* Lippincott, Philadelphia, 1968.

765. **Goodman, L. S. and Gilman, A.,** in *Pharmacological Basis of Therapeutics,* 4th ed., Macmillan, New York, 1970.

766. **Oleson, K. H., Sigurd, B., and Steiness, E.,** Leth bumetamide, a new potent diuretic. *Acta Med. Scand.,* 193, 119, 1973.

767. **Dale, E. and Spivey, S. H.,** Serum proteins of women utilising combination oral or long-acting injectable progestational contraceptives. *Contraception,* 4, 241, 1976.

768. **Stringer, M. D., Steadman, C. A., and Kakke, V. V.,** Gemfibrozil in hyperlipidaemic patients with peripheral arterial disease: some undiscovered actions. *Curr. Med. Res. Opin.,* 12, 207, 1990.

769. **Martin, E. W.,** in *Hazards of Medication,* Lippincott, Philadelphia, 1971.

770. **Dellaportas, D. I., et al.,** Chronic toxicity in epileptic patients receiving single-drug treatment. *Br. Med. J.,* 285, 409, 1982.

771. **Tarnøky, A. L.,** Genetic and drug-induced variation in serum albumin. *Adv. Clin. Chem.,* 21, 101, 1980.

772. **Keyser, J. W.,** *Human Plasma Proteins. Their Investigation in Pathological Conditions,* 2nd ed., John Wiley & Sons, Chichester, 1987, 60.

773. **Kander, G.,** *Arch. Exp. Pathol. Pharmakol.,* 20, 411, 1886, quoted by Watson, D., Albumin and globulin fractions in blood. *Adv. Clin. Chem.,* 8, 265, 1965.

774. **Lewith, S.,** *Arch. Exp. Pathol. Pharmakol.,* 24, 1, 1888, quoted by Watson, D., Albumin and globulin fractions in blood. *Adv. Clin. Chem.,* 8, 265, 1965.

775. **Howe, P. E.,** The use of sodium sulphate as the globulin precipitant in the determination of proteins in blood. *J. Biol. Chem.,* 49, 93, 1921.

776. **Howe, P. E.,** The relative precipitating capacity of certain salts when applied to blood serum or plasma, and the influence of the cation in the precipitation. *J. Biol. Chem.,* 57, 241, 1923.

777. **Bartholomew, R. J. and Deleney, A.,** Spectrophotometric studies and analytical application of the protein error of some indicators. *Proc. Aust. Assoc. Clin. Biochem.,* 1, 64, 1966.

778. **Northam, B. E. and Widdowson, G. M.,** Determination of serum albumin by auto analyser using bromcresol green. *Assoc. Clin. Biochem. Technol. Bull.,* 11, 1967.

779. **Webster, D., Bignall, A. H. C., and Attwood, E. C.,** An assessment of the suitability of bromcresol green for the determination of serum albumin. *Clin. Chim. Acta,* 53, 101, 1974.

780. **Webster, D.,** A study of the interaction of bromcresol green with isolated serum protein fractions. *Clin. Chim. Acta,* 53, 109, 1974.

781. **Doumas, B. T. and Biggs, H. T.,** Determination of serum albumin. *Stand. Methods Clin. Chem.,* 7, 175, 1972.

782. **Louderback, A., Mealey, E. H., and Taylor, N. A.,** A new dye-binding technic using bromcresol purple for determination of albumin in serum. *Clin. Chem.,* 14, 793, 1968.

783. **Pinnell, A. and Northam, B. E.,** New automated dye-binding method for serum albumin determination with bromcresol purple. *Clin. Chem.,* 24, 80, 1978.

784. **Wells, F. E., Addison, G. M., and Postlethwaite, R. J.,** Albumin analysis in serum of haemodialysis patients: discrepancies between bromcresol purple, bromcresol green and innumoassay. *Ann. Clin. Biochem.,* 22, 304, 1985.

785. **Hobbs, J. R., et al.,** The human serum standard IFCC 74/1. *Clin. Chim. Acta,* 98, 179, 1979.

786. **Hill, P. G.,** The measurement of albumin in serum and plasma. *Ann. Clin. Biochem.,* 22, 565, 1985.

787. **McMurray, J. R.,** in *"Varleys" Clinical Biochemistry,* Gowenlock, A. H., Ed., William Heinemann Medical Books, London, 1988, 411.

788. International Federation of Clinical Chemistry Education Division Expert Panel on Quantities and Units, *Clin. Chim. Acta,* 190, S51, 1990.

789. **Leonard, P. J., Persaud, J., and Motwani, R.,** The estimation of plasma albumin by BCG dye binding on the Technicon SMA 12/60. *Clin. Chim. Acta,* 35, 409, 1975.

790. **Calvo, R., Carlos, R., and Erill, S.,** Underestimation of albumin content by bromcresol green induced by drug displacer and uraemia. *Int. J. Clin. Pharmacol. Ther. Toxicol.,* 23, 76, 1985.

791. **Beng, C. G. and Lim, L. L.,** An improved automated method for determination of serum albumin using bromcresol green. *Am. J. Clin. Pathol.,* 59, 14, 1973.

792. **Bonvicini, P., et al.,** Heparin interferes with albumin determination by dye-binding methods. *Clin. Chem.,* 25, 1459, 1979.

793. **Perry, P. W. and Doumas, B. T.,** Effect of heparin on albumin determination by dye-binding methods. *Clin. Chem.,* 25, 1520, 1979.

794. **Hill, P. G. and Wells, T. N. G.,** Bromcresol purple and the measurement of albumin. Falsely high plasma albumin concentrations eliminated by increased ionic strength. *Ann. Clin. Biochem.,* 20, 264, 1983.

795. **Werner, M., Tolls, R. E., and Hultin, J. V.,** Influence of sex and age on the normal range of eleven serum constituents. *Z. Klin. Chem. Klin. Biochem.,* 8, 105, 1970.

796. **Steinmetz, J., et al.,** in *Reference Values in Human Chemistry,* Siest, G., Ed., S. Karger, Basel, 1973, 193.

797. **Lyngbye, J. and Krøll, J.,** Quantitative immunoelectrophoresis of proteins in serum from a normal population: season, age, and sex related variations. *Clin. Chem.,* 17, 495, 1971.

798. **Lewinski, J.,** *Arch. F.D. Physiol.,* 100, 611, 1903, quoted by Trevorrow, V., et al., *J. Lab. Clin. Med.,* 27, 471, 1941/42.

799. **Reinhold, J. G.,** Total protein, albumin, and globulin. *Stand. Methods Clin. Chem.,* 88, 1, 1953.

800. **Henry, R. J.,** in *Clinical Chemistry. Principles and Technics,* 1st ed., Harper & Row, New York, 1964, 224.

801. **Wooton, I. D. P.,** *Micro Methods in Clinical Chemistry,* 4th ed., J. and A. Churchill, London, 1964, 3.

802. **Richterich, R.,** *Clinical Chemistry Theory and Practice,* translated from the 2nd German ed., Raymand, S. and Wilkinson, J. H., Eds., S. Karger, Basel, 1969, 249.

803. **Henry, R. J., Cannon, J. C., and Winkleman, J. W.,** in *Clinical Chemistry Principles and Technics,* 2nd ed., Harper & Row, New York, 1974, 455.

804. **Haas, R. G.,** in *Paediatric Clinical Chemistry Reference (Normal Values),* 3rd ed., American Association of Clinical Chemists, Washington, D.C., 1989, 38.

805. **Karrlsson, B., et al.,** Postnatal changes of alpha-foetoprotein, albumin and total protein in human serum. *Acta Paediatr. Scand.,* 61, 133, 1972.

806. **Fleetwood, J. A., Reading, R. F., and Ellis, R. D.,** in *Paediatric Clinical Chemistry Reference (Normal Values),* 3rd ed., American Association of Clinical Chemists, Washington, D.C., 1989, 41.

807. **Wingerd, J. and Sponzilli, E.,** Concentration of serum protein fractions in white women. Effect of age weight tonsillectomy and other factors. *Clin. Chem.,* 23, 1310, 1977.

808. **Das, I.,** Raised C-reactive protein levels in serum from smokers. *Clin. Chim. Acta,* 153, 9, 1985.

809. **Settlage, D. F., et al.,** A quantitative analysis of serum proteins during treatment with oral contraceptive steroids. *Contraception,* 1, 101, 1970.

810. **Briggs, M. H. and Briggs, M.,** Effects of oral ethinylestradiol on serum proteins in normal women. *Contraception,* 3, 381, 1971.

811. **Jelic-Ivanovac, Z., et al.,** Effects of some anti-inflammatory drugs on 12 blood constituents: protocol for the study of in vivo effects of drugs. *Clin. Chem.,* 31, 1141, 1985.

812. **Stringer, M. D., Steadmen, C. A., and Kakkar, V. V.,** Gemfibrozil in hyperlipidaemic patients with peripheral arterial disease: some undisclosed action. *Curr. Med. Res. Opin.,* 12, 207, 1990.

813. **Gilbert, A. and Hersher M.,** Sur les variations de la cholemie physiologique. *La Presse Medicale,* 27, 209, 1906.

814. **van den Bergh, A. A. H. and Snapper, J.,** Die Farbstoffe des Blutserums. *Dtch. Arch. Klin. Med.,* 113, 540, 1913, quoted by Koch, T. R. and Do, B. T., *Sel. Methods Clin. Chem.,* 9, 113, 1982.

815. **Winkelman, J., Cannon, D. C., and Jacobs, S. L.,** in *Clinical Chemistry — Principles and Technics,* 2nd ed., Henry, R. J., Cannon, D. C., and Winkelman, J. W., Harper & Row, New York, 1974, 1043.

816. **Billing, B. H., Haslam, R., and Wald, N.,** Tech. Bull. No. 22. Bilirubin standards and the determination of bilirubin by manual and Technicon Autoanalyser methods. *Ann. Clin. Biochem.,* 8, 21, 1971.
817. **Jendrassik, L. and Gróf, P.,** Vereinfachte Photometrishe Methoden sur Bestimmdag des Blutbilirubin. *Biochem. Z.,* 297, 81, 1938.
818. **Michäelson, M.,** Bilirubin determination in serum and urine. *Scand. J. Clin. Lab. Invest.,* 13 (Suppl.), 56, 1961.
819. **Michäelson, M., Nosslin, B., and Sjohn, S.,** Plasma bilirubin determination in the new born infant. *Paediatrics,* 35, 925, 1965.
820. **Turnell, D.,** The calibration of total bilirubin assays. *Ann. Clin. Biochem.,* 22, 217, 1985.
821. **Meites, S. and Hogg, C. K.,** Direct spectrophotometry of total serum bilirubin in the newborn. *Clin. Chem.,* 6, 421, 1960.
822. **Henry, R. J.,** in *Clinical Chemistry — Principles and Technics,* 1st ed., Harper & Row, New York, 1964, 591.
823. **Wells, F. E.,** in *"Varleys" Practical Clinical Biochemistry,* 6th ed., Gowenlock, A. L. Eds., William Heinemann Medical Books, London, 1988, 720.
824. **Fraser, C. G.,** *Interpretation of Clinical Chemistry Data,* Blackwell Scientific, Oxford, 1986.
825. **Blijenberg, B. G., et al.,** Surveys of neonatal bilirubin. An evaluation. *J. Clin. Chem. Clin. Biochem.,* 22, 609, 1984.
826. **Engel, M.,** Eine Methode zur Quantitatisen Bestimmung des Bilirubins im Vollblut undim Hämoglobonhaltigen Plasma und Serum. *Z. Physiol. Chem.,* 259, 75, 1939.
827. **Watson, D.,** A note on the haemoglobin error in some non-precipitation diazo-methods for bilirubin determination. *Clin. Chim. Acta,* 5, 613, 1960.
828. **Powell, W. N.,** A method for the quantitative determination of serum bilirubin with the photoelectric colorimeter. *Am. J. Clin. Pathol.,* (Technical Section, Vol. 1), 8, 55, 1944.
829. **Sims, F. M. and Horn, C.,** Some observations on Powell's method for the determination of serum bilirubin. *Am. J. Clin. Pathol.,* 29, 412, 1958.
830. **Lathe, G. H. and Ruthven, C. R. J.,** Factors affecting the rate of coupling of bilirubin in the Van den Bergh reaction. *J. Clin. Pathol.,* 11, 155, 1958.
831. **Laurence, K. M. and Abbott, A. L.,** A micromethod for the estimation of serum bilirubin. *J. Clin. Pathol.,* 9, 270, 1956.
832. **Schull-Lees, H. and Li P. K.,** Mechanism of interference by haemoglobin in the determination of total bilirubin. I. Method of Malloy-Evelyn. *Clin. Chem.,* 26, 22, 1980.
833. **Andrewes, C. H.,** An unexplained diazo-colour reaction in uraemic sera. *Lancet,* i, 590, 1924.
834. **Harrison, G. A. and Bromfield, R. J.,** The cause of Andrewe's diazo test for renal insufficiency. *Biochem. J.,* 22, 43, 1928.
835. **Stone, W. J., McKinney, T., and Warnock, L. G.,** Spurious hyperbilirubinaemia in ureamic patients on propanolol therapy. *Clin. Chem.,* 25, 1761, 1979.
836. **Crowley, L. V.,** Interference with certain chemical analyses caused by dextran. *Am. J. Clin. Pathol.,* 51, 425, 1969.
837. **Notler, D.,** in *Interpretation of Clinical Laboratory Tests,* Siest, G., et al., Eds., Biomedical Publishers, Foster City, CA, 1985, 151.
838. **Cremer, R. J., Perryman, P. W., and Richards, D. H.,** Influence of light on the hyperbilirubinaemia of infants. *Lancet,* i, 1094, 1958.
839. **Gilbert, A. and Herscher, M.,** Sur la teneur de sang normal en bilirubin. *Compt. Rend. Soc. Biol. (Paris),* 58, 899, 1905.
840. **Broun, G. O., et al.,** Blood pigments in pernicious anaemia. *J. Clin. Invest.,* 1, 295, 1925.
841. **Perkin, F. S.,** Blood bilirubin. Estimation and clinical significance. *Arch. Int. Med.,* 40, 195, 1927.
842. **Felscher, B. F., Rickard, D., and Redeker, A. G.,** The reciprocal relation between calorie intake and the degree of hyperbilirubinaemia in Gilbert's syndrome. *N. Engl. J. Med.,* 283, 170, 1970.
843. **Owens, D. and Sherlock, S.,** Diagnosis of Gilbert's syndrome: role of reduced calorie intake test. *Br. Med. J.,* 3, 559, 1973.
844. **Dawson, J., et al.,** Gilbert's syndrome: evidence of morphological heterogenicity. *Gut,* 20, 848, 1979.
845. **Gollan, J. L., Bateman, C., and Billing, B. H.,** Effect of dietary composition on the unconjugated hyperbilirubinaemia of Gilbert's syndrome. *Gut,* 17, 335, 1976.
846. **Broderson, R., Flodgaard, H., and Jacobson, J.,** Periodical weekly variation of serum bilirubin concentration in women. *Scand. J. Clin. Lab. Invest.,* 24, 227, 1969.
847. **Werner, M., et al.,** Influence of sex and age on the normal range of eleven serum constituents. *Z. Klin. Chem. Klin. Biochem.,* 8, 105, 1970.
848. **Rosenthal, P., Pincus, M., and Fink, D.,** Sex- and age-related differences in bilirubin concentrations in serum. *Clin. Chem.,* 30, 1380, 1984.
849. **Vaughan, J. M. and Haslewood, G. A. D.,** The normal level of plasma bilirubin. *Lancet,* 31, 920, 1937.
850. **Bailey, A., Robinson, D., and Dawson, A. M.,** Does Gilbert's disease exist? *Lancet,* i, 931, 1977.
851. **Owens, D. and Evans, J.,** Population studies on Gilbert's syndrome. *J. Med. Genet.,* 12, 152, 1975.

852. **Morrison, B., et al.,** Intra-individual variation in commonly analysed constituents. *Clin. Chem.,* 25, 1799, 1979.

853. **Haas, R. G.,** in *Paediatric Clinical Chemistry Reference (Normal) Values,* 3rd ed., Meites, S., Ed., AACC Press, Washington, DC, 1989, 69.

854. **Clayton, B. E., Jenkins, P., and Round, J. M.,** in *Paediatric Chemical Pathology,* Blackwell Scientific, Oxford, 1980, 38.

855. **Meites, S.,** Bilirubin, direct reacting and total, modified Malloy-Evelyn method, *Sel. Methods Clin. Chem.,* 9, 122, 1982.

856. **Anttolainen, I., Simila, G., and Wallgren, E. I.,** Effect of seasonal variation in daylight on bilirubin level in premature infants. *Arch. Dis. Child.,* 50, 156, 1975.

857. **Malageau, P.,** in *Reference Values in Human Chemistry,* S. Karger, Basel, 1973, 13.

858. **Nosslin, B.,** The direct diazo reaction of bile pigments in serum. Experimental and clinical studies. *Scand. J. Clin. Invest.,* 12 (Suppl. 49), 160, 1960.

859. **Davidson, A. R., et al.,** Reduced calorie intake and nicotinic acid provocation tests in the diagnosis of Gilbert's syndrome. *Br. Med. J.,* 2, 480, 1975.

860. **Sutherland, J. M. and Keller, W. H.,** Novobiocin and neonatal hyperbilirubinaemia. *Am. J. Dis. Child.,* 101, 447, 1961.

861. **Hargreaves, T. and Holton, B.,** Jaundice of the newborn due to novobiocin. *Lancet,* i, 839, 1962.

862. **Finland, M. and Nichols, R. L.,** Current therapeutics CXIV Novobiocin. *Practitioner,* 179, 84, 1957.

863. **Fekerty, F. R.,** Gastrointestinal complications of antibiotic therapy. *JAMA,* 203, 210, 1968.

864. **Johnson, W. J.,** in *Renal Function Tests,* Duarte, C. G., Ed., Little, Brown, Boston, 1980, 90.

865. **Strauss, H.,** *Die chronischen Nierenentzündungen,* Berlin, 1902, referred to by Möller, E., McIntosch, J. F., and Van Slyke, D. D., *J. Clin. Invest.,* 61, 427, 1928.

866. **Widal, F. and Javel, A.,** *Compt. Rend. Soc. Biol.,* ivii, 301, 1904, referred to by Möller, E., McIntosch, J. F., and Van Slyke, D. D., *J. Clin. Invest.,* 61, 427, 1928.

867. **DiGordio, J.,** in *Clinical Chemistry. Principles and Technics,* Henry, R. J., Cannon, D. C., and Winkelman, J. W., Eds., Harper & Row, New York, 1974, 504.

868. **Taylor, A. J. and Vadgama, P.,** Analytical reviews in clinical biochemistry: the estimation of urea. *Ann. Clin. Biochem.,* 29, 245, 1992.

869. **Marshall, E. K., Jr.,** A new method for the determination of urea in blood, *J. Biol. Chem.,* 15, 487, 1913.

870. **Conway, E. J.,** An absorption apparatus for the microdetermination of certain volatile substances. I. The microdermination of ammonia. *Biochem. J.,* 27, 430, 1933.

871. **Fawcett, J. K. and Scott, J. E.,** A rapid and precise method for the determination of urea. *J. Clin. Pathol.,* 13, 156, 1960.

872. **Schales, O.,** Urea nitrogen. *Stand. Methods Clin. Chem.,* 1, 118, 1953.

873. **Sampson, E. J. and Baird, M. A.,** Chemical inhibition used as a kinetic urease/glutamate dehydrogenase method for urea in serum. *Clin. Chem.,* 25, 1721, 1979.

874. **Lespinas, F., et al.,** Enzymic urea assay; a new colorimetric method based on hydrogen peroxide measurement. *Clin. Chem.,* 35, 654, 1989.

875. **Fearon, W. R.,** The carbamide diacetyl reaction: a test for citrulline. *Biochem. J.,* 33, 902, 1939.

876. **Haslam, R. H.,** Tech. Bull. No. 9, Assoc. of Clinical Biochemists, London, 1966.

877. **Morin, L. G. and Prox, J.,** An improved diacetyl aminobenzaldehyde procedure for determining urea. *Clin. Chim. Acta,* 47, 27, 1973.

878. **Jung, D., et al.,** New colorimetric reaction for end-point, continuous flow, and kinetic measurement of urea. *Clin. Chem.,* 21, 1721, 1975.

879. **Peters, J. P. and Van Slyke, D. D.,** in *Quantitative Clinical Chemistry, Vol. 2, Methods,* Bailliere Tyndall, London, 1932, 357.

880. **Sampson, E. J., et al.,** A coupled-enzyme equilibrium method for measuring urea in serum. Optimization and evaluation of the AACC Study Group on Urea. Candidate reference method. *Clin. Chem.,* 26, 816, 1980.

881. **Marsh, W. H., Fingerhut, B., and Kirsch, E.,** Determination of urea nitrogen with the diacetyl method and an automatic dialysis apparatus. *Am. J. Clin. Pathol.,* 28, 681, 1957.

882. **Zilva, J. F. and London, D. R.,** Blood urea estimation in uraemia. *Lancet,* ii, 730, 1962.

883. **Searcy, R. L., et al.,** Blood-urea estimation in uraemia. *Lancet,* ii, 1114, 1962.

884. **Hall, S. M. and Preston, I. W.,** The effect of the patients acid-base balance on azostix strip estimation of blood urea. *Ann. Clin. Biochem.,* 9, 208, 1972.

885. **Fales, F. W.,** Urea in serum. Direct diacetyl monoxime method. *Sel. Methods Clin. Chem.,* 9, 365, 1982.

886. **Shull, B., Cheng, C.-S., and Rahill, W. J.,** Effect of haemolysis on values obtained for urea nitrogen in plasma. *Clin. Chem.,* 19, 1226, 1973.

887. **Lequang, N. T., et al.,** Improved dye procedure for determining urea concentration by using *o*-phthaldehyde and naphthyethylene diamine. *Clin. Chem.,* 33, 192, 1987.

888. **Kaplan, A.,** Urea nitrogen and urinary ammonia. *Sel. Methods Clin. Chem.,* 5, 245, 1965.

889. **Addis, T.,** An error in the urease method for the determination of urea. *Proc. Soc. Exp. Biol. Med.,* 25, 365, 1928.

890. **Addis, T., et al.,** The relation between the serum urea concentration and the protein consumption of normal individuals. *J. Clin. Invest.,* 26, 869, 1947.

891. **King, E. J. and Allott, E. N.,** in *Recent Advances in Clinical Pathology,* 1st ed., Dyke, S. C., Ed., J. and A. Churchill, London, 1947, 215.

892. **Sunderman, F. W., Jr.,** Drug interference in clinical biochemistry. *Crit. Rev. Clin. Lab. Sci.,* 1, 417, 1970.

893. **Kaplan, A. and Teng, L. L.,** Urea in serum, urease-Bertholet method. *Sel. Methods Clin. Chem.,* 9, 357, 1982.

894. **Wooton, I. D. P.,** in *Micro Analysis in Medical Biochemistry,* 4th ed., J. and A. Churchill, London, 1964, 90.

895. **Bolleter, W. T., Bushman, C. J., and Tidwell, P. W.,** Spectrophotometric determination of ammonia as indophenol. *Anal. Chem.,* 33, 592, 1961.

896. **Levitt, P. E., Jones, R., and Samuell, C. T.,** Positive interference by cotrimoxazole in the *o*-phthaldehyde method for plasma urea, in *Proc. ACB National Meeting,* Association of Clinical Biochemists, London, 1991, 97.

897. **Wu, H.,** Separate analysis of the corpuscles and the plasma. *J. Biol. Chem.,* 51, 22, 1922.

898. **Ralls, J. O.,** Urea is not equally distributed between the water of the blood cells and that of the plasma. *J. Biol. Chem.,* 151, 529, 1943.

899. **Sacre, M. and Walker, G.,** Measurement of blood glucose level. *Lancet,* i, 1034, 1968.

900. **Dagnall, P., Fackerell, R., and Weston, P.,** Measurement of blood glucose levels. *Lancet,* i, 860, 1968.

901. **Keyser, J. W. and Walters, W. E.,** Measurement of blood-glucose and blood-urea. *Lancet,* ii, 50, 1968.

902. **MacKay, E. M. and MacKay, L. L.,** The concentration of urea in the blood of normal individuals. *J. Clin. Invest.,* 4, 295, 1927.

903. **Haralambie, G.,** in *Reference Values in Human Chemistry,* Siest, G., Ed., S. Karger, Basel, 1973, 249.

904. **Statland, B. E., Winkel, P., and Shaper, A. G.,** Factors contributing to intra-individual variation of serum constituents. I. Within day variation of serum constituents in healthy subjects. *Clin. Chem.,* 19, 1374, 1973.

905. **Lellough, J. and Claude, J. R.,** in *Reference Values in Human Chemistry,* Siest, G., Ed., S. Karger, Basel, 1973, 100.

906. **Tazi, A. and Bagrel, A.,** in *Interpretation of Clinical Laboratory Tests,* Siest, G., et al., Eds., Biomedical Publishers, Foster City, CA, 1985, 451.

907. **Lewis, W. H. and Alving, A. S.,** Changes with age of the renal function in adult men *Amer. J. Physiol.,* 123, 500, 1938.

908. **Pryce, W. H. and Wooton, I. D. P.,** Population Studies in Clinical Biochemistry *Proc. Ass. Clin. Biochem.,* 3, 62, 1964.

909. **Tietz, N. W.,** in *Fundamentals of Clinical Chemistry,* W. B. Saunders, 1970.

910. **Kaplan, L. A. and Pesce, A. J.,** in *Clinical Chemistry Theory Analysis and Correlation* 1st edit. pub C.V. Mosby St. Louis 1984.

911. **Fraser, C. G.,** Desirable performance standards for clinical chemistry tests *Adv. Clin. Chem.,* 23, 300, 1983.

912. **Josephson, B., Fürst, P., and Järnmark, O.,** Age variation in the concentration of nonprotein nitrogen, creatinine and urea in blood of infants and children *Acta Paed. Scand.* Suppl., 135, 111, 1962.

913. **Appleton, C.,** in *Paediatric Clinical Chemistry. Reference (Normal) Values,* 3rd ed., Meites, S., Ed., Washington, AACC Press, 1989, 278.

914. **Haas, R. G.,** in *Paediatric Clinical Chemistry Reference (Normal) Values,* 3rd ed., Meites, S., Ed., AACC Press, Washington, D.C., 1989, 279.

915. **McCance, R. A. and Widdowson, E. M.,** Blood urea in the first nine days of life. *Lancet,* i, 707, 1947.

916. **Pincus, J. B., et al.,** A study of plasma values of sodium, potassium, chloride, carbon dioxide, carbon dioxide tension, sugar, urea and the protein base-binding power, pH and haematocrit in prematures in the first day of life. *Paediatrics,* 18, 39, 1956.

917. **Thomas, J. L. and Reichelderfer, T. E.,** Premature infants. Analysis of serum during the first seven weeks. *Clin. Chem.,* 22, 272, 1968.

918. **Slemon, M. and Morriss, W.,** The nonprotein nitrogen and urea in the maternal and the fetal blood at the time of birth. *Bull. Johns Hopkins Hosp.,* 27, 343, 1916.

919. **Bunker, C. W. O. and Mundell, J. J.,** The value of blood chemistry in pregnancy. *JAMA,* 83, 836, 1924.

920. **Peters, J. P. and Van Slyke, D. D.,** in *Quantitative Clinical Chemistry Vol. 1, Interpretations,* 1st ed., Bailliere Tyndall, London, 1932, 288.

921. **Peters, J. P. and Van Slyke, D. D.,** in *Quantitative Clinical Chemistry Vol. 1, Interpretations,* 2nd ed., Bailliere Tyndall, London, 1946, 666.

922. **Sims, E. A. H. and Krantz, K. E.,** Serial studies of renal function during pregnancy and the puerperium in normal women. *J. Clin. Invest.,* 37, 1764, 1958.

923. **Elliot, J. F. and O'Kell, R. T. O.,** Normal clinical chemistry values for pregnant women at term. *Clin. Chem.,* 17, 156, 1971.

924. **Lellough, J., et al.,** The relationships between smoking and levels of serum urea and uric acid. *J. Chr. Dis.,* 22, 9, 1969.

925. **Spencer, K.,** Analytical reviews in clinical chemistry: the estimation of creatinine. *Ann. Clin. Biochem.,* 23, 1, 1986.

926. **Cook, J. G. H.,** Tech. Bull. No. 36. Factors influencing the assay of creatinine. *Ann. Clin. Biochem.,* 12, 219, 1975.

927. **Narayanan, S. and Appleton, H. D.,** Creatinine: a review. *Clin. Chem.,* 26, 1119, 1980.

928. **McLaughlan, D. M.,** in *"Varleys" Practical Clinical Biochemistry,* 6th ed., Gowenlock, A. L., Ed., William Heinemann Medical Books, London, 1988, 350.

929. **Jaffé, M.,** Ueber den Niederschlag welchen Picrinsäure in Normalen Harn erzeugt und über eine neue Reaction des Kreatinins, *Z. Physiol. Chem.,* 10, 391, 1886, referred to by Cook, J. G. H., *Ann. Clin. Biochem.,* 12, 319, 1975.

930. **Folin, O.,** On the determination of creatinine and creatine in blood milk and tissues. *J. Biol. Chem.,* 17, 475, 1914.

931. **Owen, J. A., et al.,** The determination of creatinine in plasma or serum and in urine: a critical examination. *Biochem. J.,* 58, 426, 1954.

932. **Masson, P., Ohlsson, P., and Björkhem, I.,** Combined enzymeic-Jaffé method for determination of creatinine in serum. *Clin. Chem.,* 27, 18, 1981.

933. **Miller, B. F. and Dubos, R.,** Determination by a specific enzymatic method of the creatinine content of blood and urine from normal and nephrotic individuals. *J. Biol. Chem.,* 121, 457, 1937.

934. **Janes, P. K., Feld, R. D., and Johnson, G. F.,** An enzymic reaction-rate assay for serum creatinine with a centrifugal analyser. *Clin. Chem.,* 28, 114, 1982.

935. **Fossati, P., Prencipe, L., and Berti, G.,** Enzymic creatinine assay: a new colorimetric method based on hydrogen peroxide measurement. *Clin. Chem.,* 29, 1494, 1983.

936. **Tanganelli, E., et al.,** Enzymic assay of creatinine in serum and urine with creatinine imino-hydrolase and glutamate dehydrogenase. *Clin. Chem.,* 28, 1461, 1982.

937. **Sugita, O., et al.,** Reference values of serum and urine creatinine and of creatinine clearance by a new enzymic method. *Ann. Clin. Biochem.,* 29, 523, 1992.

938. **Rosano, T. G., et al.,** Candidate reference method for determining creatinine in serum: method development and interlaboratory validation. *Clin. Chem.,* 36, 1951, 1990.

939. **Börner, V., et al.,** Referenzwer für Kreatinin im Serum ermittert mit einer spezifischen enzymatischen Methode. *J. Clin. Chem. Clin. Biochem.,* 17, 679, 1979.

940. **Chasson, A. L., Grady, H. J., and Stanley, M. A.,** Determination of creatinine by means of automatic chemical analysis. *Am. J. Clin. Pathol.,* 35, 83, 1961.

941. **DiGorgio, J.,** in *Clinical Chemistry Principles and Technics,* 2nd ed., Henry, R. J., Cannon, D. C., and Winkleman, J. W., Eds., Harper & Row, New York, 1974, 550.

942. **Tausskey, H. H.,** A procedure increasing the specificity of the Jaffé reaction for the determination of creatine and creatinine in urine and plasma. *Clin. Chim. Acta,* 1, 210, 1956.

943. **Munz, E., Bernt, E., and Wahlefeld, A. W.,** An evaluation of a fully enzymatic method for creatinine. *Z. Klin. Chem. Klin. Biochem.,* 12, 259, 1974.

944. **Weber, J. A. and Van Zanten, A. P.,** Interferences in current methods for measurement of creatinine. *Clin. Chem.,* 37, 695, 1991.

945. **Lustgarten, J. A. and Wenk, R. E.,** Simple rapid kinetic method for serum creatinine measurement. *Clin. Chem.,* 18, 1419, 1972.

946. **Knight, D. R. and Trainer, T. D.,** Negligible effect of bilirubin on serum creatinine measurement by the kinetic-Jaffé method. *Clin. Chem.,* 24, 1851, 1978.

947. **Daugherty, N. A., Hammond, K. B., and Osberg, I. M.,** Bilirubin interference with the kinetic-Jaffé method for serum creatinine. *Clin. Chem.,* 24, 392, 1978.

948. **Dorwart, W. V.,** Bilirubin interference in kinetic creatinine determination. *Clin. Chem.,* 25, 196, 1979.

949. **Soldin, S. J., Henderson, L., and Hill, J. G.,** The effect of bilirubin and ketones on reaction rate methods for the measurement of creatinine. *Clin. Biochem.,* 11, 82, 1978.

950. **Knapp, M. L. and Hadid, O.,** Investigations into negative interference by jaundiced plasma in kinetic Jaffé method for plasma creatinine determination. *Ann. Clin. Biochem.,* 24, 85, 1987.

951. **Osberg, I. M. and Hammond, K. B.,** A Solution to the problem of bilirubin interference with the kinetic Jaffé method for serum creatinine. *Clin. Chem.,* 24, 1196, 1978.

952. **Scott, P. H.,** Measurement of plasma creatinine in the newborn. *Proc. Assoc. of Clinical Biochemists National Meet., Glasgow, U.K. May 13–17, 1991,* Association of Clinical Biochemists, London, 1991, 113.

953. **Aberhalden, E. and Kanen, E.,** Uber die Anhydridstrukter des Proteine. *Hoppe-Seylers Zeitschrift für Physiolosche Chimie,* 139, 181, 1924.

954. **de Haan, J. B.,** Creatinine in serum and plasma. Direct microdetermination by kinetics. *Anal. Lett.,* 5, 815, 1972.

955. **Price, C. P. and Spencer, K.,** in *Methods in Laboratory Medicine, Vol. 1, Centrifugal Analysers in Clinical Chemistry,* Praeger, New York, 1980, 237.

956. **Jaynes, P. K., et al.,** Interference of some monoclonal IgMs in discrete serum creatinine analysis. *Clin. Chem.,* 28, 1580, 1982.

957. **Datta, P., Graham, G., and Schoen, I.,** A paraprotein phenomenon evidenced by interference with creatinine determination in sera of multiple myeloma patients. *Clin. Chem.,* 30, 968, 1984.

958. **Fabini, D. L. and Ertingshausen, G.,** Automated reaction-rate method for determination of serum creatinine with the Centrifichem. *Clin. Chem.,* 17, 696, 1971.

959. **Blass, K. G. and Ng, D. S. K.,** Reactivity of aceto acetate with alkaline picrate: an interference of the Jaffé reaction. *Clin. Biochem.,* 21, 39, 1988.

960. **Larsen, K.,** Creatinine assay by a reaction-kinetic principle. *Clin. Chim. Acta,* 41, 209, 1972.

961. **Baba, S. and Baba, T.,** Iwanaga effect of acetohexamide (a sulphonylurea hypoglycaemic agent) in blood plasma on creatinine assay in clinical laboratory tests. *Chem. Pharm. Bull. (Tokyo),* 27, 139, 1979.

962. **Roach, N. A., Kroll, M. H., and Elin, R. J.,** Interference with sulphonylurea drugs with the Jaffé method for creatinine. *Clin. Chim. Acta,* 151, 301, 1985.

963. **Van Steirteghem, A. C., Robertson, E. A., and Young, D. S.,** Influence of large doses of ascorbic acid on laboratory test results. *Clin. Chem.,* 24, 54, 1978.

964. **Tillson, E. K. and Schuchatdt, G. S.,** The determination of creatinine in plasma and urine in the presence of large amounts of phenol red. *J. Lab. Clin. Med.,* 41, 312, 1953.

965. **Swain, R. R. and Briggs, S. L.,** Positive interference with the Jaffé reaction by cephalosporin antibiotics. *Clin. Chem.,* 23, 1340, 1977.

966. **Saah, A. J., Koch, T. R., and Drusano, G. L.,** Cefoxitin falsely elevates creatinine levels. *JAMA,* 247, 205, 1982.

967. **Bruns, D. E.,** Lactulose interference in the alkaline picrate assay for creatinine. *Clin. Chem.,* 34, 2592, 1988.

968. **Maddocks, J., et al.,** Effect of methyl dopa on creatinine estimation. *Lancet,* i, 157, 1973.

969. **De Leacy-Brown, N. N. and Claque, A. E.,** Nitromethane interferes in assay of creatinine by the Jaffé reaction. *Clin. Chem.,* 35, 1772, 1989.

970. **Kroll, M. H., Nealon, L., and Vogel, M. A.,** How certain drugs interfere negatively with the Jaffé reaction for creatinine. *Clin. Chem.,* 31, 306, 198.

971. **Sundberg, M. W., et al.,** An enzymic creatinine assay and a direct ammonia assay in coated thin films. *Clin. Chem.,* 29, 645, 1983.

972. **Couttie, K., Earle, J., and Coakley, J.,** Evaluation of single-slide creatinine method with Kodak Ectochem 700 shows positive interference from lignocaine metabolites. *Clin. Chem.,* 33, 1674, 1987.

973. **Roberts, R. T., Alexander, N. M., and Keiner, M. J.,** Definitive liquid-chromatographic demonstration that *N*-ethyl glycine is the metabolite of lidocaine that interferes in the Kodak sarcosine-oxidase-coupled method for creatinine. *Clin. Chem.,* 34, 2569, 1988.

974. **Kenny, D.,** A study of interferences in routine methods for creatinine measurement. *Scand. J. Clin. Lab. Invest.,* 53 (Suppl. 212), 43, 1993.

975. **Pearce, C. J. and Bosomworth, M. P.,** Storage of heparinised blood. *Ann. Clin. Biochem.,* 28, 112, 1991.

976. **Laessig, R. H., et al.,** Changes in serum chemical values as a result of prolonged contact with the clot. *Am. J. Clin. Pathol.,* 66, 598, 1976.

977. **Rehak, N. N. and Chiang, B. T.,** Storage of whole blood: effect of temperature on the measured concentration of analytes in serum. *Clin. Chem.,* 34, 2111, 1988.

978. **Simpson, W. G.,** Plasma creatinine and the effect of delay in separation of samples. *Ann. Clin. Biochem.,* 29, 307, 1992.

979. **Harrison, S. P.,** Delay in separation of blood samples. *Ann. Clin. Biochem.,* 30, 108, 1993.

980. **Rapoport, A. and Husdan, H.,** Endogenous creatinine clearance and serum creatinine in the clinical assessment of kidney function. *Can. Med. Assoc. J.,* 99, 149, 1968.

981. **Pasternak, A. and Kuhlbäck, B.,** Diurnal variation of serum and urine creatine and creatinine. *Scand. J. Lab. Clin. Invest.,* 27, 1, 1971.

982. **Camera, A. A., et al.,** The twenty-four hourly endogenous creatinine clearance as a clinical measure of the functional state of the kidneys. *J. Lab. Clin. Med.,* 37, 743, 1951.

983. **Jacobson, F. K., et al.,** Pronounced increase in serum creatinine concentration after eating cooked meat. *Br. Med. J.,* 1, 1049, 1979.

984. **Houet, O.,** in *Interpretation of Clinical Laboratory Tests,* Siest, G., Ed., Biomedical Publishers, Foster City, CA, 1985, 231.

985. **Gettler, A. O. and St. George, A. V.,** The value of modern blood chemistry to the clinician. *JAMA,* 17, 2033, 1918.

986. **Plass, E. D.,** Placental transmission: creatinine and creatine in the whole blood and plasma of mother and foetus. *Bull. Johns Hopkins Hosp.,* 28, 137, 1917.

987. **Gardner, M. D. and Scott, R.,** Age and sex related reference ranges for eight plasma constituents derived from randomly selected adults in a Scottish new town. *J. Clin. Pathol.,* 33, 380, 1980.

988. **Tobias, G. J., et al.,** Endogenous creatinine clearance. A valuable clinical test of glomerular filtration and a prognostic guide in chronic renal disease, *N. Engl. J. Med.,* 266, 317, 1962.

989. **Savoury, D. J.,** Reference ranges for serum creatinine in infants children and adolescents. *Ann. Clin. Biochem.,* 27, 99, 1990.

990. **Haas, R. G.,** in *Paediatric Clinical Chemistry Reference (Normal Values),* Meites, S., Ed., American Association of Clinical Chemists, Washington, D.C., 1989, 110.

991. **Donckerwolcke, R. A. M. G., et al.,** Serum creatinine values in healthy children. *Acta Paediatr. Scand.,* 59, 399, 1970.

992. **Schwartz, G. J., Hancock, G. B., and Spitzer, A.,** Plasma creatinine and urea concentrations in children: normal values for age and sex. *J. Paediatr.,* 88, 828, 1976.

993. **Stonestreet, B. S. and Oh, W.,** Plasma creatinine levels in low-birth-weight infants during the first three months of life. *Paediatrics,* 61, 788, 1978.

994. **Feldman, H. and Guignard, J.-P.,** Plasma creatinine in the first month of life. *Arch. Dis. Child.,* 57, 123, 1982.

995. **Rudd, P. T., Hughes, E. A., and Placzek, M. M.,** Hodses reference ranges for plasma creatinine in the first month of life. *Arch. Dis. Child.,* 58, 212, 1983.

996. **Kuhlbäck, B. and Widholm, O.,** Plasma creatinine in normal pregnancy. *Scand. J. Clin. Lab. Invest.,* 18, 654, 1966.

997. **Perrone, R. D., Madias, N. E., and Levey, A. S.,** Serum creatinine as an index of renal function: new insights into old concepts. *Clin. Chem.,* 38, 1933, 1992.

998. **Bagrel, A., et al.,** in *Drug Effects on Laboratory Test Results,* Siest, G., Ed., Nijhoff, The Hague, 1980, 201.

999. **Wyngaarden, J. B. and Kelley, W. N.,** in *Metabolic Basis of Inherited Disease,* 5th ed., Stanbury, J. S., Ed., McGraw-Hill, New York, 1983, 917.

1000. **Folin, O. and Denis, W.,** A new (colorimetric) method for the determination of uric acid in blood. *J. Biol. Chem.,* 11, 265, 1912.

1001. **Benedict, S. R. and Hitchcock, E. H.,** On the colorimetric estimation of uric acid in urine. *J. Biol. Chem.,* 20, 619, 1915.

1002. **Benedict, S. R.,** The determination of uric acid. *J. Biol. Chem.,* 51, 187, 1922.

1003. **Watts, R. W. E.,** Tech. Bull. No. 31, Determination of uric acid in blood and urine. *Ann. Clin. Biochem.,* 11, 103, 1974.

1004. **Natelson, S.,** Uric acid. *Stand. Methods Clin. Chem.,* 1, 123, 1953.

1005. **McLaughlan, D. M.,** in *"Varleys" Practical Clinical Biochemistry,* Gowenlock, A. H., Ed., William Heinemann Medical Books, London, 1988, 356.

1006. **Praetorius, E.,** An enzymatic method for the determination of uric acid by ultra violet spectrophotometry. *Scand. J. Clin. Lab. Invest.,* 1, 222, 1949.

1007. **Duncan, P. H., et al.,** A candidate reference method for uric acid in serum. Optimisation and evaluation. *Clin. Chem.,* 28, 284, 1982.

1008. **Lous, P. and Sylvest, O.,** A comparison of three methods utilising different principles for the determination of uric acid in biological fluids. *Scand. J. Clin. Lab. Invest.,* 6, 40, 1954.

1009. **Alper, C. and Seitchikkern, J.,** Comparison of the Archibald-Kern and Stransky colorimetric procedures and the Praetorius enzymatic procedure for the determination of uric acid. *Clin. Chem.,* 3, 95, 1957.

1010. **Kanabrocki, E. L., et al.,** Comparison of plasma uric acid levels obtained with five different methods. *Clin. Chem.,* 3, 156, 1957.

1011. **Archibald, R. M.,** Colorimetric measurement of uric acid. *Clin. Chem.,* 3, 102, 1957.

1012. **Caraway, W. T. and Marable, H.,** Comparison of carbonate and uricase-carbonate method for the determination of uric acid in serum. *Clin. Chem.,* 12, 18, 1966.

1013. **DiGorgio, J.,** in *Clinical Chemistry Principles and Technics,* 2nd ed., Henry, R. J., Cannon, D. C., Winkleman, J. W., Eds., Harper & Row, New York, 1974, 541.

1014. **James, D. R. and Price, C. P.,** Problems associated with the measurement of uric acid using two enzyme-mediated reaction systems. *Ann. Clin. Biochem.,* 21, 405, 1984.

1015. **Fossati, P., Prencipe, L., and Berti, G.,** Use of 3, 5, dichloro-2-hydroxybenzenesulphonic acid/4-aminophenazone system in direct enzymic assay of uric acid in serum and urine. *Clin. Chem.,* 26, 227, 1980.

1016. **Majkic-Singh, N., et al.,** Evaluation of the enzymatic assay of serum uric acid with 2, 2′-azino-di(3-ethylbenzthiazolino-6-sulphonate) (ABTS) as chromogen. *Ann. Clin. Biochem.,* 21, 504, 1984.

1017. **Kageyama, N.,** A direct colorimetric determination of uric acid in serum and urine with a uricase-catalase system. *Clin. Chem. Acta,* 31, 421, 1971.

1018. **Hullin, D. A. and McGrane, M. T. G.,** Effect of bilirubin on uricase-peroxidase coupled reactions. Implication for urate measurement in clinical samples and external quality control schemes. *Ann. Clin. Biochem.,* 28, 98, 1991.

1019. **Trivedi, R. C., et al.,** New enzymatic method for serum uric acid at 500 nm. *Clin. Chem.,* 24, 1908, 1978.

1020. **Patel, C. P.,** Semimicromethod for determination of serum uric acid using EDTA-hydrazine. *Clin. Chem.,* 14, 764, 1968.

1021. **Potter, J. L.,** Xanthine interference in the Kodak "Ektachem" determination of uric acid. *Clin. Chem.,* 33, 1265, 1987.

1022. **Cawein, M. J. and Hewins, J.,** False rise in serum uric acid after L-dopa. *N. Engl. J. Med.,* 281, 1489, 1969.

1023. **Bierer, D. W. and Quebbermann, A. J.,** Interference of levodopa and its metabolites with colorimetry of uric acid. *Clin. Chem.,* 27, 756, 1981.
1024. **Sanders, G. T. B., Pasman, A. J., and Hoek, F. J.,** Determination of uric acid with uricase and peroxidase. *Clin. Chim. Acta,* 101, 299, 1980.
1025. **Matheke, M. L., Kessler, G., and Chan, K.-M.,** Interference of the chemotherapeutic agent eptopside with the direct phosphotungstate method for uric acid. *Clin. Chem.,* 33, 2109, 1987.
1026. **O'Sullivan, J. B., Francis, J. O., and Kantor, N.,** Comparison of a colorimetric (automated) with an enzymatic (manual) uric acid procedure. *Clin. Chem.,* 11, 427, 1965.
1027. **Brown, R. A. and Freier, E. F.,** Evaluation of an improved automated carbonate procedure for serum urate. *Clin. Biochem.,* 1, 154, 1967.
1028. **Beetham, R. and Sanders, P. G.,** Calibrant solutions for continuous-flow urate analysis: interference by formaldehyde. *Ann. Clin. Biochem.,* 17, 323, 1980.
1029. **Wilding, P. and Heath, D. A.,** Effect of paracetamol on uric acid determination. *Ann. Clin. Biochem.,* 12, 142, 1975.
1030. **Smith, M. and Payne, R. B.,** Re-examination of effect of paracetamol on serum uric acid measured by phosphotungstate reaction. *Ann. Clin. Biochem.,* 16, 96, 1979.
1031. **Caraway, W. T.,** Chemical and diagnostic specificity of laboratory tests. *Am. J. Clin. Pathol.,* 37, 445, 1962.
1032. **Hubsch, G.,** in *Interpretations of Clinical Laboratory Tests,* Siest, G., et al., Biomedical Publishers, Foster City, CA, 1985, 428.
1033. **Folin, O. and Trimble, H.,** A system of blood analysis supplement. V. Improvements in the quantity and method of preparing the uric acid reagent. *J. Biol. Chem.,* 60, 473, 1924.
1034. **Gomolianska, M.,** Decomposition of uric acid in blood. *Biochem. J.,* 22, 1301, 1928.
1035. **Blauch, M. and Koch, F. C.,** Application of the uricase method to the study of changes in vitro in the uric acid content of certain mammalian bloods. *J. Biol. Chem.,* 130, 455, 1939.
1036. **Buchanan, M. J., Isdale, I. C., and Rose, B. S.,** Serum uric acid estimation. Chemical and enzymatic methods compared. *Ann. Rheum. Dis.,* 24, 285, 1965.
1037. **Lennox, W. G.,** A study of the retention of uric acid during fasting. *J. Biol. Chem.,* 66, 521, 1925.
1038. **Hoeffel-Moriaty, M.,** The effect of fasting on the metabolism of epileptic children. *Am. J. Dis. Child.,* 28, 16, 1924.
1039. **Steinmetz, J., et al.,** Influence of food intake on biochemical parameters, in *Reference Values in Human Biochemistry,* Siest, G., Ed., S. Karger, Basel, 1973, 193.
1040. **Seegmiller, J. E., et al.,** Uric acid production in gout. *J. Clin. Invest.,* 40, 1304, 1961.
1041. **Rakestraw, N. W.,** Chemical factors in fatigue. I. The effect of muscular exercise on certain common blood constituents. *J. Biol. Chem.,* 47, 565, 1921.
1042. **Levine, S. A., Gordon, B., and Derick, C. L.,** Some changes in the chemical composition of the blood following a marathon race. *JAMA,* 82, 1778, 1924.
1043. **Nicholls, J., Miller, A. T., and Hiatt, E. P.,** Influence of muscular exercise on uric acid excretion in man. *J. Appl. Physiol.,* 51, 501, 1950.
1044. **Zachau-Christiansen, B.,** The rise in the serum uric acid during muscular exercise. *Scand. J. Clin. Lab. Invest.,* 11, 57, 1959.
1045. **Becker, K. L. and Goldstein, R. A.,** Hyperuricaemia in healthy men: intermittent elevation and the effects of sunlight. *Am. J. Clin. Nutr.,* 25, 453, 1972.
1046. **Newcome, D. S.,** in *Inherited Biochemical Disorders and Uric Acid Metabolism,* H. M. and M. Aylesbury, University Park Press, Baltimore, 1975, 3.
1047. **Wyngaarden, J. B. and Kelley, W. N.,** in *Metabolic Basis of Inherited Disease,* 5th ed., Stanbury, J. S., Ed., McGraw-Hill, New York 1983, 936.
1048. **Hall, A. P., et al.,** Epidemiology of gout and hyperuricaemia. A long term population study. *Am. J. Med.,* 42, 27, 1967.
1049. **Ryckewaert, A.,** Pathogenie de la goutte. *Rev. Franc. Etud. Clin. Biol.,* 11, 664, 1966.
1050. **Prior, I. A., et al.,** Hyperuricaemia gout and diabetic abnormality in Polynesian people. *Lancet,* i, 333, 1966.
1051. **Harlan, W. R., Huntley, J. C., and Leaverton, P. E.,** Physiologic determinants of serum urate levels in adolescence. *Paediatrics,* 63, 569, 1979.
1052. **Griebsch, A. and Zollner, N.,** Plasmaharnsäure in Süddeutchland. Vergleich mit Bestimmungen vor sehr Jahren. *Z. Klin. Chem. Klin. Biochem.,* 11, 348, 1973.
1053. **Pobert, A. J. and Hewitt, J. V.,** Gout and hyperuricaemia in rural and urban populations. *Ann. Rheum. Dis.,* 21, 154, 1962.
1054. **Anon.,** Uric acid and the psyche. *JAMA,* 208, 1180, 1969.
1055. **Takala, J., et al.,** Diuretics and hyperuricaemia in the elderly. *Scand. J. Rheum.,* 17, 155, 1988.
1056. **Mikklesen, W. M., Dodge, H. J., and Valkenburg, H.,** The distribution of serum uric acid values in a population unselected as to gout or hyperuricaemia. *Am. J. Med.,* 39, 242, 1965.

1057. **Haas, R. G.,** in *Paediatric Clinical Chemistry Reference (Normal Values),* Meites, S., Ed., American Association of Clinical Chemists, Washington, D.C., 1989, 284.

1058. **Marks, J. F., et al.,** Uric acid levels in full term and low birth weight infants. *J. Paediatr.,* 73, 609, 1968.

1059. **Monkus, E., et al.,** Concentration of uric acid in the serum of neonatal infants and their mothers. *Am. J. Obstet. Gynecol.,* 108, 91, 1970.

1060. **Peters, J. P. and Van Slyke, D. D.,** in *Qualitative Clinical Chemistry, Vol. 1. Interpretations,* Bailliere Tyndall, London, 1932.

1061. **Harding, V. J., Allin, K. D., and Van Wyck, H. B.,** Nonprotein nitrogen and uric acid values in blood in pregnancy. *J. Obstet. Gynaecol. Br. Emp.,* 31, 595, 1924.

1062. **Boyle, J. A., et al.,** Serum uric acid levels in normal pregnancy with observations on the renal excretion of urate in pregnancy. *J. Clin. Pathol.,* 19, 501, 1966.

1063. **Dunlop, W. and Davison, J. M.,** The effect of normal pregnancy upon the renal handling of uric acid. *Br. J. Obstet. Gynaecol.,* 84, 13, 1977.

1064. **Acheson, R. M. and O'Brien, W. M.,** Dependence of serum-uric-acid on haemoglobin and other factors in the general population. *Lancet,* ii, 777, 1966.

1065. **Acheson, R. M., Florey, C. du V.,** Body weight, ABO blood groups and altitude of domicile as determinants of serum-uric-acid in military recruits in four countries. *Lancet,* ii, 391, 1969.

1066. **Bengtsson, C. and Tibblin, E.,** Serum uric acid levels in women. An epidemiological survey with special reference to women with high uric acid values. *Acta Med. Scand.,* 196, 93, 1974.

1067. **Garrod, A. B.,** in *The Nature and Treatment of Gout and Rheumatic Gout,* Walton and Maberley, 1863, 251, quoted by Wyngaarden, J. B. and Kelley, W. N., *Metabolic Basis of Inherited Disease,* 5th ed., Stanbury, J. S., Ed., McGraw-Hill, New York, 1983, 983.

1068. **Lieber, C. S., et al.,** Interrelation of uric acid and ethanol metabolism in man. *J. Clin. Invest.,* 41, 1863, 1962.

1069. **Baker, B. M., et al.,** Alcohol consumption and gout. *Med. J. Aust.,* 1, 1213, 1967.

1070. **Newcome, D. S.,** Ethanol metabolism and uric acid. *Metabolism,* 21, 1193, 1972.

1071. **Nicolaier, A. and Dohrn, M.,** Ueber die Wirkung von Chinolincarbosäure und ihrer Derivate auf die Ausscheidung den Harnsäure. *Deut. Arch. Klin. Med.* 93, 331, 1908, quoted by Wyngaarden, J. B. and Kelley, W. N., *Gout and Hyperuricaemia,* Grune and Stratton, New York, 1976.

1072. **Bartels, E. C.,** Allopurinol (xanthine oxidase inhibitor) in the treatment of gout. *JAMA,* 198, 708, 1966.

1073. **Fine, M. S. and Chace, A. F.,** The influence of salicylate upon the uric acid concentration of blood. *J. Biol. Chem.,* 21, 371, 1915.

1074. **Salome, E. G.,** *Med. Jahrb. Wien.,* 1885, p. 463, quoted by Wyngaarden, J. B. and Kelley, W. N., *Gout and Hyperuricaemia,* Grune and Stratton, New York, 1976.

1075. **Graysel, A. I., Liddle, L., and Seegmiller, J. E.,** Diagnostic significance of hyperuricaemia in arthritis. *N. Engl. J. Med.,* 265, 763, 1961.

1076. **Yü, T. F. and Gutman, A. B.,** Study of the paradoxical effects of salicylate in low, intermediate and high dosage on the renal mechanism for excretion of urate in man. *J. Clin. Invest.,* 38, 1298, 1959.

1077. **Dresse, A., et al.,** Uricosuric properties of diflunisal in man. *Br. J. Clin. Pharmacol.,* 7, 267, 1979.

1078. **Meffin, P. J., et al.,** Diflunisal disposition and hypouricaemic response in osteoarthritis. *Clin. Pharmacol. Ther.,* 33, 813, 1983.

1079. **Huskisson, E. C., et al.,** Treatment of rheumatoid arthritis with fenoprofen: comparison with aspirin. *Br. Med. J.,* i, 176, 1974.

1080. **Goldfarb, S., Walker, B. R., and Agus, Z. S.,** The uricosuric effect of oxaprocin in humans. *J. Clin. Pharmacol.,* 25, 144, 1985.

1081. **Broekhuysen, J., et al.,** Effect of oxametacin on endogenous uric acid clearance rate in healthy volunteers. *Eur. J. Clin. Pharmacol.,* 24, 671, 1983.

1082. **Murphy, J. E.,** Piroxican in the treatment of acute gout. A multicentre open study in general practice. *J. Int. Med. Res.,* 7, 517, 1979.

1083. **Gutman, A. B. and Yü, T. F.,** Effects of adrenocorticalhormone (ACTH) in gout. *Am. J. Med.,* 9, 24, 1950.

1084. **Nichols, A., Snaith, M. L., and Scott, J. T.,** Effect of oestrogen therapy on plasma and urinary levels of uric acid. *Br. Med. J.,* i, 449, 1973.

1085. **Albert, M. and Stansell, M. J.,** Vascular symptomatic relief during administration of ethylchlorophenoxy isobutyrate (clifibrate). *Metabolism,* 18, 635, 1969.

1086. **Lisch, H. J., Sailer, S., and Bruansteiner, H.,** Comparison of the effects of halofenate (MK-185) and clofibrate on plasma lipid and uric acid concentration in hyperlipoproteinaemic patients. *Atherosclerosis,* 21, 391, 1975.

1087. **Stringer, M. D., Steadman, C. A., and Kakkar, V. V.,** Gemfibrozil in hyperlipidaemic patients with peripheral arterial disease: some undiscovered actions. *Curr. Med. Res. Opin.,* 12, 207, 1990.

1088. **Stein, H. B., Hasen, A., and Fox, I. H.,** Ascorbic acid-induced uricosuria. *Ann. Int. Med.,* 84, 385, 1976.

1089. **Yü T. F., Berger, L., and Gutman, A. B.,** Hypoglycaemic and uricosuric properties of acetohexamide and hydroxyhexamide. *Metabolism,* 17, 309, 1968.

1090. **Leary, W. P., et al.,** Captopril once daily as monotherapy in patients with hyperuricaemia and essential hypertension. *Lancet,* ii, 156, 1985.
1091. **Sougin-Mibashan, R. and Horwitz, M.,** The uricosuric action of ethyl bis coumacetate. *Lancet,* i, 1191, 1955.
1092. **Thompson, G. R., Mikkelson, W. M., and Willis, P. W., III,** The uricosuric effect of certain oral anticoagulant drugs. *Arthritis Rheum.,* 2, 383, 1959.
1093. **Christensen, F.,** Uricosuric effect of dicoumarol. *Acta Med. Scand.,* 175, 461, 1964.
1094. **Batt, A. M., Siest, G., and Khudjet el Khil, R.,** in *Drug Interference and Drug Measurement in Clinical Chemistry,* Siest, G. and Young, D. S., Eds., S. Karger, Basel, 1976, 33.
1095. **Faris, H. M. and Potts, D. W.,** Aziocillin and serum uric acid. *Ann. Int. Med.,* 98, 414, 1983.
1096. **Malý, J. and Nádvorníková-Schück, O.,** The effect of prednisone and azothiaprine (Imuran) on renal excretion of uric acid. *Int. J. Clin. Pharmacol. Ther. Toxicol.,* 20, 44, 1982.
1097. **Healey, L. A., Harrison, M., and Decker, J. L.,** Uricosuric effect of chlorprothixene. *N. Engl. J. Med.,* 272, 526, 1965.
1098. **Skeith, M. D., Healey, L. A., and Cutler, R. E.,** Urate excretion during mannitol and glucose diuresis. *J. Lab. Clin. Med.,* 70, 213, 1967.
1099. **Yú, T., Kaung, C., and Gutman, A. B.,** Effect of glycine loading on plasma and urinary uric acid and amino acid in normal and gouty subjects. *Am. J. Med.,* 49, 352, 1970.
1100. **Krakoff, I. H.,** Clinical pharmacology of drugs which influence uric acid production and excretion. *Clin. Pharmacol. Ther.,* 8, 124, 1967.
1101. **Dohrn, M.,** Uber die Wirkung des Atophans, mit einem Beitrag zur Theorie der Gicht. *Z. Klin. Med.,* 74, 445, 1912, quoted by Peters, J. P. and Van Slyke, D. D., *Qualitative Clinical Chemistry, Vol 1., Interpretations,* Bailliere Tyndall, London, 1932, 437.
1102. **Steele, T. H.,** Evidence for altered renal urate reabsorption during changes in volume of the extracellular fluid. *J. Lab. Clin. Med.,* 74, 288, 1969.
1103. **Calabresi, P. and Turner, R. W.,** Beneficial effects of triacetyl azauridine in psoriasis and mycosis fungoides. *Ann. Int. Med.,* 64, 352, 1966.
1104. **Mudge, G. H.,** Uricosuric action of cholecystographic agents. A possible factor in nephrotoxicity. *N. Engl. J. Med.,* 284, 929, 1971.
1105. **Berglund, G., et al.,** Antihypertensive effect and side-effects of bendroflumethiazol and propanolol. *Acta Med. Scand.,* 199, 499, 1976.
1106. **Fagard, R., Amery, A., and Deplaen, J. F.,** Relative value of beta blockers and thiazides for initiating antihypertensive therapy. Beta blockers or thiazides in hypertension. *Acta Cardiol.,* 31, 411, 1976.
1107. **Kjeldsen, S. E., et al.,** The effect on HDL cholesterol of oxprenol and atenolol. *Scand. J. Clin. Lab. Invest.,* 42, 449, 1982.
1108. **Postlethwaite, A. E., Bartel, A. G., and Kelley, W. N.,** Hyperuricaemia due to ethambutol. *N. Engl. J. Med.,* 286, 761, 1972.
1109. **Narang, R. K., et al.,** Hyperuricaemia induced by ethambutol. *Br. J. Dis. Chest.,* 77, 403, 1983.
1110. **Khanan, B. K. and Gupta, V. P.,** Ethambutol-induced hyperuricaemia. *Tubercule,* 65, 195, 1984.
1111. **Ayvazian, J. H. and Ayvazian, L. F.,** A study of the hyperuricaemia induced by hydrochlorthiazide and acetolamide separately and in combination. *J. Clin. Invest.,* 40, 1961, 1961.
1112. **Demartini, F., et al.,** Effect of chlorthiazide on the renal excretion of uric acid. *Am. J. Med.,* 32, 572, 1962.
1113. **Russell, R. P., Lindeman, R. D., and Prescott, L. F.,** Metabolism and hypotensive effects of ethacrynic acid. Comparative study with hydrochlorthiazide. *Lancet,* i, 947, 1964.
1114. **Roberts, C. J. C., et al.,** Effect of pietamide, bumetamide and furesemide on electrolye and urate excretion in normal subjects. *Br. J. Clin. Pharmacol.,* 6, 129, 1978.
1115. **Bengtsson, C.,** Comparison between alprenolol and chlorthalidone as hypertensive agents. *Acta Med. Scand.,* 191, 433, 1972.
1116. **Dollery, C. T., Parry, E. H. O., and Young, D. S.,** Diuretic and hypotensive properties of ethacrynic acid: a comparison with hydrochlorthiazide. *Lancet,* i, 947, 1964.
1117. **Jackson, W. P. U. and Nellen, M.,** Effect of frusemide on carbohydrate metabolism, blood pressure and other modalities: a comparison with chlorthiazide. *Br. Med. J.,* ii, 333, 1966.
1118. **Godwin, T. F. and Gunton, R. W.,** Clinical trial of a new diuretic furosemide: comparison with hydrochlorthiazide and mercaptomerin. *Can. Med. Assoc. J.,* 93, 1296, 1965.
1119. **Lowe, J., et al.,** Adverse reactions to frusemide in hospital patients. *Br. Med. J.,* ii, 360, 1979.
1120. **Larsson, R., et al.,** The effects of cimetidine (Tagamet) on renal function in patients with renal failure. *Acta Med. Scand.,* 208, 27, 1980.
1121. **Al Hujaj, M. and Schönthal, M.,** Hyperuricaemia and levodopa. *N. Engl. J. Med.,* 285, 859, 1971.
1122. **Jonas, S.,** Hyperuricaemia and levodopa. *N. Engl. J. Med.,* 285, 1489, 1971.
1123. **Honda, H. and Gindin, R. A.,** Gout while receiving levodopa for parkinsonism. *JAMA,* 219, 55, 1972.
1124. **Perheentupa, J. and Raivio, K.,** Fructose-induced hyperuricaemia. *Lancet,* ii, 528, 1967.

1125. **Stirpe, F., et al.,** Fructose-induced hyperuricaemia. *Lancet,* ii, 1319, 1970.
1126. **Curreri, P. W. and Pruitt, B. A.,** Absence of fructose-induced hyperuricaemia in men. *Lancet,* i, 839, 1970.
1127. **Sahebjami, H. and Scalettar, R.,** Effects of fructose infusion on lactate and uric acid metabolism. *Lancet,* i, 366, 1971.
1128. **Heukenkamp, P.-U. and Zöllner, N.,** Fructose-induced hyperuricaemia *Lancet,* i, 808, 1971.
1129. **Maaze, R. I., Shue, G. L., and Jackson, S. H.,** Renal dysfunction associated with methoxyflurane anaesthesia. A randomised, prospective clinical evaluation. *JAMA,* 216, 278, 1971.
1130. **Black, G. W. and Keilty, S. R.,** Renal function following methoxyflurane anaesthesia. *Br. J. Anaesth.,* 45, 353, 1973.
1131. **Robertson, G. S. and Hamilton, W. F. D.,** Methoxyflurane and renal function. *Br. J. Anaesth.,* 45, 55, 1973.
1132. **Robertson, G. S. and Hamilton, W. F. D.,** Changes in serum uric acid related to the dose of methoxyflurane. *Br. J. Anaesth.,* 46, 54, 1974.
1133. **Berge, K. G., et al.,** Hypercholesterolaemia and nicotinic acid. A long-term study. *Am. J. Med.,* 31, 25, 1961.
1134. **Solomon, H. M. and Thomas, G. B.,** Oral glucose tolerance, plasma insulin and uric acid excretion in man during chronic administration of nicotinic acid. *Metabolism,* 20, 1031, 1971.
1135. **Becker, M. A., et al.,** The effect of nicotinic acid on human purine metabolism. *Clin. Res.,* 21, 616, 1973.
1136. **Gershon, S. L. and Fox, I. H.,** Pharmacological effects of nicotinic acid on human purine metabolism, *J. Lab. Clin. Med.,* 84, 179, 1974.
1137. **Stapleton, F. B., et al.,** Hyperuricaemia due to high-dose pancreatic extract therapy in cystic fibrosis. *N. Engl. J. Med.,* 295, 246, 1976.
1138. **Davidson, G. P., et al.,** Iatrogenic hyperuricaemia in children with cystic fibrosis. *J. Paediatr.,* 93, 976, 1978.
1139. **Morita, Y., et al.,** Theophylline increases serum uric acid levels. *J. Allergy Clin. Immunol.,* 74, 707, 1984.
1140. **Shepherd, J. and Packard, C. J.,** in *Human Plasma Lipoproteins,* De Gruyder, Berlin, 1989, 55.
1141. **Carlson, L. A. and Böttinger, L. E.,** Ischaemic heart disease in relation to fasting values of plasma triglycerides and cholesterol. Stockholm prospective study. *Lancet,* i, 865, 1976.
1142. **Soloni, F.,** Simplified manual micromethod for determination of serum triglycerides. *Clin. Chem.,* 17, 529, 1971.
1143. **Rice, E. W.,** Triglycerides ("neutral fat") in serum. *Stand. Methods Clin. Chem.,* 6, 215, 1970.
1144. **Baculo, G. and David, H.,** Quantitative determination of serum triglyceride by the use of enzymes. *Clin. Chem.,* 19, 476, 1973.
1145. **Gowland, E.,** in *"Varleys" Practical Clinical Chemistry,* Gowenlock, A. H., Ed., William Heinemann Medical Books, London, 1988, 466.
1146. **Carlström, S. and Christensson, B.,** Plasma glycerol concentration in patients with myocardial ischaemia and arrhythmias. *Br. Heart J.,* 33, 884, 1971.
1147. **Elin, R. J.,** The variability of glycerol concentration in human serum. *Clin. Chem.,* 29, 1174, 1983.
1148. **Ter Welle, H. F., Baartscheer, T., and Fiolet, J. W. T.,** Influence of free glycerol on enzymic evaluation of triglycerides. *Clin. Chem.,* 30, 1102, 1984.
1149. **Neri, B. P. and Frings, C. S.,** Improved method for determination of triglycerides in serum. *Clin. Chem.,* 19, 1201, 1973.
1150. **Steinmetz, J.,** Triglycerides, in *Interpretations of Clinical Laboratory Tests,* Siest, G., et al., Biomedical Publishers, Foster City, CA, 1985, 413.
1151. **Zilva, J. F., Pennall, P. R., and Mayne, P. D.,** in *Clinical Chemistry in Diagnosis and Treatment,* 5th ed., Edward Arnold, London, 1988.
1152. **Bachorik, P. S.,** Collection of blood samples for lipoprotein analysis. *Sel. Methods Clin. Chem.,* 10, 87, 1983.
1153. **Tan, M. H., et al.,** Effect of posture on serum lipids. *N. Engl. J. Med.,* 289, 416, 1973.
1154. **Henry, R. J.,** in *Clinical Chemistry. Principles and Technics,* 1st ed., Harper & Row, New York, 1964, 865.
1155. **Henny, J., et al.,** Comparaison des valeurs obtenus sur serum ou plasma heparinised pour les examens biochimique courants. *Ann. Biol. Chem.,* 34, 383, 1976.
1156. Laboratory Methods Committee of the Lipid Research Clinics Program, Cholesterol and triglyceride concentrations in serum and plasma. *Clin. Chem.,* 23, 60, 1977.
1157. **Tiffany, T. O., et al.,** Clinical evaluation of kinetic enzymic fixed-time and integral analysis of serum triglycerides. *Clin. Chem.,* 20, 476, 1974.
1158. **Ryder, K., et al.,** Effect of dry-skin products on ectochem triglyceride results. *Clin. Chem.,* 32, 1410, 1986.
1159. **Von Mühlfellner, O., et al.,** Uber die haltbarkeit von plasmalipiden unter verschiedenen lagerungsbedingungen. *Z. Klin. Chem. Klin. Biochem.,* 10, 37, 1972.
1160. **Schwertner, H. A. and Friedman, H. S.,** Changes in lipid values and lipoprotein patterns of serum samples contaminated with bacteria. *Am. J. Clin. Pathol.,* 59, 829, 1973.
1161. **Olefsky, J. M., Crapo, P., and Reaven, G. M.,** Post-prandial plasma triglyceride and cholesterol responses to a low-fat meal. *Am. J. Clin. Nutr.,* 29, 535, 1976.
1162. **Kuo, P. T. and Bassett, D. R.,** Dietary sugar in the production of hypertriglyceridaemia. *Ann. Int. Med.,* 62, 1199, 1965.

1163. **Schiele, G., et al.,** Acute dietary effect on diurnal plasma lipids in normal subjects. *Atherosclerosis,* 26, 525, 1977.
1164. **DenBesten, L., et al.,** The different effects on the serum lipids and faecal steroids of high carbohydrate diets given orally or intravenously. *J. Clin. Invest.,* 52, 1384, 1973.
1165. **Cohen, H. and Goldberg, C.,** Effect of physical exercise on alimentary lipaemia. *Br. Med. J.,* ii, 509, 1960.
1166. **Nikkilä, E. A. and Konttinen, A.,** Effect of physical activity on postprandial levels of fats in serum. *Lancet,* i, 1151, 1962.
1167. **Sannerstedt, R., Sanbar, S. S., and Conway, J.,** Metabolic effects of exercise in patients with type IV hyperlipoproteinaemia. *Am. J. Cardiol.,* 25, 642, 1970.
1168. **Holloszy, J. O., et al.,** Effect of a six month program of endurance exercise on the serum lipid. *Am. J. Cardiol.,* 14, 753, 1964.
1169. **Hoffman, A. A., Nelson, W. R., and Goss, F. A.,** Effects of an exercise program on plasma lipids of senior Air Force officers. *Am. J. Cardiol.,* 20, 516, 1967.
1170. **Björntorp, P., et al.,** Carbohydrate and lipid metabolism in middle-aged physically well-trained men. *Metabolism,* 21, 1037, 1972.
1171. **Hurter, R., et al.,** Some immediate and long-term effects of exercise on the plasma-lipids. *Lancet,* ii, 671, 1972.
1130. **Wood, P. D., et al.,** Plasma lipoprotein distribution in male and female runners. *Ann. N.Y. Acad. Sci.,* 301, 748, 1977.
1173. **Lehtonen, A. and Viikari, J.,** The effect of vigorous activity at work on serum lipids with special reference to serum high-density lipoprotein cholesterol. *Acta Physiol. Scand.,* 104, 117, 1978.
1174. **Fuller, J. H., et al.,** Possible seasonal variation of plasma lipids in healthy populations. *Clin. Chim. Acta,* 52, 305, 1974.
1175. **Carlson, L. A. and Lindstedt, S.,** The Stockholm prospective study. I. The initial values for plasma lipid. *Acta Med. Scand.,* 493 (Suppl.), 35, 1969.
1176. **Romon, M., et al.,** Increased triglyceride levels in shift workers. *Am. J. Med.,* 93, 259, 1992.
1177. **Lewis, B.,** in *The Hyperlipidaemias. Clinical and Laboratory Practice,* Blackwell Scientific, Oxford, 1976.
1178. **Carlson, L. A.,** Serum lipids in normal men. *Acta Med. Scand.,* 167, 377, 1960.
1179. **Christensen, N. C., et al.,** Serum triglyceride values in healthy adults. *Scand. J. Clin. Lab. Invest.,* 23, 355, 1969.
1180. **Claude, J. R. and Lellough, J.,** A study of several biological parameters measured in a large population of a single profession. I. Distribution and concept of "normal values", in *Reference Values in Human Biochemistry,* Siest, G., Ed., S. Karger, Basel, 1973, 88.
1181. **Cooper, G. R.,** Introduction to analysis of cholesterol, triglyceride, and lipoprotein cholesterol. Reference values and conditions for analysis. *Sel. Methods Clin. Chem.,* 9, 157, 1982.
1182. **Steinmetz, J.,** in *Interpretation of Clinical Laboratory Tests,* Siest, G., et al., Eds., Biomedical Publishers, Foster City, CA, 1985, 424.
1183. **Elveback, L. R., Weidman, W. H., and Ellefson, R. D.,** Day-to-day variability and analytic error in determination of lipid in children. *Mayo Clin. Proc.,* 55, 267, 1980.
1184. **Haas, R. G.,** in *Paediatric Clinical Chemistry Reference (Normal Values),* Meites, S., Ed., American Association of Clinical Chemists, Washington, D.C., 1989, 268.
1185. **Tyroler, H., et al.,** Black-white differences in serum lipids and lipoproteins in Evans County. *Prev. Med.,* 4, 541, 1975.
1186. **Fredrichs, R., et al.,** Serum cholesterol and triglyceride levels in 33,446 children from a biracial community. *Circulation,* 54, 302, 1976.
1187. **Christensen, B., et al.,** Plasma cholesterol and triglyceride distribution in 13,663 children and adolescents: the prevalence study of the Lipid Research Clinics program. *Paediatr. Res.,* 14, 194, 1980.
1188. **Brody, S. and Carlson, L. A.,** Plasma lipid concentration in the newborn with special reference to the distribution of the different lipid fractions. *Clin. Chim. Acta,* 7, 694, 1962.
1189. **Tsang, R. C., Fallat, R. W., and Glueck, C. J.,** Cholesterol at birth and age. I. Comparison of normal and hypercholesterolaemic neonates. *Paediatrics,* 53, 458, 1974.
1190. **Carlson, L. A. and Hardell, L.,** Sex differences in serum lipid and lipoprotein of blood. *Eur. J. Clin. Invest.,* 7, 133, 1977.
1191. **Kontinnen, A., Pyörälä, T., and Carpén, E.,** Serum lipid patterns in normal pregnancy and pre-eclampsia. *J. Obstet. Gynaecol. Br. Common.,* 71, 453, 1964.
1192. **Cramer, K., Aurell, M., and Pehrson, S.,** Serum lipid and lipoprotein during pregnancy. *Clin. Chim. Acta,* 10, 470, 1964.
1193. **Svanborg, A. and Vikrot, O.,** Plasma lipid fractions, including individual phospholipid at various stages of pregnancy. *Acta Med. Scand.,* 178, 615, 1965.
1194. **Darmady, J. and Postle, A. D.,** Lipid metabolism in pregnancy. *Br. J. Obstet. Gynaecol.,* 89, 211, 1982.

1195. **Ginsberg, H., et al.,** Moderate ethanol ingestion and plasma triglyceride levels: a study in normal and hypertriglyceridemic patients. *Ann. Int. Med.,* 80, 143, 1974.

1196. **Chait, A., et al.,** Clinical and metabolic study of alcoholic hyperlipaemia. *Lancet,* ii, 62, 1972.

1197. **Whitfield, J. B., et al.,** Effects of age and sex on biochemical responses to drinking habits. *Med. J. Austr.,* ii, 629, 1978.

1198. **Allen, J. K. and Adena, M. A.,** The association between plasma cholesterol high-density-lipoprotein, triglycerides and uric acid in ethanol consumers. *Ann. Clin. Biochem.,* 22, 62, 1985.

1199. **Ferrari, C., et al.,** Effect of short term clofibrate administration on glucose tolerance and insulin secretion in patients with chemical diabetes or triglyceridaemia. *Metabolism,* 26, 129, 1977.

1200. **Series, J. J., et al.,** Effect of combined therapy with benzafibrate and cholestyramine on low-density lipoprotein metabolism. *Metabolism,* 38, 153, 1989.

1201. **Franceschini, G., et al.,** Plasma lipoprotein changes after treatment with pravastatin and gemfibrosil in patients with familial hypercholesterolaemia. *J. Lab. Clin. Med.,* 114, 250, 1989.

1202. **Goldsmith, G. A.,** Niacin: antipellagra factor, hypercholesterolaemic agent. *JAMA,* 194, 167, 1965.

1203. **Dujovne, C. A., et al.,** One year trials with halofenate, clofibrate, and placebo. *Clin. Pharmacol. Ther.,* 19, 352, 1976.

1204. **Mitchell, W. D.,** A comparison of the effect of clofibrate and thyroxine on serum lipid in three hypothyroid subjects. *Clin. Chim. Acta,* 35, 429, 1971.

1205. **Feldman, E. B. and Carter, A. C.,** Reduction of serum triglycerides in patients treated with sodium D-thyroxine. *Metabolism,* 12, 1132, 1963.

1206. **Howard, R. P., Brusco, O. J., and Furman, R. H.,** Effect of cholestyramine administration on serum lipids and on nitrogen balance in familial hypercholesterolaemia. *J. Lab. Clin. Med.,* 68, 12, 1966.

1207. **Fallon, H. J. and Woods, J. W.,** Cholestyramine therapy of hyperlipidaemia. *Clin. Res.,* 15, 73, 1967.

1208. **Berkowitz, D.,** Selective blood lipid reduction in newer pharmacological agents. *Am. J. Cardiol.,* 12, 834, 1963.

1209. **Weitzel, A., et al.,** Cholestyramine effect on plasma triglyceride in normolipidaemic patients. *Proc. Soc. Exp. Biol.,* 130, 149, 1969.

1210. **Henkin, Y., Como, J. A., and Oberman, A.,** Secondary dyslipidaemia. *JAMA,* 267, 961, 1992.

1211. **Sokoloff, B., et al.,** Aging, atherosclerosis and ascorbic acid metabolism. *J. Am. Germ. Soc.,* 14, 1239, 1966.

1212. **Cěrně, O. and Ginter, E.,** Blood lipids and vitamin C status. *Lancet,* i, 1055, 1978.

1213. **Politi, A., Poggio, G., and Margiolta, A.,** Can amioderone induce hyperglycaemia and hypertriglyceridaemia? *Br. Med. J.,* 288, 285, 1984.

1214. **Fogari, R., et al.,** Plasma lipids during chronic antihypertensive therapy with different-B-blockers. *J. Cardiol. Pharmacol.,* 14 (Suppl. 7), 528, 1989.

1215. **Terent, A., Ribacke, M., and Carlson, L. A.,** Long-term effect of pindolol on lipids and lipoproteins in men with newly diagnosed hypertension. *Eur. J. Clin. Pharmacol.,* 36, 347, 1989.

1216. **Bell, G. D., Whitney, B., and Dowling, R. H.,** Gallstone dissolution in man using chenodeoxycholic acid. *Lancet,* ii, 1213, 1972.

1217. **Doar, J. W. H. and Wynn, V.,** Serum lipid levels during oral contraceptive and glucocorticoid administration. *J. Clin. Pathol.,* 3 (Suppl.), 55, 1970.

1218. **Jefferys, D. B., Lessof, M. H., and Mattock, M. B.,** Corticosteroid treatment, serum lipids and coronary arterial disease. *Postgrad. Med. J.,* 56, 491, 1980.

1219. **Luciano, A. A., Wallace, R. B., and Sherman, B. M.,** Effect of danazol on plasma lipid and lipoprotein levels in normal women. *Atherosclerosis,* 43, 133, 1982.

1220. **Fähraeus, L., et al.,** Profound alteration of lipoprotein metabolism during danazol treatment in premenopausal women. *Fertil. Steril.,* 42, 52, 1984.

1221. **Ames, R. P. and Hill, P.,** Increase in serum-lipids during treatment of hypertension with chlorthalidone. *Lancet,* i, 721, 1976.

1222. **Schnaper, M., et al.,** Chlorthalidone and serum cholesterol. *Lancet,* ii, 295, 1977.

1223. **Veterans Administration Cooperative Study Group on Antihypertensive Agents,** Comparison of propanolol and hydrochlorthiazide for the initial treatment of hypertension. II. Results of long-term therapy. *JAMA,* 248, 2004, 1982.

1224. **Chandler, B. and Lewis, P. T.,** Efficacy and tolerability of enalapril and its effect on serum lipids in patients with mild uncomplicated essential hypertension. *Curr. Ther. Res.,* 43, 1143, 1988.

1225. **Caren, R. and Corbo, L.,** Depression of plasma lipid fractions and inhibition of platelet aggregation by action of glucagon. *Metabolism,* 20, 1057, 1971.

1226. **Sasaki, J., Funakoski, M., and Arawawa, K.,** Lipids and apolipoproteins in patients treated with major tranquillisors. *Clin. Pharmacol. Ther.,* 37, 684, 1985.

1227. **Thompson, P. D., et al.,** Contrasting effect of testosterone and stanazotol on serum lipoprotein. *JAMA,* 261, 1165, 1989.

1228. **Foldes, F. F. and Murphy, A. J.,** Distribution of cholesterol, cholesterol esters and phospholipid phosphorus in normal blood. *Proc. Soc. Exp. Biol. Med.,* 62, 215, 1946.

1229. **Wybenga, D. R. and Inkpen, J. A.,** in *Clinical Chemistry. Principles and Technics,* 2nd ed., Henry, R. J., Cannon, J. C., and Winkelman, J. W., Eds., Harper & Row, New York, 1974.

1230. **Keys, A., et al.,** Lessons from serum cholesterol studies in Japan, Hawaii, and Los Angeles. *Ann. Int. Med.,* 48, 83, 1958.

1231. **Bloor, W. R.,** A method for the determination of fat in small amounts of blood. *J. Biol. Chem.,* 17, 377, 1914.

1232. **Schoenheimer, R. and Sperry, W. M.,** A micromethod for the determination of free and combined cholesterol. *J. Biol. Chem.,* 106, 745, 1934.

1233. **Webster, D.,** The chromatographic separation of ester and free cholesterol in blood. *Clin. Chim. Acta,* 8, 19, 1963.

1234. **Abell, L. L., et al.,** A simplified method for the estimation of total cholesterol in serum and demonstration of its specificity. *J. Biol. Chem.,* 195, 357, 1952.

1235. **Zak, B.,** Cholesterol methodology: a review. *Clin. Chem.,* 23, 1201, 1977.

1236. **Richmond, W.,** Analytical reviews in clinical chemistry: the quantitative analysis of cholesterol. *Ann. Clin. Biochem.,* 29, 577, 1992.

1237. **Sperry, W. M. and Webb, M. A.,** A revision of the Schoenheimer-Sperry method for cholesterol determination. *J. Biol. Chem.,* 187, 97, 1950.

1238. **Zlatkis, A., Zak, B., and Boyle, A. J.,** A new method for the direct determination of serum cholesterol. *J. Lab. Clin. Med.,* 41, 486, 1953.

1239. **Tonks, D. B.,** The estimation of cholesterol in serum: a classification and critical review of methods. *Clin. Biochem.,* 1, 12, 1967.

1240. **Richardson, R. W., Setchell, K. D. R., and Woodman, D. D.,** An improved method for the estimation of serum cholesterol. *Clin. Chim. Acta,* 31, 403, 1971.

1241. **Watson, D.,** A simple method for the determination of serum cholesterol. *Clin. Chim. Acta,* 5, 637, 1960.

1242. **Wybenga, D. R., et al.,** Direct Manual Determination of serum Total Cholesterol with a Single Stable Reagent. *Clin. Chem.,* 16, 980, 1970.

1243. **Stadtman, T. C.,** Preparation and assay of cholesterol and ergosterol in *Methods in Enzymology III,* Colowick, S. P. and Kaplan, N. O., Eds., Academic Press, New York, 1957, 392.

1244. **Flegg, H. M.,** An Investigation of the Determination of Serum Cholesterol by an Enzymatic Method. *Ann. Clin. Biochem.,* 10, 79, 1973.

1245. **Allain, C. C., et al.,** Enzymatic Determination of Total Serum Cholesterol. *Clin. Chem.,* 20, 470, 1974.

1246. **Richmond, W.,** Preparation and properties of a cholesterol oxidase from *Nocardia* sp. and its application to the enzymatic assay of total cholesterol in serum. *Clin. Chem.,* 19, 1350, 1973.

1247. **Wentz, P. W., Cross, R. E., and Savory, J.,** An integrated approach to lipid profiling: enzymatic determination of cholesterol and triglycerides with a centrifugal analyser of total and free cholesterol in serum. *Clin. Chem.,* 22, 188, 1976.

1248. **Lie, R. F., et al.,** Cholesterol oxidase-based determination by continuous-flow analysis of total and free cholesterol in serum. *Clin. Chem.,* 22, 1627, 1976.

1249. **Richmond, W.,** Use of cholesterol oxidase for assay of total and free cholesterol in serum by continuous flow analysis. *Clin. Chem.,* 22, 1579, 1976.

1250. **Cooper, G. R., et al.,** Chemical characteristics and sources of error of an enzymatic cholesterol method. *Clin. Chem.,* 25, 1074, 1979.

1251. **Derks, H. J. G. M., Van Heiningen, A., and Koedan, H. C.,** Gas-chromatographic determination of cholesterol in serum: candidate reference method. *Clin. Chem.,* 31, 691, 1985.

1252. **Warnick, G. R., et al.,** Evaluation of portable analysers for lipid analysis with emphasis on cholesterol screening, in *Proc. IXth Int. Symp. on Drugs Affecting Lipid Metabolism,* Florence, Italy, 1986.

1253. **MacManus, B. M., et al.,** Feasibility and impact of cholesterol screening: experiences with Reflotron in the community and the work place, in *Int. Symp. on Cholesterol Control in Cardiac Disease,* Milan, Italy, 1987.

1254. **Boerma, G. J. M., et al.,** Revised calibration of Reflotron cholesterol assay evaluated. *Clin. Chem.,* 34, 1124, 1988.

1255. **Nelson, L. M. and Fraser, C. G.,** Cholesterol assays with the Boehringer Reflotron: a laboratory, in-ward and outpatient clinical evaluation. *Ann. Clin. Biochem.,* 24. Suppl. 2, 91, 1987.

1256. **Siedel, J., et al.,** Reagent for the enzymatic determination of serum total cholesterol with improved lipolytic efficiency. *Clin. Chem.,* 29, 1075, 1983.

1257. **Svensson, L., et al.,** A possible model for accuracy control of determination of serum cholesterol with use of reference method. A NORDKEM project. *Scand. J. Lab. Clin. Invest.,* 42, 99, 1982.

1258. **Blank, D. W., et al.,** The method of determination must be considered in interpreting blood cholesterol levels. *JAMA,* 256, 2867, 1986.

1259. **Kroll, M. H., et al.,** Bias between enzymatic methods and the reference method for cholesterol. *Clin. Chem.,* 34, 131, 1988.

1260. **Laboratory Standardisation Panel of the National Cholesterol Education Program,** Report on current state of blood cholesterol measurement in clinical laboratories in the United States. *Clin. Chem.,* 34, 193, 1988.

1261. **Anon.,** Medical news campaign seeks to increase U.S. cholesterol consciousness. *JAMA,* 255, 1097, 1986.

1262. National Institutes of Health. Consensus Development Conference, lowering blood cholesterol to prevent heart disease. *JAMA,* 253, 2080, 1985.

1263. **Kroll, M. H., Ruddel, M., and Elin, R. J.,** Analytical bias for cholesterol and the percent of the population deemed at risk for coronary heart disease. *Clin. Chem.,* 34, 2009, 1988.

1264. **Boyd, J. C.,** Accuracy in cholesterol assays. *Clin. Chem.,* 34, 2194, 1988.

1265. **Hainline, A., Jr., et al.,** Accuracy and comparability of long-term measurement of cholesterol. *Clin. Chem.,* 32, 611, 1986.

1266. **Hainline, A., Jr., et al.,** Quality control of lipid measurements in epidemiological studies: the U.S. Air Force's HEART program. *Clin. Chem.,* 31, 261, 1985.

1267. **Broughton, P. M. G. and Buckley, B. M.,** The need for better plasma cholesterol assays. *Ann. Clin. Biochem.,* 22, 547, 1985.

1268. **Moore, R. V. and Boyle, E., Jr.,** Errors associated with the direct measurement of human serum cholesterol using the $FeCl_3$ color reagent. *Clin. Chem.,* 9, 156, 1963.

1269. **Heachel, R., et al.,** Comparison of 9 methods for the determination of cholesterol. *J. Clin. Chem. Clin. Biochem.,* 17, 553, 1979.

1270. **Witte, D. L., Barrett, D. A., II, and Wycoff, D. A.,** Evaluation of an enzymatic procedure for determination of serum cholesterol with the Abbott ABA 100. *Clin. Chem.,* 20, 1282, 1974.

1271. Technicon Instrument Corporation Method No. SF4 0040 FC6.

1272. **Pesce, M. A. and Bodourian, S. H.,** Interference with the enzymic measurement of cholesterol in serum by the use of five reagent kits. *Clin. Chem.,* 23, 757, 1977.

1273. **Richmond, W.,** Use of cholesterol oxidase for assay of total and free cholesterol in serum by continuous-flow analysis. *Clin. Chem.,* 22, 1579, 1976.

1274. **Spain, M. A. and Wu, A. H. B.,** Bilirubin interference with determination of uric acid, cholesterol and triglyceride in commercial peroxidase-coupled assays and the effect of ferricyanide. *Clin. Chem.,* 32, 518, 1986.

1275. **Artiss, J. D., McEnroe, R. J., and Zak, B.,** Bilirubin interference in a peroxidase-coupled procedure for creatinine: elimination by bilirubin oxidase. *Clin. Chem.,* 30, 1389, 1984.

1276. **Small, N., et al.,** Cholesterol analysis on the Lipotrend. *Assoc. Clin. Biochem. Newssheet,* 341, 28, 1991.

1277. **Henry, R. J.,** *Clinical Chemistry Principles and Technics,* 1st. ed., Harper & Row, New York, 1964.

1278. **Rice, E. W.,** Interference of nitrate and nitrite in the iron-sulphuric acid cholesterol reaction. *Clin. Chim. Acta,* 14, 278, 1966.

1279. **Poon, R. and Hinberg, I.,** Sodium azide lowers cholesterol reading with "Reflectron". *Clin. Chem.,* 36, 1252, 1990.

1280. **Rice, E. W. and Lukasiewicz, D. B.,** Interference of bromide in the Zak ferric chloride-sulphuric acid cholesterol method and means of eliminating this interference. *Clin. Chem.,* 3, 160, 1957.

1281. **Jeliać-Ivanović, Z., et al.,** Interference by analgesic and antirheumatic drugs in 25 common laboratory assays. *J. Clin. Chem. Clin. Biochem.,* 23, 287, 1985.

1282. **Kupke, I. R., et al.,** Differences in lipid and lipoprotein concentrations of capillary and venous blood samples. *Clin. Chim. Acta,* 97, 279, 1979.

1283. **Alzofon, J., Tilton, K. A., and Haley, N. J.,** Enzymic determination of cholesterol in plasma obtained by finger stick. *Clin. Chem.,* 31, 168, 1985.

1284. **Greenland, P., et al.,** Blood cholesterol concentration: fingerstick plasma vs venous serum sampling. *Clin. Chem.,* 36, 628, 1990.

1285. **Koeselman, H. B., Lewis, B., and Pilkington, T. R. E.,** The effect of venous occusion on the level of serum cholesterol. *J. Athero. Res.,* 1, 85, 1961.

1286. **Sperry, W. M. and Schoenheimer, R.,** A comparison of serum, heparinized plasma and oxalated plasma in regard to cholesterol content. *J. Biol. Chem.,* 110, 655, 1935.

1287. **Grande, F., Amatuzio, D. S., and Wada, S.,** Cholesterol measurement in serum and plasma. *Clin. Chem.,* 10, 619, 1964.

1288. **Bachorik, P. S.,** Collection of samples for lipoprotein analysis. *Clin. Chem.,* 28, 1375, 1982.

1289. **Cloey, T., et al.,** Re-evaluation of serum-plasma differences in total cholesterol concentration. *JAMA,* 263, 2788, 1990.

1290. **Wickus, G. G. and Dukerscheim, R. O.,** Serum-plasma differences in total cholesterol: what correction factor should be used. *JAMA,* 257, 234, 1992.

1291. **Briggs, C. J., Anderson, D., and Muirhead, R. A.,** Interference by thimerosal in cholesterol estimation by the CHOD-PAP method. *Ann. Clin. Biochem.,* 21, 146, 1984.

1292. **Grafmetter, D., et al.,** The effect of storage on levels of cholesterol in serum as measured by a simple direct method. *Clin. Chim. Acta,* 16, 33, 1967.

1293. **Crawford, N.,** The determination of serum a- and b-lipoprotein cholesterol. *Clin. Chim. Acta,* 4, 494, 1959.

1294. **Wood, P. D., et al.,** Effects of sample aging on total cholesterol values determined by the automated ferric chloride-sulphuric acid and Liebermann-Burchard procedures. *Clin. Chem.,* 26, 592, 1980.

1295. **Keys, A., Anderson, J. T., and Mickelson, M.,** Serum cholesterol in men in basal and nonbasal states. *Science,* 123, 29, 1956.

1296. **Linder, M. C.,** Nutrition and metabolism of fats, in *Nutritional Biochemistry and Metabolism with Clinical Applications,* Linder, M. C., Ed., Elsevier, Amsterdam, 1985.

1297. **Huang, C. T. L., Gopalakrishna, G. S., and Nichols, B. L.,** Fiber, intestinal sterols and colonic cancer. *Am. J. Nutr.,* 31, 516, 1978.

1298. **Jenkins, D. J. A., et al.,** Effect of pectin, guar gum and wheat fibre on serum cholesterol. *Lancet,* i, 1116, 1975.

1299. **Truswell, A. S. and Kay, R. M.,** Absence of effect of bran on serum lipids. *Lancet,* i, 922, 1975.

1300. **Keys, A., Grande, F., and Anderson, J. T.,** Fiber and pectin in the diet and serum cholesterol concentration in man. *Proc. Soc. Exp. Biol. Med.,* 106, 555, 1961.

1301. **Boyd, C. A. R.,** Dietary bran, guar, and blood cholesterol: a role for hydroxycitrate? *Lancet,* i, 1345, 1985.

1302. **Kirby, R. W., et al.,** Oat-bran intake selectively lowers serum low-density lipoprotein cholesterol concentration of hypercholesterolaemic men. *Am. J. Clin. Nutr.,* 34, 824, 1981.

1303. **Anderson, J. W., et al.,** Hypocholesterolaemic effects of oat bran and bean intake for hypercholesterolaemic men. *Am. J. Clin. Nutr.,* 40, 1146, 1984.

1304. **Van Horn, L. V., et al.,** Serum lipid response to oat product intake with a fat modified diet. *J. Am. Diet. Assoc.,* 86, 759, 1986.

1305. **Swain, J. F., et al.,** Comparison of the effects of oat bran and low-fiber wheat on serum lipoprotein levels and blood pressure. *N. Engl. J. Med.,* 322, 147, 1990.

1306. Correspondence. Oat bran and serum cholesterol. *N. Engl. J. Med.,* 322, 1747, 1990.

1307. **Birkeland, K. L., et al.,** Oat bran and serum cholesterol. *N. Engl. J. Med.,* 322, 1749, 1990.

1308. **Kinsell, L. W., et al.,** Dietary modification of serum cholesterol and phospholipid levels. *J. Clin. Endocrinol.,* 12, 909, 1952.

1309. **Mancini, M., et al.,** Studies on the mechanism of carbohydrate-induced lipaemia in normal men. *Atherosclerosis,* 17, 445, 1973.

1310. **Keys, A., et al.,** American Heart Association Monograph No. 29. Coronary heart disease in seven countries. *Circulation* 41 (Suppl. 1), 1–1, 1970.

1311. **Thorogood, M., et al.,** Dietary intake and plasma lipid levels: lessons from a study of the diet of health concious groups. *Br. Med. J.,* 300, 1297, 1990.

1312. **Hegsted, D. M., et al.,** Quantitative effect of dietary fat on serum cholesterol in man. *Am. J. Clin. Nutr.,* 17, 281, 1965.

1312a. **Stoker, D. J., Wynn, V., and Robertson, G.,** Effect of posture on plasma cholesterol level. *Br. Med. J.,* i, 336, 1966.

1313. **Grundy, S. M.,** Transmonounsaturated fatty acids and serum cholesterol levels. *N. Engl. J. Med.,* 323, 480, 1990.

1314. **Mensink, R. B. and Katan, M. B.,** Effect of a diet enriched with monosaturated or polyunsaturated fatty acids on level of low-density and high-density lipoprotein cholesterol in healthy women and men. *N. Engl. J. Med.,* 321, 436, 1989.

1315. **Mensink, R. B. and Katan, M. B.,** Effect of dietary transfatty acid on high-density and low-density lipoprotein cholesterol levels in healthy subjects. *N. Engl. J. Med.,* 323, 439, 1990.

1316. **Gotto, A. M.,** Cholesterol intake and serum cholesterol level. *N. Engl. J. Med.,* 324, 912, 1991.

1317. **Kern, F., Jr.,** Normal plasma cholesterol in an 88-year-old man who eats 25 eggs per day — mechanism of adaption. *N. Engl. J. Med.,* 324, 896, 1991.

1318. **Shekelle, R. B., et al.,** Diet, serum cholesterol and death from coronary heart disease. The Western Electric study. *N. Engl. J. Med.,* 304, 65, 1981.

1319. **Thelle, D. S., Arnesen, E., and Førde, O. H.,** The Tromsø heart study. Does coffee raise serum cholesterol? *N. Engl. J. Med.,* 308, 1454, 1983.

1320. **Arnesen, E., Førde, O. H., and Thelle, D. S.,** Coffee and serum cholesterol. *Br. Med. J.,* 288, 1960, 1984.

1321. **Bønan, K., et al.,** Coffee and cholesterol. Is it all in the brewing? The Tromsø study. *Br. Med. J.,* 297, 1103, 1988.

1322. **Bak, A. A. A. and Grobbee, D. H.,** The effect on serum cholesterol levels of coffee brewed by filtering or boiling. *N. Engl. J. Med.,* 321, 1432, 1989.

1323. **Thelle, D. S., Heyden, S., and Fodor, J. G.,** Coffee and cholesterol in epidemiological and in experimental studies. *Atherosclerosis,* 67, 97, 1987.

1324. **Campbell, D. E.,** Influence of several physical activities on serum cholesterol concentrations in young men. *J. Lipid Res.,* 6, 478, 1965.

1324a. **Bordia, A. and Bansal, H. C.,** Essential oil of garlic in prevention of atherosclerosis. *Lancet,* ii, 1491, 1973.

1325. **Carlson, L. A. and Fröberg, S. O.,** Lipid and glucose levels during a ten-day period of low-calorie intake and exercise in man. *Metabolism,* 16, 624, 1967.

1325a. **Jain, A. K., et al.,** Can garlic reduce levels of serum lipids? A controlled clinical study. *Am. J. Med.,* 94, 632, 1993.

1326. **Wood, P. D. and Haskell, W. L.,** The effect of exercise on plasma high density lipoprotein. *Lipids,* 14, 417, 1979.

1326a. **Sabate, J., et al.,** Effects of walnuts on serum lipid levels and blood pressure in normal men. *N. Engl. J. Med.,* 328, 603, 1993.

1327. **Thomas, C. B., Holljes, H. W. D., and Eisenberg, F. F.,** Observations on seasonal variation in total serum cholesterol level among healthy young prisoners. *Ann. Int. Med.,* 54, 413, 1961.

1328. **Thomson, E. M. and Kight, M. A.,** Effect of high environmental temperature on basal metabolism and concentrations of serum protein-bound iodine and total cholesterol. *Am. J. Clin. Nutr.,* 13, 219, 1963.

1329. **Bleiler, R. E., et al.,** A seasonal variation of cholesterol in serum of men and women. *Am. J. Clin. Nutr.,* 12, 12, 1963.

1330. **Doyle, J. T., Kinch, S. H., and Brown, D. F.,** Seasonal variation in serum cholesterol concentration. *J. Chr. Dis.,* 18, 657, 1965.

1331. **Fyfe, T., et al.,** Seasonal variation in serum lipids and incidence and mortality of ischaemic heart disease. *J. Athero. Res.,* 8, 591, 1968.

1332. **Thompson, G. R.,** in *A Handbook of Hyperlipaemia,* Current Science, London, 1989, 18.

1333. **Friedman, M., Rosenman, R. H., and Carroll, V.,** Changes in the serum cholesterol and blood clotting time in men subjected to cyclic occupational stress. *Circulation,* 17, 852, 1958.

1334. **Grundy, S. M. and Griffin, A. C.,** Effects of periodic mental stress on cholesterol levels. *Circulation,* 25, 798, 1962.

1335. **Zarafonetis, C. J. D., et al.,** Lipid mobilisation as a consequence of surgical stress. *Am. J. Med. Sci.,* 237, 418, 1959.

1336. **Gonalonus, G. R.,** quoted by Oliver, M. P. and Boyd, G. S., *Clin. Sci.,* 12, 217, 1953.

1337. **Oliver, M. F. and Boyd, G. S.,** Changes in the plasma lipids during the menstrual cycle. *Clin. Sci.,* 12, 217, 1953.

1338. **Aldercreutz, H. and Tallqvist, G.,** Variations in the serum cholesterol and haematocrit values in normal women during the menstrual cycle. *Scand. J. Clin. Invest.,* 11, 1, 1959.

1339. **Duboff, G. S. and Stevenson, W. W.,** An ultra micro-method for the estimation of serum cholesterol. *Clin. Chem.,* 8, 105, 1962.

1340. **Woodman, D. D.,** An investigation of serum lipids in health and disease with special reference to the role of lecithin cholesterol acyl transferase. Master's thesis, Council for National Academic Awards, London, 1974.

1341. **Lewis, B.,** in *The Hyperlipidaemias — Clinical and Laboratory Practice,* Blackwell Scientific, Oxford, 1976, 131.

1342. **Shaper, A. G. and Jones, K. W.,** Serum cholesterol, diet, and coronary heart disease in Africans and Asians in Uganda. *Lancet,* ii, 534, 1959.

1343. **Leonard, P. J.,** The effect of age and sex on biochemical parameters in blood of healthy subjects, in *Reference Values in Human Biochemistry,* Siest, G., Ed., S. Karger, Basel, 1973, 134.

1344. **Thelle, D. S., et al.,** Blood lipids in middle aged British men. *Br. Heart J.,* 49, 205, 1983.

1345. **Stamler, J.,** Life styles, major risk factors, proof and public policies. *Circulation,* 58, 3, 1978.

1346. **Beaglehole, R., et al.,** Serum cholesterol, diet and the decline in coronary heart disease mortality. *Prev. Med.,* 8, 538, 1979.

1347. **National Center for Health Statistics, National Heart, Lung and Blood Institute Collaborative Lipid Group,** Trends in serum cholesterol levels among U.S. adults aged 20 to 74 years. Data from the National Health and Nutrition Examination Survey 1960 to 1980. *JAMA,* 257, 937, 1987.

1348. **Bruger, M. and Somach, I.,** The diurnal variation of the cholesterol content of blood. *J. Biol. Chem.,* 97, 23, 1932.

1349. **Sperry, W. M.,** The concentration of total cholesterol in blood serum. *J. Biol. Chem.,* 117, 391, 1937.

1350. **Chandler, H. L., et al.,** Spontaneous and induced variation in serum lipoproteins. *Circulation,* 8, 723, 1953.

1351. **Anderson, J. T. and Keys, A.,** Cholesterol in serum and lipoprotein fractions. *Clin. Chem.,* 2, 145, 1956.

1352. **Shapiro, W., Estes, E. H., and Hilderman, H. L.,** Diurnal variability of serum cholesterol at normal and reduced levels. *J. Lab. Clin. Med.,* 54, 213, 1959.

1353. **Demacker, P. N. M., et al.,** Intraindividual variation of serum cholesterol. *Atherosclerosis,* 45, 259, 1982.

1354. **Keys, A.,** Introductory statement. *Ann. N.Y. Acad. Sci.,* 134, 505, 1966.

1355. **Morrison, L. M., Gonzales, W. T., and Hall, L.,** The significance of cholesterol variation in human blood serum. *J. Lab. Clin. Med.,* 34, 1473, 1949.

1356. **Friedlander, Y., Kark, J. D., and Stein, Y.,** Variability of plasma lipids and lipoproteins. The Jerusalem lipid research study. *Clin. Chem.,* 31, 1121, 1985.

1357. **Bronte-Stewart, B., Keys, A., and Brock, J. F.,** Serum cholesterol, diet, and coronary heart disease. An interracial survey in the Cape Peninsula. *Lancet,* ii, 1103, 1955.

1358. **Harnung, R.,** *Deut. Med. Wohnschr.* 52, 1849, 1926, quoted by Rafstedt, S., *Acta Paediatr. Scand.,* 44 (Suppl.), 102, 1955.

1359. **Rafstedt, S.,** Studies of serum lipids and lipoproteins in infancy and childhood. *Acta Paediatr. Scand.,* 44 (Suppl.), 102, 1955.

1360. **Persson, B. and Gentz, J.,** The pattern of blood lipids, glycerol and ketone bodies during the neonatal period, infancy and childhood. *Acta Paediatr. Scand.,* 55, 353, 1966.

1361. **Darmady, J. M., Fosbrooke, A. S., and Lloyd, J. K.,** Prospective study of serum cholesterol levels during the first year of life. *Br. Med. J.,* ii, 685, 1972.

1362. **Haas, R. G.,** in *Paediatric Clinical Chemistry Reference (Normal Values),* 3rd ed., Meites, S. Ed., American Association of Clinical Chemists, Washington, D.C., 1989, 94.

1363. **Herrman, E.,** *J. Biol. Zeitschr.* 43, 47, 1912, quoted by Rafstedt, S. *Acta Paediatr. Scand.,* 44 (Suppl.), 102, 1955.

1364. **Kleeberg, J. and Polishuk, W. Z.,** Lipid determinations in maternal and foetal blood. *J. Obstet. Gynaecol. Br. Common.,* 70, 701, 1963.

1365. **Glueck, C. J., et al.,** Neonatal familial type II hyperlipoproteinaemia: cord blood cholesterol in 1800 births. *Metabolism,* 20, 597, 1971.

1366. **Mishkel, M. A.,** Neonatal plasma lipids as measured in cord blood. *Can. Med. Assoc. J.,* 111, 775, 1974.

1367. **Kaplan, A. and Lee, V. F.,** Serum lipid levels in infants and mothers at parturition. *Clin. Chim. Acta,* 12, 258, 1965.

1368. **von Studnitz, W.,** Studies on serum lipids and lipoproteins in pregnancy. *Scand. J. Clin. Lab. Invest.,* 7, 329, 1955.

1369. **Peters, J. P., Heinemann, M., and Man, E. B.,** The lipids of serum in pregnancy, *J. Clin. Invest.,* 30, 388, 1951.

1370. **Tanner, J. M.,** The relation between serum cholesterol and physique in healthy young men. *J. Physiol.,* 115, 371, 1951.

1371. **Keys, A. and Fidanza, F.,** Serum cholesterol and relative body weight of coronary patients in different populations. *Circulation,* 22, 1091, 1960.

1372. **Fischer, R. A.,** Serum cholesterol in a military population. *J. Am. Diet. Assoc.,* 42, 511, 1963.

1373. **Thelle, D. S., et al.,** Blood lipids in middle-aged British men. *Br. Heart J.,* 49, 205, 1983.

1374. **Nanas, S., et al.,** The role of relative weight in the positive association between age and serum cholesterol in men and women. *J. Chron. Dis.,* 40, 887, 1987.

1375. **Wynder, E. L., Harris, R. E., and Haley, N. J.,** Population screening for plasma cholesterol: community-based results from Connecticut. *Am. Heart J.,* 117, 649, 1989.

1376. **Starr, P.,** Comparative clinical and biochemical effects of dextro- and levo-isomers of thyroxine. *Arch. Int. Med.,* 101, 722, 1958.

1377. **Greene, R., Pearce, J. F. and Rideout, D. F.,** Effect of *d*-thyroxine on serum cholesterol. *Br. Med. J.,* i, 1572, 1961.

1378. **Samuel, P. and Steiner, A.,** Effect of neomycin on serum cholesterol level of man. *Proc. Soc. Exp. Biol. Med.,* 100, 193, 1959.

1379. **Samuel, P. and Waithe, W. I.,** Reduction of serum cholesterol concentration by neomycin, para-amino acid and other bacterial drugs in man. *Circulation,* 24, 578, 1961.

1380. **Eyssen, H., Evrard, E., and Vanderhaaghe, H.,** Cholesterol-lowering effects of *N*-methylated neomycin and basic antibiotics. *J. Lab. Clin. Med.,* 68, 753, 1966.

1381. **Parsons, W. B.,** Treatment of hypercholesterolaemia by nicotinic acid. *Arch. Int. Med.,* 107, 639, 1961.

1382. **Miller, O. N., Hamilton, J. G. and Goldsmith, G. A.,** Investigation of the mechanism of action of nicotinic acid on serum lipid levels in man. *Am. J. Clin. Nutr.,* 8, 480, 1960.

1383. **Goldsmith, G. A.,** Therapy of hypercholesterolaemia. *Am. J. Dig. Dis.,* 9, 651, 1964.

1384. **Wiersinga, W. M. et al.,** An increase in plasma cholesterol independent of thyroid function during long-term amioderone therapy. A dose-dependent relationship. *Ann. Int. Med.,* 114, 128, 1991.

1385. **Miller, N. E. and Nestel, P. J.,** Altered bile acid metabolism during treatment with phenobarbitone. *Clin. Sci.,* 45, 257, 1973.

1386. **Pelkonen, R., Fogelholm, R., and Nikkalau, E. A.,** Increase in serum cholesterol during phenytoin treatment. *Br. Med. J.,* 10, 85, 1975.

1387. **Pederson, L.,** Biliary lipids during vitamin C feeding in healthy persons. *Scand. J. Gastroenterol.,* 10, 311, 1975.

1388. **Kallner, A.,** Serum bile acids in man during vitamin C supplementation and restriction. *Acta Med. Scand.,* 202, 283, 1977.

1389. **Spittle, C. R.,** Atherosclerosis and vitamin C. *Lancet,* ii, 1280, 1971.

1390. **Haskell, C. M., et al.,** L-asparaginase. Therapeutic and toxic effects in patients with neoplastic disease. *N. Engl. J. Med.,* 281, 1028, 1969.

1391. **Stern, M. P., et al.,** Adrenocortical steroid treatment of rheumatic disease. Effects on lipid metabolism. *Arch. Int. Med.,* 132, 97, 1973.

1392. **Mälkönen, M., Manninen, V., and Hirvonen, E.,** Effects of danazol and lyrestrenol on serum lipoproteins in endometriosis. *Clin. Pharmacol. Ther.,* 28, 602, 1980.

1393. **Luciano, A. A., et al.,** Effects of danazol on plasma lipid and lipoprotein levels in healthy men and women with endometriosis. *Am. J. Obstet. Gynecol.,* 145, 422, 1983.

1394. **Mazzaferri, E. and Skillman, T. G.,** Diazepan (Valium®) and thyroid function: a double-blind, placebo controlled study in normal volunteers showing no drug effect. *Am. J. Med. Sci.,* 257, 388, 1969.

1395. **Goldman, A. I., et al.,** Serum lipoprotein levels during chlorthalidone therapy. A Veterans Administration–National Heart, Lung, and Blood Institute co-operative study on antihypertensive therapy; mild hypertension. *JAMA,* 244, 1691, 1980.

1396. **Grimm, R. H., et al.,** Effects of thiazide diuretics on plasma lipids and lipoproteins in mildly hypertensive patients. *Ann. Int. Med.,* 94, 7, 1981.

1397. **Sirtori, C. R., Bolme, P., and Azarnoff, D. L.,** Metabolic response to acute and chronic L-dopa administration in patients with parkinsonism. *N. Engl. J. Med.,* 287, 729, 1972.

1398. **Bolton, C. H., et al.,** Enzyme induction and serum lipoprotein lipids: a study of glutethimide in normal subjects. *Clin. Sci.,* 58, 419, 1980.

1399. **Nanyam, B. V.,** Isoniazid-induced reduction in serum cholesterol. *Chest,* 84, 120, 1983.

1400. **Barton, G. M. G., Freeman, P. R., and Lawson, J. P.,** Oral contraceptives and serum lipids. *J. Obstet. Br. Common.,* 77, 551, 1970.

1401. **Hennekens, C. H., et al.,** Oral contraceptive use and fasting triglyceride, plasma cholesterol and H.D.L. cholesterol. *Circulation,* 60, 486, 1079.

1402. **Knopp, R. H. et al.,** Oral contraceptive and post menopausal estrogen effects on lipoprotein, triglycerides, and cholesterol in an adult female population: relationship to estrogen and progestrin potency. *J. Clin. Endocrinol. Metab.,* 53, 1123, 1981.

1403. **Eckstein, P., et al.,** Clinical and laboratory findings in a trial of norgestrol, a low-dose progestogen only contraceptive. *Br. Med. J.,* 3, 195, 1972.

1404. **Levene, R. A.,** Steattorhea induced by para-aminosalicylic acid. *Ann. Int. Med.,* 68, 1265, 1968.

1405. **Ames, R. P. and Peacock, P. B.,** Serum cholesterol during treatment of hypertension with diuretic drugs. *Arch. Int. Med.,* 144, 710, 1984.

1406. **Merimee, T. J. and Tyson, J. E.,** Stabilisation of plasma glucose during fasting. *N. Engl. J. Med.,* 291, 1275, 1974.

1407. **World Health Organization Expert Committee on Diabetes Mellitus,** Technical Report Series 646. Second report. WHO, Geneva, 1980, 9.

1408. **Reid, E. W.,** A method for the estimation of sugar in blood. *J. Physiol.,* 20, 316, 1896.

1409. **Burrin, J. and Price, C. P.,** Review article: measurement of blood glucose. *Ann. Clin. Biochem.,* 22, 327, 1985.

1410. **Nelson, N. A.,,** A photometric adaption of the Somogyi method for the determination of glucose. *J. Biol. Chem.,* 153, 375, 1944.

1411. **Hultman, E.,** Rapid specific method for the determination of aldosaccharides in blood. *Nature,* 183, 108, 1959.

1412. **Ceriotti, G. and Frank, A.,** An improved procedure for blood glucose determination with o-toluidine. *Clin Chim. Acta,* 24, 311, 1969.

1413. **Ceriotti, G.,** Blood glucose determination without deproteinisation with the use of o-toluidine in dilute acetic acid. *Clin. Chem.,* 17, 440, 1971.

1414. **Zender, R.,** Une micro-methode automatique pour l'analyses quantitative des aldohexoses dans les liquides biologiques par l'o toluidine. *Clin. Chim. Acta,* 8, 351, 1968.

1415. **Hiller, A., Linder, G. C., and Van Slyke, D. D.,** The reducing substances in blood. *J. Biol. Chem.,* 64, 625, 1925.

1416. **Keilin, D. and Hawtree, E. F.,** The use of glucose oxidase (notatin) for the determination of glucose in biological material and for the study of glucose-producing systems by manometric methods. *Biochem. J.,* 42, 230, 1948.

1417. **Froesh, E. R. and Renold, A. E.,** Specific enzymatic determination of glucose in blood and urine using glucose-oxidase. *Diabetes,* 5, 1, 1956.

1418. **Sunderman, F. W., Jr. and Sunderman, F. W.,** Measurement of glucose in blood, serum, and plasma by means of a glucose oxidase-catalase enzyme system. *Am. J. Clin. Pathol.,* 36, 75, 1961.

1419. **Huggett, A. and Nixon, D. A.,** Use of glucose oxidase, peroxidase and o-dianisidine in determination of blood and urinary glucose. *Lancet,* ii, 368, 1957.

1420. **Barham, D. and Trinder, P.,** An improved colour reagent for the determination of blood glucose by the oxidase system. *Analyst,* 97, 142, 1972.

1421. **Trinder, P.,** Determination of glucose in blood using glucose oxidase with an alternative oxygen accepter. *Ann. Clin. Biochem.,* 6, 24, 1969.

1422. **Sharp, P. et al.,** Effect of two sulphonylureas on glucose determination by enzymic methods. *Clin. Chim. Acta,* 36, 93, 1972.

1423. **Kaafman-Raab, I., et al.,** Interference by acetaminophen in the glucose oxidase-peroxidase method for glucose determination. *Clin. Chem.,* 22, 1729, 1976.

1424. **Farrance, I. and Aldous, J.,** Paracetamol interference with YSI glucose analyser. *Clin. Chem.,* 27, 782, 1981.

1425. **Farah, D. A., et al.,** Paracetamol interference with blood glucose: a potentially fatal phenomenon. *Br. Med. J.,* 285, 172, 1982.

1426. **Richardson, T.,** A modification of Trinders autoanalyser method for glucose. *Ann. Clin. Biochem.,* 14, 223, 1977.

1427. **Passey, R. B., et al.,** Evaluation and comparison of 10 glucose methods and the reference method recommended in the proposal product class standard (1974). *Clin. Chem.,* 23, 131, 1977.

1428. **Passey, R. B., et al.,** Evaluation and comparison of 10 glucose methods and the reference method recommended in the proposed product class standard (1974). *Sel. Methods Clin. Chem.,* 8, 9, 1977.

1429. **Gaspart, E.,** in *Interpretation of Clinical Laboratory Tests,* Siest, G. et al., Eds., Biomedical Publishers, Foster City, CA 1985, 253.

1430. **McLauchlan, D. M.,** in *"Varleys" Practical Clinical Biochemistry,* 6th ed., Gowenlock, A. H. Ed., William Heinemann Medical Books, London, 1988, 327.

1431. **Cooper, G. R. and McDaniel, V.,** The determination of glucose by the ortho-toluidine method (Filtrate and direct procedure). *Stand. Methods Clin. Chem.,* 6, 159, 1970.

1432. **Barash, P., Hodnett, W., and Young, D. S.,** Measuring glucose with dextran present. *N. Engl. J. Med.,* 280, 1481, 1969.

1433. **Pennock, C. A., et al.,** A comparison of autoanalyser methods for the estimation of glucose in blood. *Clin. Chim. Acta,* 48, 193, 1973.

1434. **White-Stevens, R. H.,** Interference by ascorbic acid in test system involving peroxidase. I. Reversible indicators and the effects of copper, iron and mercury. *Clin. Chem.,* 28, 521, 1982.

1435. **Neese, J. W.,** Glucose. Direct hexokinase method. *Sel. Methods Clin. Chem.,* 9, 241, 1982.

1436. **Zalme, E. and Knowles, H. C., Jr.,** A plea for plasma sugar. *Diabetes,* 14, 165, 1965.

1437. **Varley, H., Gowenlock, A. H., and Bell, M.,** *Practical Clinical Biochemistry,* 5th ed., William Heinemann Medical Books, London, 1980, 408.

1438. **Ruiter, J., Weinberg, F., and Morrison, H.,** The stability of glucose in serum. *Clin. Chem.,* 9, 356, 1963.

1439. **De Pasqua, A., et al.,** Errors in blood glucose determination. *Lancet,* ii, 1165, 1984.

1440. **Meites, S. and Saniel-Banrey, K.,** Preservation, distribution and assay of glucose in blood, with special reference to the newborn. *Clin. Chem.,* 25, 531, 1979.

1441. **Chan, A. Y. W., Swaminathan, R., and Cackram, C. S.,** Effectiveness of sodium fluoride as a preservative of glucose in blood. *Clin. Chem.,* 35, 315, 1989.

1442. **Clark, A. J. L., et al.,** Capillary tubes for blood sampling. *Diabetologia,* 23, 539, 1982.

1443. **Chan, A. Y. W., et al.,** Handling of blood specimens for glucose analysis. *J. Clin. Chem. Clin. Biochem.,* 28, 181, 1990.

1444. **Burrin, J. M. and Alberti, K. G. M. M.,** What is blood glucose: can it be measured? *Diabetic Med.,* 7, 199, 1990.

1445. **Giampistro, O., Navelesi, R., and Buzzigoli, G.,** Decrease in plasma glucose concentration during storage at −20°. *Clin. Chem.,* 26, 1710, 1980.

1446. **Lloyd, B., Burrin, J., and Smythe, P.,** Enzymic fluorimetric continuous flow assays for blood glucose, lactate, pyruvate, alanine, glycerol and 3-hydroxy butyrate. *Clin. Chem.,* 24, 1724, 1978.

1447. **Barreau, P. B. and Buttery, J. E.,** The effect of the haematocrit value on the determination of glucose levels by reagent strip methods. *Med. J. Aust.,* 147, 286, 1987.

1448. **Doumas, B. T., et al.,** Difference between values for plasma and serum in tests performed with the Ectochem 700 XR analyser and evaluation of "plasma separator" tubes (PST). *Clin. Chem.,* 35, 151, 1989.

1449. **Peters, J. P. and Van Slyke, D. D.,** *Quantitative Clinical Chemistry, Vol. 1. Interpretations,* Bailliere Tyndall, London, 1932, 107–112.

1450. **Jenkins, D. J. A., et al.,** Unabsorbable carbohydrate and diabetes. Decreased post prandial hyperglycaemia. *Lancet,* ii, 172, 1976.

1451. **Torsdottir, I., et al.,** Dietary guar gum effects on post prandial blood glucose, insulin and hydroxyproline in humans. *J. Nutr.,* 119, 1925, 1989.

1452. **Iwaoka, T., et al.,** The effect of low and high NaCl diets on oral glucose tolerance. *Klin. Wochenschr.,* 66, 724, 1988.

1453. **Chopra, R. N., et al.,** in *Chopra's Indigenous Drugs of India,* Calcutta, 1958, 494, quoted by Jain, J. C., Vyas, C. R., and Mahatma, O. P., *Lancet,* ii, 1471, 1973.

1454. **Jain, R. C., Vyas, C. R., and Mahatma, O. P.,** Hypoglycaemic action of onion and garlic. *Lancet,* ii, 1471, 1973.

1455. **Klachko, D. M., et al.,** Blood glucose levels during walking in normal and diabetic subjects. *Diabetes,* 21, 89, 1972.

1456. **Udassin, R., Shoenfeld, Y., and Shapiro, Y.,** Serum glucose and lactic acid concentration during prolonged and strenuous exercise in men. *Am. J. Phys. Med. Rehabil.,* 56, 249, 1977.

1457. **Suarez, L. and Barrett-Connor, E.,** Seasonal variation in fasting plasma glucose level in man. *Diabetologia,* 22, 250, 1982.

1458. **Campbell, I. T., Jarrett, R. J., and Keen, H.,** Diurnal and seasonal variation in oral glucose tolerance studies in the Antarctic. *Diabetologia,* 11, 139, 1975.

1459. **Picón-Roátegui, E.,** Intravenous glucose tolerance at sea level and at altitudes. *J. Clin. Endocrinol. Metab.,* 23, 1256, 1963.

1460. **De Lauture, H., et al.,** Concentrations of cholesterol, uric acid, urea, glucose and creatinine in a population of 50,000 active individuals. *Proc. 2nd Int. Colloquium Automatisation and Prospective Biology,* S. Karger, Basel, 1973, 141.

1461. **Report of a Working Party appointed by the College of General Practitioners,** Glucose tolerance and glycosuria in the general population. *Br. Med. J.,* ii, 655, 1963.

1462. **Jarrett, R. J. and Keen, H.,** Further observations on the diurnal variation in oral glucose tolerance. *Br. Med. J.,* iv, 334, 1970.

1463. **Grabner, W., et al.,** Untersuchungen zur circadianen rhythmik der glucose toleranz. *Klin. Wochenschr.,* 53, 773, 1975.

1464. **Roberts, H. J.,** Afternoon glucose tolerance testing: a key to the pathogenesis, early diagnosis and prognosis of diabetic hyperinsulinism. *J. Am. Germ. Assoc.,* 12, 423, 1964.

1465. **Hodkinson, H. M.,** in *Biochemical Diagnosis of the Elderly,* Chapman and Hall, London, 1977, 78.

1466. **O'Sullivan, J. B., et al.,** Effect of age on carbohydrate metabolism. *J. Clin. Endocrinol. Metab.,* 33, 619, 1971.

1467. **Haas, R. G.,** in *Paediatric Clinical Chemistry Reference (Normal values),* Meites S., Ed., American Association of Clinical Chemists, Washington, D.C., 1989, 136.

1468. **Lockitch, G. and Halstead, A. C.,** in *Paediatric Clinical Chemistry Reference (Normal values),* Meites, S., Ed., American Association of Clinical Chemists, Washington, D.C., 1989, 135.

1469. **Brown, M. J.,** The sugar content of the blood in normal and undernourished children and the effect of fat on the absorption of carbohydrate. *Qt. J. Med.,* 18, 175, 1925.

1470. **Srinivasan, G., et al.,** Plasma glucose in normal neonates. A new look. *J. Paediatr.,* 109, 114, 1986.

1471. **Heck, L. J. and Erenberg, A.,** Serum glucose levels in neonates during the first 48 hours of life. *J. Paediatr.,* 110, 119, 1987.

1472. **Bleicher, S. J., O'Sullivan, J. B., and Freinkel, N.,** Carbohydrate metabolism in pregnancy. *N. Engl. J. Med.,* 271, 866, 1964.

1473. **Tyson, J. E. and Merimee, T. J.,** Some physiologic effects of protein ingestion in pregnancy. *Am. J. Obstet. Gynecol.,* 107, 797, 1970.

1474. **Lind, T., Billewicz, W. Z., and Brown, G. A.,** A serial study of changes occurring in the oral glucose tolerance test during pregnancy. *J. Obstet. Gynaecol. Br. Common.,* 80, 1033, 1973.

1475. **National Diabetes Data Group,** Classification and diagnosis of diabetes mellitus and other categories of glucose intolerance. *Diabetes,* 28, 1039, 1979.

1476. **Gershberg, H., Javier, Z., and Hulse, M.,** Glucose tolerance in women receiving an ovulatory suppressant. *Diabetes,* 13, 278, 1964.

1477. **Peterson, W. F., Steel, M. W., Jr., and Coyne, R. V.,** Analysis of the effect of ovulatory suppressants on glucose tolerance. *Am. J. Obstet. Gynecol.,* 95, 484, 1966.

1478. **Wynn, V. and Doar, J. W. H.,** Some effects of oral contraceptives on carbohydrate metabolism. *Lancet,* ii, 715, 1966.

1479. **Halling, G. R., Michals, E. L., and Paulson, C. A.,** Glucose intolerance during ethyndiol diacetate-mestranol therapy. *Metabolism,* 16, 465, 1967.

1480. **Klein, J. P.,** Diphenyl hydantoin intoxication associated with hyperglycaemia. *J. Paediatr.,* 69, 413, 1966.

1481. **Peters, B. H. and Samaan, N. A.,** Hyperglycaemia with relative hypoinsulinism in diphenyl hydantoin toxicity. *N. Engl. J. Med.,* 281, 91, 1969.

1482. **Brogden, R. N., Speight, T. M., and Avery, G. S.,** Levodopa: a review of its pharmacological properties and therapeutic use with particular reference to parkinsonism. *Drugs,* 2, 262, 1971.

1483. **Langrall, H. M. and Joseph, C.,** Status of the clinical evaluation of levodopa in the treatment of Parkinson's disease and syndrome. *Clin. Pharmacol. Ther.,* 12, 323, 1971.

1484. **Massie, B., et al.,** Diltazem and propanolol in mild to moderate hypertension as monotherapy or with hydrochlorthiazide. *Ann. Int. Med.,* 107, 150, 1987.

1485. **Abrason, E. A., Arky, R. A., and Woebar, K. A.,** Effects of propanolol on the hormonal and metabolic responses to insulin in induced hypoglycaemia. *Lancet,* ii, 1388, 1966.

1486. **Deacon, S. P. and Barnet, D.,** Comparison of atenolol and propanolol during insulin-induced hypoglycaemia. *Br. Med. J.,* ii, 272, 1976.

1487. **Newman, R. J.,** Comparison of proponolol metoprolol and acebutolol on insulin-induced hypoglycaemia in healthy volunteers. *Br. Med. J.,* ii, 447, 1976.

1488. **Wilkins, R. W.,** New drugs for the treatment of hypertension. *Ann. Int. Med.,* 50, 1, 1959.

1489. **Goldner, M. G., Zarowitz, H., and Akgun, S.,** Hyperglycaemia and glycosuria due to thiazide derivatives administered in diabetes mellitus. *N. Engl. J. Med.,* 262, 403, 1960.

1490. **Sugar, S. J. N.,** Diabetic acidosis during chlorthiazide therapy. *JAMA,* 175, 618, 1961.

1491. **Hollis, W. C.,** Aggravation of diabetes mellitus during treatment with chlorthiazide. *JAMA,* 176, 947, 1961.

1492. **Wolff, F. W., Parmley, W. W., and White, K.,** Drug-induced diabetes. Diabetogenic activity of long term administration of benzothiazines. *JAMA,* 183, 568, 1963.

1493. **Brackenbridge, A., et al.,** Glucose tolerance in hypertensive patients on long-term diuretic therapy. *Lancet,* i, 61, 1969.

1494. **Wilson, G. M.,** Diuretics. *Br. Med. J.,* i, 285, 1963.

1495. **Senior, B., et al.,** Benzothiazines and neonatal hypoglycaemia. *Lancet,* ii, 377, 1976.

1496. **Andersen, O. O. and Persson, I.,** Carbohydrate metabolism during treatment with chlorthalidone and ethacrynic acid. *Br. Med. J.,* ii, 798, 1968.

1497. **Spino, M., et al.,** Adverse biochemical and clinical consequences of furosemide administration. *Can. Med. Assoc. J.,* 118, 1513, 1978.

1498. **Thonnard-Neuman, E.,** Phenothiazines and diabetes in hospitalised women. *Am. J. Psychiatry,* 124, 978, 1968.

1499. **Peters, J. P. and Van Slyke, D. D.,** in *Qualitative Clinical Chemistry, Vol. 1, Interpretations,* 1st ed., Bailliere Tyndall, London, 1932.

1500. **Peters, J. P. and Van Slyke, D. D.,** in *Qualitative Clinical Chemistry, Vol. 1, Interpretations,* 2nd ed., Bailliere Tyndall, London, 1946.

1501. **Charles, S., et. al.,** Hyperglycaemic effect of nifedipine. *Br. Med. J.,* 283, 19, 1981.

1502. **Donnelly, T. and Harrower, A. D. B.,** Effect of nifedipine on glucose tolerance and insulin secretion in diabetic and nondiabetic patients. *Curr. Med. Res. Opin.,* 6, 690, 1980.

1503. **Giugliano, D., et al.,** Impairment if insulin secretion in man by nifedipine. *Eur. J. Clin. Pharmacol.,* 18, 393, 1980.

1504. **Langmead, F.,** Salicylate poisoning in children. *Lancet,* i, 1822, 1906.

1505. **Olmstead, J. G. M. and Aldrich, C. A.,** Acidosis in methyl salicylate poisoning: report of 2 cases and review of the literature. *JAMA,* 90, 1438, 1928.

1506. **Severinghaus, E. L. and Meyer, O. O.,** Glycosuria and recovery following methyl salicylate therapy. *Ann. Int. Med.,* 3, 1147, 1930.

1507. **Morris, N. and Graham, S.,** The value of alkali in salicylate therapy. *Ann. Dis. Child.,* 6, 273, 1931.

1508. **Segar, W. E. and Holliday, M. A.,** Physiologic abnormalities of salicylate intoxication. *N. Engl. J. Med.,* 259, 1191, 1958.

1509. **Kaye, R., et al.,** Antipyretics in patients with juvenile diabetes mellitus. *Am. J. Dis. Child.,* 112, 52, 1966.

1510. **Limbeck, G. A., et al.,** Salicylates and hypoglycaemia. *Am. J. Dis. Child.,* 109, 165, 1965.

1511. **Mortimer, E. A., Jr., and Lapour, M. L.,** Varicella and hypoglycaemia possibly due to salicylates. *Am. J. Dis. Child.,* 103, 91, 1962.

1512. **Barnett, H. L., et al.,** Salicylate intoxication in infants and children. *J. Paediatr.,* 21, 214, 1942.

INDEX

A

Accuracy
  in albumin measurement, 144
  in alkaline phosphatase measurement, 96–97
  in bilirubin measurement, 158
  in cholesterol measurement, 241–242
  in creatinine measurement, 185
  defined, 5
  in glucose measurement, 268–269
  in inorganic phosphate measurement, 43–44
  in potassium measurement, 68
  in protein measurement, 130
  in sodium measurement, 68
  in triglyceride measurement, 225–226
  in urate measurement, 199–200
  in urea measurement, 170–171
ACE, see Angiotensin-converting enzyme
Acebutolol, 278
Acetazolamide, 86, 221
Acetoacetate, 116–117, 186
Acetohexamide, 187, 217, 277
Acetyl salicylic acid, 201
Acidosis, 48
Acid phosphatase, 6
ACTH, see Adrenocorticotrophic hormone
Adenine, 199
ADH, see Antidiuretic hormone
Adosterone antagonists, 87, see also specific types
Adrenalin, 14, 59–60
Adrenocorticoids, 279, see also specific types
Adrenocorticotrophic hormone (ACTH), 6, 277
Age, 13–14, see also Children; Elderly
  albumin and, 148, 152
  alkaline phosphatase and, 102–105
  aminotransferase and, 120, 124–125
  bilirubin and, 164–165
  calcium and, 28–31
  cholesterol and, 257–258
  creatinine and, 191, 194–196
  drugs and, 12
  glucose and, 275, 277
  inorganic phosphate and, 53–56
  proteins and, 138–139, 141
  triglycerides and, 230, 233
  urate and, 206–210, 220
  urea and, 175, 179
Alanine aminotransferase, see Glutamic-pyruvic
     transaminase (GPT)
Albumin, 143–155
  accuracy in measurement of, 144
  age and, 148, 152
  alkaline phosphatase and, 111
  analytic considerations in measurement of,
    143–144
  anticoagulants and, 146

  between-day variation in, 148
  bilirubin and, 143, 145
  body weight and, 151
  calcium and, 143
  in children, 148, 152
  collection of, 145–146
  drugs and, 143, 146, 153, 155
  dye-binding methods and, 143–145
  environmental changes and, 147
  exercise and, 10
  gender differences in, 149–150
  in healthy subjects, 148–151
  hemolysis and, 144–145
  interference in analysis of, 144–145
  intraindividual differences in, 148, 151
  lipemia and, 145
  meals and, 147
  menstrual cycle and, 11
  in neonates, 148, 152
  physiologic changes and, 146–147
  posture and, 146–147
  preanalytic error and, 145–146
  precision in measurement of, 144
  in pregnancy, 34, 151, 153
  proteins and, 129
  racial differences in, 148
  seasonal variation in, 147
  smoking and, 10, 151, 154–155
  stability of, 146
  standardization and, 144
  stress and, 147
  temperature and, 146
  units of, 144
  venous stasis and, 146
  within-individual variation in, 148
Alcohol, 8, 10–11, 13
  aminotransferase and, 122–123
  bilirubin and, 159
  breakdown of, 6
  cholesterol and, 261
  potassium and, 78, 81
  sodium and, 78, 81
  triglycerides and, 234–235
  urate and, 211
Aldolase, 13
Aldosterone
  exercise and, 10
  menstrual cycle and, 11
  potassium and, 82, 85, 88
  sodium and, 82, 85, 88
Alkaline phosphatase, 95–113
  age and, 102–105
  albumin and, 111
  analytic considerations in measurement of, 95–97
  anticoagulants and, 98
  bed rest and, 100

I

Ibuprofen, 90, 153, 216
Immobilization, 22, 100
Imprecision, 5
Indirect-reacting (unconjugated, free) bilirubin, 157
Indomethacin
　creatinine and, 193
　potassium and, 90
　sodium and, 90
　urate and, 201, 215–216
Inorganic phosphate, 43–65
　acidosis and, 48
　age and, 53–56
　alkalosis and, 48
　analytic considerations in measurement of, 43–44
　anticoagulants and, 45–46
　bilirubin and, 44
　blindness and, 56, 59
　blood pressure and, 56, 59
　body weight and, 56
　in children, 53–56
　contamination and, 46
　diet and, 47
　diurnal variation in, 52–53
　drugs and, 59–65
　exercise and, 47–48
　gender differences in, 49–51
　in healthy subjects, 48–56
　hemolysis and, 44–45
　interference in analysis of, 44–45
　intraindividual differences in, 48–53
　meals and, 47
　menstrual cycle and, 47
　in neonates, 56–58
　physiologic changes and, 47–48
　preanalytic error and, 45–46
　in pregnancy, 56, 58
　racial differences in, 56, 58
　stability of, 46
　sunlight and, 48
　temperature and, 46–47
　units of, 44
　within-individual variation in, 48–53
Insulin, 9
　exercise and, 10
　glucose and, 276, 279
　inorganic phosphate and, 61
　proteins and, 138
Interference, 5
　in albumin analysis, 144–145
　in alkaline phosphatase analysis, 97
　in aminotransferase analysis, 116–117
　in bilirubin analysis, 5, 158–159
　in calcium analysis, 18–19
　in cholesterol analysis, 242–244
　in creatinine analysis, 185–189
　in inorganic phosphate analysis, 44–45
　in potassium analysis, 69–70
　in protein analysis, 130–132
　in sodium analysis, 69–70

in triglycerides analysis, 226
in urate analysis, 200–202
in urea analysis, 171–172
Interleukin-2, 38
Intraindividual differences
　in albumin, 148, 151
　in alkaline phosphatase, 100–102
　in aminotransferase, 120
　in bilirubin, 161–164
　in cholesterol, 252–256
　in creatinine, 190–191, 193
　in glucose, 273
　in inorganic phosphate, 48–53
　in potassium, 74–76
　in proteins, 135
　in sodium, 74–76
　in urate, 204–208
　in urea, 174–175, 179
Ion exchange resins, 235, 262, see also specific types
Ion-selective electrodes (ISEs), 67–68, 71
Iron, 11
Iron saccharate, 61
ISEs, see Ion-selective electrodes
Isoniazid, 61, 82, 264
Isoniazide, 166
Isopropanol, 159

J

Jaffe reaction, 183, 186–188

K

Katal, 4
Keto acids, 115, 186–187, see also specific types
Ketoconazole, 89
Ketosteroids, 15, see also specific types

L

Lactate, 11, 78
Lactate dehydrogenase (LDH), 6, 13
Lactate dehydrogenase (LDH) inhibitors, 118, see
　also specific types
Lactic dehydrogenase, 115
Lactulose, 89, 187
LDH, see Lactate dehydrogenase
LH, see Luteinizing hormone
Licorice, 38, 89
Life style, 14, see also Alcohol; Diet; Smoking
Lipase, 227
Lipemia
　albumin and, 145
　aminotransferase and, 116
　cholesterol and, 242–243
　creatinine and, 186
　interference and, 5
　proteins and, 131
　urea and, 171
Lipid-lowering drugs, 217, 235, see also specific types
Lipid phosphate, 43